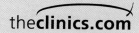

RADIOLOGIC CLINICS
OF NORTH AMERICA

Update on Radiologic Evaluation of Common Malignancies

Guest Editors
HEDVIG HRICAK, MD, PhD
DAVID M. PANICEK, MD

January 2007 • Volume 45 • Number 1

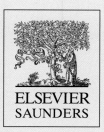

**ELSEVIER
SAUNDERS**

An imprint of Elsevier, Inc
PHILADELPHIA LONDON TORONTO MONTREAL SYDNEY TOKYO

W.B. SAUNDERS COMPANY
A Division of Elsevier Inc.

1600 John F. Kennedy Boulevard • Suite 1800 • Philadelphia, Pennsylvania 19103-2899

http://www.theclinics.com

RADIOLOGIC CLINICS OF NORTH AMERICA Volume 45, Number 1
January 2007 ISSN 0033-8389, ISBN 1-4160-4788-3; 978-1-4160-4788-9

Editor: Barton Dudlick

Reprints: For copies of 100 or more, of articles in this publication, please contact the Commercial Reprints Department, Elsevier Inc., 360 Park Avenue South, New York, New York 10010-1710. Tel.: (+1) 212-633-3813; Fax: (+1) 212-462-1935; E-mail: reprints@elsevier.com.

Radiologic Clinics of North America (ISSN 0033-8389) is published bimonthly in January, March, May, July, September, and November by Elsevier Inc., 360 Park Avenue South, New York, NY 10010-1710. Business and editorial offices: 1600 John F. Kenedy Boulevard, Suite 1800, Philadelphia, Pennsylvania 19103-2899. Customer Service Office: 6277 Sea Harbor Drive, Orlando, FL 32887-4800. Periodicals postage paid at New York, NY, and additional mailing offices. Subscription prices are USD 259 per year for US individuals, USD 385 per year for US institutions, USD 127 per year for US students and residents, USD 303 per year for Canadian individuals, USD 473 per year of Canadian institutions, USD 352 per year for international individuals, USD 473 per year for international institutions, and USD 171 per year for Canadian and foreign students/residents. To receive student and resident rate, orders must be accompanied by name of affiliated institution, date of term, and the signature of program/residency coordinatior on institution letterhead. Orders will be billed at individual rate until proof of status is received. Foreign air speed delivery is included in all Clinics subscriptionprices. All prices are subject to change without notice. **POSTMASTER:** Send address changes to *Radiologic Clinics of North America,* Elsevier Periodicals Customer Service, 6277 Sea Harbor Drive, Orlando, FL 32887-4800. **Customer Service: 1-800-654-2452 (US). From outside of the US, call (+1) 407-345-4000.**

Radiologic Clinics of North America also published in Greek Paschalidis Medical Publications, Athens, Greece.

Radiologic Clinics of North America is covered in *Index Medicus, EMBASE/Excerpta Medica, Current Contents/Life Sciences, Current Contents/Clinical Medicine, RSNA Index to Imaging Literature, BIOSIS, Science Citation Index,* and *ISI/BIOMED.*

Printed in the United States of America.

RADIOLOGIC CLINICS OF NORTH AMERICA JANUARY 2007

GOAL STATEMENT

The goal of the *Radiologic Clinics of North America* is to keep practicing radiologists and radiology residents up to date with current clinical practice in radiology by providing timely articles reviewing the state of the art in patient care.

ACCREDITATION

The *Radiologic Clinics of North America* is planned and implemented in accordance with the Essential Areas and Policies of the Accreditation Council for Continuing Medical Education (ACCME) through the joint sponsorship of the University of Virginia School of Medicine and Elsevier. The University of Virginia School of Medicine is accredited by the ACCME to provide continuing medical education for physicians.

The University of Virginia School of Medicine designates this educational activity for a maximum of 15 *AMA PRA Category 1 Credits™*. Physicians should only claim credit commensurate with the extent of their participation in the activity.

The American Medical Association has determined that physicians not licensed in the US who participate in this CME activity are eligible for 15 *AMA PRA Category 1 Credits™*.

Credit can be earned by reading the text material, taking the CME examination online at http://www.theclinics.com/home/cme, and completing the evaluation. After taking the test, you will be required to review any and all incorrect answers. Following completion of the test and evaluation, your credit will be awarded and you may print your certificate.

FACULTY DISCLOSURE/CONFLICT OF INTEREST

The University of Virginia School of Medicine, as an ACCME accredited provider, endorses and strives to comply with the Accreditation Council for Continuing Medical Education (ACCME) Standards of Commercial Support, Commonwealth of Virginia statutes, University of Virginia policies and procedures, and associated federal and private regulations and guidelines on the need for disclosure and monitoring of proprietary and financial interests that may affect the scientific integrity and balance of content delivered in continuing medical education activities under our auspices.

The University of Virginia School of Medicine requires that all CME activities accredited through this institution be developed independently and be scientifically rigorous, balanced and objective in the presentation/ discussion of its content, theories and practices.

All authors/editors participating in an accredited CME activity are expected to disclose to the readers relevant financial relationships with commercial entities occurring within the past 12 months (such as grants or research support, employee, consultant, stock holder, member of speakers bureau, etc.). The University of Virginia School of Medicine will employ appropriate mechanisms to resolve potential conflicts of interest to maintain the standards of fair and balanced education to the reader. Questions about specific strategies can be directed to the Office of Continuing Medical Education, University of Virginia School of Medicine, Charlottesville, Virginia.

The authors/editors listed below have identified no financial or professional relationships for themselves or their spouse/partner:
Tim Akhurst, MD; Oguz Akin, MD; Adriadne Bach, MD; Lia Bartella, MD; D. David Dershaw, MD; Barton Dudlick (Acquisitions Editor); Michelle S. Ginsberg, MD; Marc J. Gollub, MD; Ravinder K. Grewal, MD; Lucy E. Hann, MD; Robert T. Heelan, MD; Hedvig Hricak, MD, PhD (Guest Editor); Sasan Karimi, MD; Nancy Lee, MD; Robert A. Lefkowitz, MD; Laura Liberman, MD, FACR; Svetlana Mironov, MD; Neeta Pandit-Taskar, MD; David M. Panicek, MD (Guest Editor); Jürgen Rademaker, MD; Lawrence H. Schwartz, MD; Clare S. Smith, MB, BCh, BAO, FRCR; and, Jingbo Zhang, MD.

The authors/editors listed below have identified the following financial or professional relationships for themselves or their spouse/partner:
Scott Gerst, MD owns stock in SafeMed, Inc.
Snehal G. Patel receives royalties for a textbook from Elsevier Science.
Hilda Stambuk, MD is a contributor/author for Amirsys.

Disclosure of Discussion of Non-FDA Approved Uses for Pharmaceutical and/or Medical Devices:
The University of Virginia School of Medicine, as an ACCME provider, requires that all authors identify and disclose any "off label" uses for pharmaceutical and medical device products. The University of Virginia School of Medicine recommends that each physician fully review all the available data on new products or procedures prior to clinical use.

TO ENROLL

To enroll in the *Radiologic Clinics of North America* Continuing Medical Education program, call customer service at 1-800-654-2452 or sign up online at http://www.theclinics.com/home/cme. The CME program is available to subscribers for an additional annual fee of $205.00.

iv

UPDATE ON RADIOLOGIC EVALUATION OF COMMON MALIGNANCIES

GUEST EDITORS

HEDVIG HRICAK, MD, PhD
Professor of Radiology, Weill Medical
College of Cornell University; Chairman,
Department of Radiology, Memorial
Sloan-Kettering Cancer Center, New York,
New York

DAVID M. PANICEK, MD
Professor of Radiology, Weill Medical College of
Cornell University; Vice Chair for Clinical Affairs,
Department of Radiology, Memorial
Sloan-Kettering Cancer Center, New York,
New York

CONTRIBUTORS

TIM AKHURST, MD
Assistant Professor of Nuclear Medicine,
Section of Nuclear Medicine, Department
of Radiology, Weill Medical College of Cornell
University, Memorial Sloan-Kettering Cancer
Center, New York, New York

OGUZ AKIN, MD
Assistant Professor of Radiology, Weill Medical
College of Cornell University; Attending
Radiologist, Department of Radiology, Memorial
Sloan-Kettering Cancer Center, New York,
New York

ARIADNE BACH, MD
Assistant Attending, Memorial Sloan-Kettering
Cancer Center; Associate Professor of Radiology,
Cornell University, Weill Medical College,
New York, New York

LIA BARTELLA, MD, FRCR
Assistant Professor of Radiology, Weill Medical
College of Cornell University; Assistant Attending
Radiologist, Breast Imaging Section, Department
of Radiology, Memorial Sloan-Kettering Cancer
Center, New York, New York

D. DAVID DERSHAW, MD, FACR
Professor of Radiology, Weill Medical College
of Cornell University; Director and Attending
Radiologist, Breast Imaging Section, Department
of Radiology, Memorial Sloan-Kettering Cancer
Center, New York, New York

SCOTT GERST, MD
Assistant Attending, Memorial Sloan-Kettering
Cancer Center; Assistant Professor of Radiology,
Cornell University, Weill Medical College,
New York, New York

MICHELLE S. GINSBERG, MD
Department of Radiology, Memorial
Sloan-Kettering Cancer Center;
Weill Medical College of Cornell University,
New York, New York

MARC J. GOLLUB, MD
Associate Professor of Radiology, and Director
of CT and GI Radiology, Department of Radiology,
Weill Medical College of Cornell University,
Memorial Sloan-Kettering Cancer Center,
New York, New York

RAVINDER K. GREWAL, MD
Department of Radiology, Memorial Sloan-
Kettering Cancer Center; Weill Medical College
of Cornell University, New York, New York

LUCY E. HANN, MD
Professor of Radiology, Weill Medical College
of Cornell University; Attending Radiologist,
Department of Radiology, Memorial Sloan-
Kettering Cancer Center, New York, New York

ROBERT T. HEELAN, MD
Department of Radiology, Memorial Sloan-
Kettering Cancer Center; Weill Medical College
of Cornell University, New York, New York

HEDVIG HRICAK, MD, PhD
Professor of Radiology, Weill Medical College
of Cornell University; Chairman, Department
of Radiology, Memorial Sloan-Kettering Cancer
Center, New York, New York

SASAN KARIMI, MD
Assistant Attending, Neuroradiology Service,
Department of Radiology, Memorial
Sloan-Kettering Cancer Center, New York, NY

NANCY LEE, MD
Assistant Attending, Department of Radiation
Oncology, Memorial Sloan-Kettering Cancer
Center, New York, NY

ROBERT A. LEFKOWITZ, MD
Associate Attending, Memorial Sloan-Kettering
Cancer Center; Associate Professor of Radiology,
Cornell University, Weill Medical College,
New York, New York

LAURA LIBERMAN, MD, FACR
Professor of Radiology, Weill Medical College of
Cornell University; and Director of Breast Imaging
Research Programs and Attending Radiologist,
Breast Imaging Section, Department of Radiology,
Memorial Sloan-Kettering Cancer Center,
New York, New York

SVETLANA MIRONOV, MD
Assistant Professor of Radiology, Weill Medical
College of Cornell University; Attending
Radiologist, Department of Radiology, Memorial
Sloan-Kettering Cancer Center, New York,
New York

NEETA PANDIT-TASKAR, MD
Assistant Professor of Radiology, Weill Medical
College of Cornell University; Attending
Radiologist, Department of Radiology, Memorial
Sloan-Kettering Cancer Center, New York,
New York

SNEHAL G. PATEL, MD
Assistant Attending,
Head and Neck Service, Department of Surgery,
Memorial Sloan-Kettering Cancer Center,
New York, NY

JÜRGEN RADEMAKER, MD
Department of Radiology, Memorial
Sloan-Kettering Cancer Center, Cornell University,
Weill Medical College, New York, New York

LAWRENCE H. SCHWARTZ, MD
Associate Professor of Radiology, Director of MRI,
Department of Radiology, Weill Medical College
of Cornell University, Memorial Sloan-Kettering
Cancer Center, New York, New York

CLARE S. SMITH, MB, BCh, BAO, FRCR
Instructor, Breast Imaging Section, Department
of Radiology, Memorial Sloan-Kettering Cancer
Center, New York, New York

HILDA E. STAMBUK, MD
Associate Attending, Neuroradiology Service,
Department of Radiology, Memorial
Sloan-Kettering Cancer Center, New York, NY

JINGBO ZHANG, MD
Assistant Attending, Memorial Sloan-Kettering
Cancer Center; Assistant Professor of Radiology,
Cornell University, Weill Medical College, New
York, New York

UPDATE ON RADIOLOGIC EVALUATION OF COMMON MALIGNANCIES

Volume 45 • Number 1 • January 2007

Contents

The diagnosis and management of lymphoma have undergone significant changes in the past 20 years. For example, new immunophenotypic and molecular methods have replaced traditional histology-based classification schemes for lymphoma. Fluorine-18-deoxyglucose (FDG) positron emission tomography (PET) has evolved into a potent staging tool and prognostic indicator in many kinds of lymphoma. The role of radiation therapy, especially in patients who have early-stage Hodgkin's disease, has changed substantially. The introduction of anti-CD 20 antibody therapy (Rituximab) has improved the treatment of B-cell lymphoma. These changes are linked with higher expectations for imaging, such as detection of more subtle lymphoma manifestations, evaluation of residual changes, and better assessment of early response. This article reviews clinical and radiologic features of both Hodgkin's disease and non-Hodgkin's lymphoma. It also describes the radiologic staging of lymphoma and the emerging role of FDG-PET for assessing lymphoma.

Colorectal cancer remains a leading cancer killer worldwide. The disease is both curable and preventable, and yet the importance of widespread screening is only now starting to be appreciated. This article reviews the variety of diagnostic tests, imaging procedures, and endoscopic examinations available to detect colorectal cancer and polyps in their early stage and also presents details on various screening options. The critical role of the radiologist is elaborated on including accurate assessment of tumor extent within the bowel wall and beyond and the detection of lymph node and distant metastases. Staging with CT, MR imaging, endorectal ultrasound, and positron emission tomography are of paramount importance in determining the most appropriate therapy and the risk of tumor recurrence and overall prognosis.

Advances in molecular genetics have expanded the understanding of renal cell tumors. Now it is understood that renal cortical tumors are a family of neoplasms with distinct cytogenetics and molecular defects, unique histopathologic features, and different malignant potentials. Imaging contributes to clinical management of patients with renal tumors in providing diagnostic information for tumor detection, characterization, staging, treatment planning, and follow-up.

Imaging has become an essential part of the clinical management of patients with ovarian cancer, contributing to tumor detection, characterization, staging, treatment planning, and follow-up. Imaging findings incorporated into the clinical impression assist in creating a treatment plan specific for an individual patient. Advances in cross-sectional imaging and nuclear medicine (PET) have yielded new insights into the evaluation of tumor prognostic factors. A multimodality approach can satisfy the complex imaging needs of a patient with ovarian cancer; however, the success of such an approach always depends on available resources and on the skills of the physicians involved.

RADIOLOGIC CLINICS OF NORTH AMERICA

Radiol Clin N Am 45 (2007) xi–xii

Preface

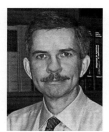
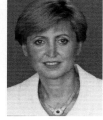

David M. Panicek, MD Hedvig Hricak, MD, PhD,
Guest Editors

David M. Panicek, MD
Department of Radiology
Memorial Sloan-Kettering Cancer Center
1275 York Avenue
New York, NY 10021, USA

E-mail address:
panicekd@mskcc.org

Hedvig Hricak, MD, PhD
Department of Radiology
Memorial Sloan-Kettering Cancer Center
1275 York Avenue
New York, NY 10021, USA

E-mail address:
hricakh@mskcc.org

Imaging has assumed a central position in the modern care of cancer patients, being essential in the detection, diagnosis, staging, response assessment, and follow-up surveillance of a wide variety of tumor types. The standard treatments of chemotherapy, surgery, and radiation therapy continue to be refined, and newer therapies, such as image-guided or image-based focal tumor ablation, continue to emerge. Decisions about which particular therapy or combination of therapies is best for a given patient often hinge on the results of imaging examinations. As cancers become increasingly common due to ever-lengthening life expectancy and to more effective therapies that result in longer lives for cancer patients, the need for effective and efficient imaging throughout the entire cancer management process will only increase.

Proper interpretation of oncologic radiologic images requires specialized knowledge about the specific radiologic manifestations and biologic behavior of a particular tumor type. If the radiology report describes abnormalities on examinations without providing a meaningful interpretation of the clinical relevance of those findings, little added value is provided. Similarly, optimal therapy response assessment requires quantification not only of changes in tumor size but of changes in tumor biology, such as those shown by dynamic contrast-enhanced CT or MRI, or by PET/SPECT imaging. If an early assessment of therapeutic response shows a suboptimal response, an appropriate change in the therapeutic regimen can be instituted, potentially sparing that patient the physical and emotional morbidities associated with a long and unsuccessful course of treatment. The informed radiologist will be able to become a more highly valued member of the cancer care team when he/she can provide the clinically relevant information in a concise manner.

The authors of this issue of the *Radiologic Clinics of North America* were chosen for their focused

doi:10.1016/j.rcl.2006.11.001

expertise in oncologic imaging. We thank these oncologic radiologists and their clinical colleagues for sharing their experience and insights to provide a comprehensive update on practical oncologic imaging. Ten of the most common cancers in the United States were selected for inclusion in this issue to provide a useful resource when interpreting imaging studies. It is our hope that readers will become better informed about the specific details of these common cancers in each of the various stages of a cancer patient's care, and as a result, maximize the vast potential of radiology to contribute to the overall control and cure of that complex disease process.

RADIOLOGIC
CLINICS
OF NORTH AMERICA

Radiol Clin N Am 45 (2007) 1–20

Oral Cavity and Oropharynx Tumors

Hilda E. Stambuk, MD[a],*, Sasan Karimi, MD[a],
Nancy Lee, MD[b], Snehal G. Patel, MD[c]

- Oral cavity
  - Screening
  - Diagnosis
  - Staging
  - Disease-specific follow-up
- Oropharynx
  - Diagnosis
  - Staging
  - Disease-specific follow-up
- Summary
- References

Cancers of the oral cavity and pharynx are the most common head and neck cancers in the United States [1]. Most tumors are squamous cell carcinomas (SCC), but other histologic types may include minor salivary gland carcinomas and, rarely, lymphomas and melanoma. For descriptive purposes, the mucosa of the oral cavity and oropharynx is divided into several anatomic sub sites (Fig. 1). The anatomic division between the oral cavity and oropharynx is artificial, and in actual practice it is not uncommon for a tumor to cross over into the oropharynx from the oral cavity and vice versa. The clinical behavior of tumors in these two locations is distinct, however. As a general rule, regional lymph node and distant metastases are more frequently observed with involvement of the oropharynx by SCC. Clinical behavior is also dictated by the histologic type of tumor; perineural spread of disease and lung metastases are features associated with adenoid cystic carcinoma of minor salivary gland origin. Clinical examination and evaluation of local extent of disease are easier in the oral cavity because the mucosa of the oral cavity is more easily accessible to clinicians for clinical inspection and palpation. It is important for clinicians and radiologists to understand these differences in clinical behavior to direct patients to appropriate imaging in the initial evaluation and subsequent follow-up of their disease. Radiologic issues pertaining to these two anatomic sites are discussed under two separate sections in this article. The focus is on SCC, but rare tumors such as adenoid cystic carcinoma are mentioned briefly where appropriate.

Oral cavity

Screening

Clinical examination of the oral cavity is superior to radiologic imaging in assessing for mucosal lesions. There is no cost-effective role for imaging in screening for index primary lesions of the oral cavity, even in selected high-risk populations. Patients who have SCC of the oral cavity are at a small but defined risk for synchronous primary tumors [2,3]. Although most of these second primary tumors occur in the oral cavity and are easily detected on clinical examination, a second primary can be missed in patients who are difficult to

[a] Department of Radiology, Memorial Sloan-Kettering Cancer Center, 1275 York Avenue, New York, NY 10021, USA
[b] Department of Radiation Oncology, Memorial Sloan-Kettering Cancer Center, 1275 York Avenue, New York, NY 10021, USA
[c] Department of Surgery, Memorial Sloan-Kettering Cancer Center, 1275 York Avenue, New York, NY 10021, USA
* Corresponding author.

doi:10.1016/j.rcl.2006.10.010

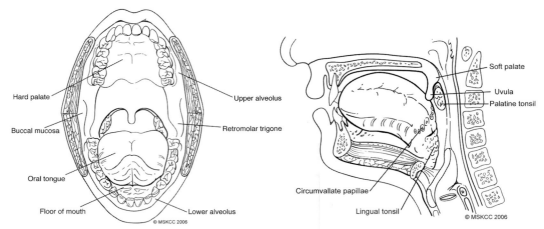

Fig. 1. The anatomic sub sites of the oral cavity, (oral tongue, floor of mouth, lower alveolus, retromolar trigone, upper alveolus, hard palate, buccal mucosa), and oropharynx (base of tongue, soft palate, palatine tonsil). (*Courtesy of* Memorial Sloan-Kettering Cancer Center, New York, NY; with permission.)

examine because of pain or trismus. The radiologist automatically should survey the upper aerodigestive tract for additional tumors when imaging studies have been ordered for staging any oral cancer. Incidental discovery of a synchronous primary tumor may result in modification of the treatment plan in a patient who is being evaluated for a known oral cavity primary (Fig. 2).

Diagnosis

Most patients who have SCC come to imaging with the diagnosis already made. The role of imaging as a diagnostic modality is limited. The radiologist should not be satisfied with identifying the tumor alone but should provide the clinician with information about the local extent and regional spread

that can impact treatment. It is important to be aware of certain common imaging characteristics that might help in differentiating benign from malignant lesions of the oral cavity (Table 1). SCC generally only mildly enhances postcontrast on CT imaging and can be subtle (Fig. 3). On MR imaging scans, SCC is isointense to muscle on T1-weighted images, tends to be of high T2 signal, and generally exhibits mild to moderate homogeneous enhancement. CT is the more common imaging modality in the evaluation of oral cavity cancers. CT imaging of the oral cavity and neck with contrast can be acquired within minutes with modern multidetector scanners, and the raw data easily can be used for coronal and sagittal reformation. CT is superior in evaluating the mandible for cortical bone invasion.

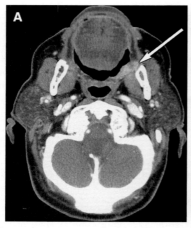
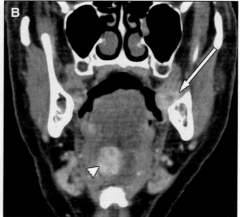

Fig. 2. (*A*) The patient presented with a clinically evident SCC of the left retromolar trigone (*arrow*) for which a CT scan of the oral cavity was performed. (*B*) Incidental right base of tongue primary cancer (*arrowhead*) was discovered at imaging.

Table 1: Imaging characteristics of benign versus malignant tumors of the oral cavity

	Benign	Malignant
Location	Generally deep	Generally superficial
Configuration	Well defined	Ill defined
Surrounding tissue	Normal or may be displaced	Invaded
Internal characteristics	Fatty, cystic or vascular ± flow voids but can be heterogeneous or solid	Solid and isodense to muscle MR imaging; T1-weighted isointense, T2-weighted hyperintense to muscle, variable enhancement
Calcifications	±	No calcifications
Bone	Not affected or regressively remodeled	Cortical invasion or destruction
Nerves	Not affected or focal lesion if benign nerve tumor	Perineural spread is generally diffuse or skips with associated oral cavity mass
FDG-PET scan	Generally no FDG uptake except in infection	+ FDG uptake except in tumors of minor salivary gland origin

MR imaging can be helpful in evaluating the full extent of medullary cavity involvement once the mandibular cortex has been violated. MR imaging is the imaging modality of choice in the evaluation of hard palate tumors, where replacement of bone marrow by tumor is more easily appreciated on precontrast T1-weighted images (Fig. 4).

CT can be limiting in the evaluation of oral cavity tumors because of beam hardening artifact from dental work. Susceptibility artifact from dental work is generally less obscuring of the underlying anatomy on MR imaging than the artifact created with CT scanning. MR imaging shows superior tumor/muscle interface and better delineates perineural spread of disease; however, it is limited by its long acquisition time. An adequate MR imaging of the oral cavity takes approximately 30 minutes to acquire, with imaging of the neck requiring another 30 minutes. Patients who have bulky tumors of the oral cavity have pooling of secretions and constant swallowing, which can render an MR imaging examination nondiagnostic.

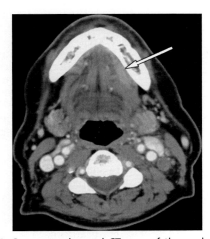

Fig. 3. Contrast-enhanced CT scan of the oral cavity. Note that tumor in left floor of mouth (*arrow*) is only mildly enhancing and relatively isodense to surrounding muscle.

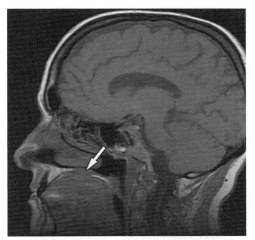

Fig. 4. Sagittal precontrast T1-weighted image shows bone marrow invasion by adjacent mucosal hard palate adenoid cystic carcinoma. The normal higher signal fatty marrow is replaced by grayish appearing tumor (*arrow*).

The presence of nodal metastases is the most significant predictor of adverse outcome in head and neck SCC [4]. Extracapsular spread of disease from a metastatic lymph node worsens the prognosis further, and these patients may benefit from more aggressive treatment [5,6]. CT shows focal nodal metastases/necrosis in "normal sized" lymph nodes and extracapsular spread of disease from lymph nodes sooner than MR imaging and before it becomes apparent on clinical examination (Fig. 5).

Staging

SCC of the oral cavity tends to spread locally with invasion of surrounding structures, and the risk and patterns of lymphatic spread to regional cervical nodes vary with the anatomic location of the primary tumor. Certain anatomic subsites, such as the oral tongue and floor of the mouth, are rich in lymphatics, and tumors of these areas have a higher risk of nodal metastases compared with other locations, such as the upper gum and hard palate. Distant metastasis is not common in patients with oral SCC, but tumors such as adenoid cystic carcinoma have a higher predilection for pulmonary metastases. Knowledge of the behavior and patterns of spread of these tumors is essential for radiologists in accurate interpretation and staging. The TNM staging system is used for epithelial tumors, including SCC and minor salivary gland carcinoma only [7].

T stage

The anatomic imaging techniques of choice for local staging are contrast-enhanced CT and MR imaging, but CT is the workhorse. MR imaging often complements CT and should be used to examine specific questions, such as perineural spread of disease. If a patient is able to lie still without swallowing or moving, MR imaging provides better delineation of tumor from muscle. MR imaging is especially useful in the evaluation of extent of involvement of the musculature of the tongue, which can be difficult to evaluate on clinical examination in an awake patient. The precise delineation of local extent of tumor not only is important for assigning T stage (Table 2) but also is crucial in treatment planning.

CT must be performed with intravenous contrast to better identify the primary tumor and help differentiate nodal metastases from adjacent vasculature. These images should be provided in axial and coronal planes in standard and bone algorithms for complete evaluation of the soft tissues and bone. MR imaging scans always should be performed with and without gadolinium intravenous contrast. The precontrast T1-weighted sequence is particularly useful in differentiating tumor from surrounding fat, detecting neurovascular bundle encasement

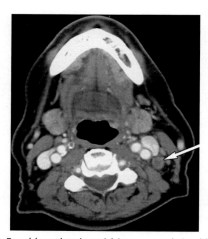

Fig. 5. Focal low density within a normal sized lymph node (*arrow*) on postcontrast CT scan indicates metastatic disease.

Table 2:	T staging of oral cavity tumors
TX	Primary tumor cannot be assessed
T0	No evidence of primary tumor
Tis	Carcinoma in situ
T1	Tumor 2 cm or less in greatest dimension
T2	Tumor more than 2 cm but not more than 4 cm in greatest dimension
T3	Tumor more than 4 cm in greatest dimension
T4a	
Lip	Tumor invades through cortical bone, inferior alveolar nerve, floor of mouth, or skin of face (ie, chin or nose)
Oral Cavity	Tumor invades through cortical bone, into deep (extrinsic) muscle of tongue (genioglossus, hyoglossus, palatoglossus, and styloglossus), maxillary sinus, or skin of face
T4b	Tumor involves masticator space, pterygoid plates, or skull base and/or encases internal carotid artery

(sublingual space), and detecting marrow involvement of the adjacent mandible and maxilla. Sagittal T2-weighted images can be helpful in assessing depth of invasion of the primary tumor of the oral tongue. The depth of invasion of the primary tumor has been shown to correlate with the risk for nodal metastases and outcome [8]. Postcontrast fat saturation T1-weighted images also can be helpful in differentiating tumor from adjacent muscle/fat and detecting perineural spread of disease. Tumors with an infiltrative border can be differentiated from those with a defined "pushing" border on imaging, and this information is helpful to clinicians in predicting outcome [9].

Advanced lip cancers that occur along the mucosal surface may abut the buccal cortex of the mandible and may require CT imaging to assess the integrity of the mandible. Imaging also may be helpful in evaluating for perineural spread of tumor, especially adenoid cystic carcinoma along the mental and inferior alveolar nerves. Otherwise, mucosal lip cancers do not require diagnostic imaging for assessment of local extension.

Most cases of oral tongue SCC are located along its lateral border or ventral surface. The prognosis of these tumors depends on their depth of invasion. Although superficial tumors are difficult to assess on radiologic imaging, involvement of the extrinsic muscles of the tongue (genioglossus, hyoglossus, palatoglossus, and styloglossus) is relatively easy to detect (Fig. 6). Another feature of interest is whether the tumor approaches or crosses the midline fibrofatty septum of the tongue. Posterior extension of an oral tongue tumor into the base of tongue should be noted because this finding has the potential to change treatment. Oral tongue SCC commonly extends into the floor of mouth. The neurovascular bundle (particularly the lingual artery and hypoglossal nerve and their branches) traverses the sublingual space and can be in close proximity to tumor (Fig. 7). Surgical excision of a lesion such as this requires sacrifice of the ipsilateral neurovascular bundle but leaves viable remnant tongue based on the intact contralateral neurovascular bundle. In contrast, if an oral tongue tumor is extensive enough to require surgical sacrifice of both neurovascular bundles (Fig. 8), the patient would require total glossectomy, which can be functionally crippling. Nonsurgical management (radiation with or without chemotherapy) should be considered in these situations. Tumors of the anterior floor of mouth can obstruct the openings of the Wharton's ducts (submandibular salivary gland ducts). Radiologically evident dilatation of Wharton's ducts should prompt a thorough search for a mucosal primary tumor in the absence of obvious calculus disease (Fig. 9).

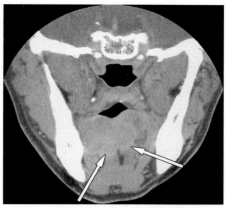

Fig. 6. CT imaging shows obvious SCC involvement of the extrinsic muscles of the tongue, including the paired genioglossus muscles (*arrows*).

Evaluation of the mandible for invasion by tumor is an important consideration in staging and treatment planning. Tumors at certain locations, such as the floor of mouth, retromolar trigone, and the lower alveolus, can invade the mandible directly. Although gross invasion is relatively easy to identify, early cortical bone loss directly adjacent to obvious tumor should be considered indicative of bone invasion (Fig. 10). If bone invasion is present, it is important for the radiologist to define its extent so that the surgeon is able to determine the extent of mandibular resection. In most situations CT is adequate for this determination, but the bone marrow may be further characterized by MR imaging if appropriate.

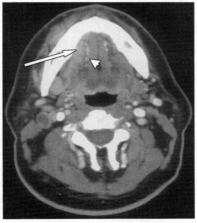

Fig. 7. CT of the oral cavity shows tumor of the right lateral tongue (*arrow*) in close proximity to but not involving the right neurovascular bundle (*arrowhead*).

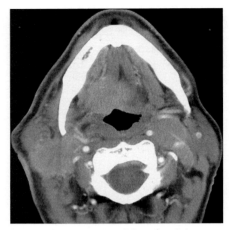

Fig. 8. Extensive tumor involving the right neurovascular bundle that would have required sacrifice of the uninvolved left neurovascular bundle and total glossectomy to achieve adequate surgical margins.

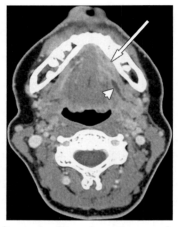

Fig. 9. Left anterior floor of mouth cancer (arrow) obstructing left Wharton's duct with subsequent ductal dilatation (arrowhead).

Resection of the involved segment of the mandible becomes necessary if there is direct invasion of the bone. On the other hand, if the primary tumor is in close proximity to but does not directly invade the mandible, marginal mandibulectomy provides an adequate surgical resection while maintaining integrity of the bone (Fig. 11). On rare occasions, segmental mandibulectomy may become necessary in the absence of direct bone invasion. Marginal resection of the mandible is technically not possible if the tumor is in close proximity to a substantial depth along its lingual (inner) cortex. Clinical examination is generally unreliable in differentiating direct tumor extension through the muscular diaphragm of the oral cavity from metastatic lymphadenopathy or an obstructed submandibular salivary gland (Fig. 12). This information has important implications in the staging and the surgical approach and should be reported clearly.

The mandible also should be evaluated in certain other situations in which mandibulotomy is required for surgical access to the primary tumor that may not necessarily be in proximity to the bone. Tumors of the posterior oral cavity and oropharynx are difficult to resect through the open mouth. The mandibular "swing" approach (mandibulotomy) can provide excellent exposure of these tumors and allow adequate resection and appropriate reconstruction of the surgical defect. A paramedian osteotomy is usually placed between the lateral incisor and canine teeth, after which the floor of mouth is incised so that the mandibular segment can be retracted laterally. Unrelated but unexpected lesions at the proposed mandibulotomy site should be recognized and reported to avoid surprises during the surgical procedure (Fig. 13).

The retromolar trigone is the part of the buccal mucosa located posterior to the last lower molar tooth along the ascending ramus of the mandible. Because the periosteum of the mandible is in close

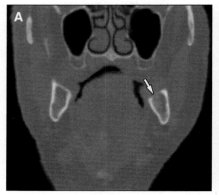

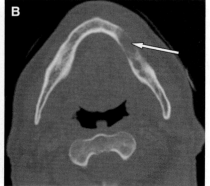

Fig. 10. (A) CT scan of the oral cavity showing early invasion of the mandibular cortex from a lower alveolar ridge SCC. (B) CT scan of the oral cavity with gross invasion of the mandible from gingival SCC.

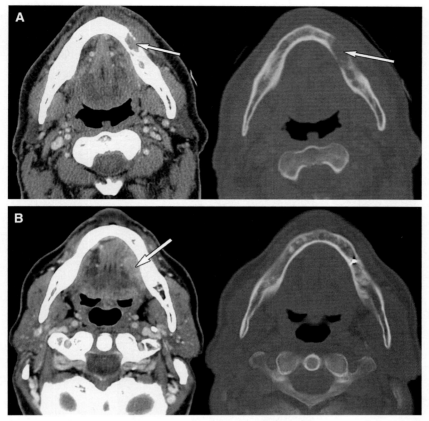

Fig. 11. The relationship of the primary tumor to the mandible determines the extent of surgical resection of the bone. (*A*) If the bone is directly invaded by tumor (*arrow*), a segmental mandibulectomy is necessary and the resultant defect may need reconstruction. (*B*) Marginal mandibulectomy involves resection of a rim of mandible to provide a surgical margin for tumors that are in close proximity but not invading bone (*arrow*). The procedure is technically feasible only if there is sufficient vertical height of bone stock and the mandibular canal with its neurovascular bundle does not get exposed or resected. The patient is at risk for stress fracture if the remnant mandible has insufficient vertical height/stock or its vascular supply is compromised.

proximity, tumors of the retromolar trigone have a higher propensity to invade bone. The pterygo-mandibular raphe is a fibrous band that runs from the hamulus of the medial pterygoid plate to the posterior end of the mylohyoid line of the mandible. The fibers of the buccinator and superior constrictor muscles interdigitate along this raphe. Once a retromolar trigone tumor infiltrates the pterygo-mandibular raphe, it has access to the buccinator muscle and buccal space, pterygoid musculature and pterygoid plates, posterior maxillary alveolar ridge, or skull base (Fig. 14). The inferior alveolar nerve is also located in close proximity to the retro-molar trigone and is at risk for direct invasion and perineural spread. Perineural spread of tumor along the inferior alveolar nerve is identified by enlargement and enhancement of the nerve more easily seen on MR imaging and widening of the bony canal on CT scan (Fig. 15).

Perineural spread of tumor is a particular feature of adenoid cystic carcinomas, which are generally submucosal in location and tend to occur on the hard palate. Tumors of the hard palate can spread along the greater and lesser palatine nerves into the pterygopalatine fossa and along V2 and the vidian nerve (Fig. 16). Radiologic evaluation of hard palate tumors should include a careful survey of these routes of spread, including the entire course of the trigeminal nerve. The submucosal extent of the lesion, involvement of the underlying bone of the hard palate, and extension into the nasal cavity or maxillary sinus also should be noted (Fig. 17).

N stage

The status of the cervical lymph nodes is the most significant predictor of outcome in patients who have SCC of the oral cavity. The risk of nodal

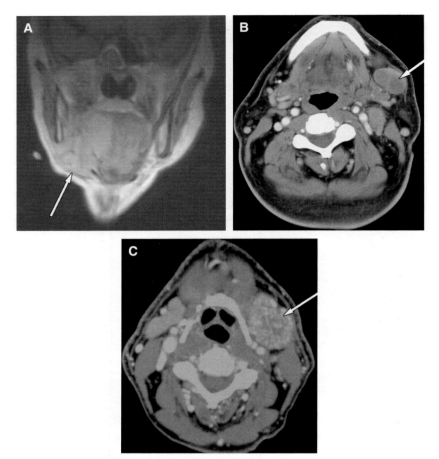

Fig. 12. Coronal imaging is helpful in delineating the relationship of the primary tumor to the lingual cortex of the mandible. It is also important to differentiate direct tumor extension through the mylohyoid muscle into the submandibular space (*A*) from a metastatic lymph node (*B*) or an enlarged submandibular gland from tumor obstructing Wharton's duct (*C*).

metastases depends on the anatomic site of the primary tumor within the oral cavity. Tumors of the oral tongue, floor of mouth, and buccal mucosa have a higher propensity to metastasize to cervical lymph nodes compared with hard palate and alveolar tumors. SCCs generally metastasize to the draining cervical lymph nodes in a predictable pattern [10]. For ease of description and consistency, the cervical lymph nodes are arbitrarily grouped into levels I-V (Fig. 18) (Table 3). Levels I-III are at highest risk for nodal metastases from oral cavity SCC. In the previously untreated neck, metastases to levels IV or V are rare in the absence of obvious lymphadenopathy at levels I-III.

Most metastatic lymph nodes from SCC are abnormally enlarged, but the size criteria for designating cervical lymph nodes as metastatic are not universally accepted. As a general rule, lymph nodes ≥1.5 cm at levels I and highest level II (jugulodigastric) and ≥1 cm at all other levels are considered

abnormal. Normal sized lymph nodes can have focal metastasis or necrosis that is more easily seen on CT than MR imaging (Fig. 19). Other radiologic features of metastatic lymphadenopathy from SCC include heterogeneous enhancement and stranding or involvement of the adjacent soft tissue if extracapsular nodal spread is present (Fig. 20). Extracapsular nodal spread is generally seen in larger lymph nodes but can be seen in small lymph nodes. The current staging system for the neck does not take into account the presence of extracapsular spread but is based on the size, number, and laterality of the metastatic lymph nodes relative to the primary tumor (Table 4).

The radiologist also should look for and report certain other features of metastatic lymphadenopathy that may be valuable in therapeutic decision making. The relationship of metastatic lymphadenopathy to the great vessels of the neck, particularly the carotid artery, is an important consideration in

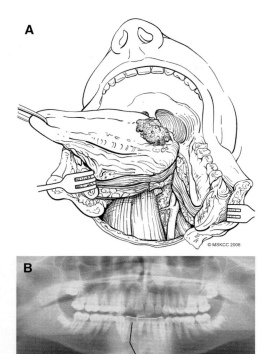

Fig. 13. (*A*) The mandibular osteotomy is placed in a paramedian location on the anterior mandible, and division of the soft tissue structures of the floor of mouth allows lateral retraction for access to the posterior oral cavity and oropharynx. (*Courtesy of Memorial Sloan Kettering Cancer Center, New York, NY; with permission.*) (*B*) Panorex shows incidental lytic lesion of the anterior mandible. Failure to recognize this lesion preoperatively places the patient at risk for poor healing and nonunion of the mandibulotomy.

determining surgical resectability. If more than 270° of the circumference of the carotid artery are surrounded by tumor, it is considered "encased" and the tumor is generally surgically unresectable. Similarly, extension of nodal disease into the prevertebral musculature is an adverse indicator of prognosis and should be reported.

M stage

Distant metastases from oral cavity SCC are rare at presentation. There is no cost-effective role for routine positron emission tomography (PET) scan in most patients who have oral SCC. Patients who present with locoregionally advanced tumor may be at higher risk for distant metastasis, especially to the lungs. Noncontrast chest CT may be indicated to assess for distant metastases in this selected group and in patients who have adenoid cystic carcinoma.

Disease-specific follow-up

The pattern of recurrence in oral cavity SCC is different from oropharyngeal SCC because nodal and distant metastases are more frequently seen in patients who have oropharyngeal SCC. Most recurrences occur at the local site or in the neck, which should be the primary focus of posttreatment surveillance. The risk for distant failure after successful treatment of oral cavity SCC is low. Patients who have multiply recurrent tumors and bulky nodal metastases may be at higher risk.

Clinical evaluation of the oral cavity for local recurrence is relatively easier than examination of oropharyngeal sites, such as the base of tongue. Conversely, submucosal and deep-seated

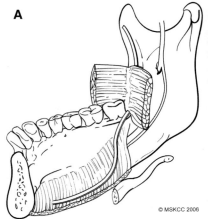

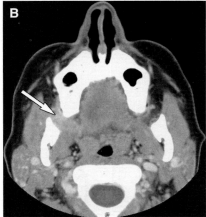

Fig. 14. (*A*) The buccinator and superior constrictor muscles interdigitate along the pterygomandibular raphe, which is attached to the medial aspect of the mandible in the vicinity of the retromolar trigone. (*Courtesy of Memorial Sloan-Kettering Cancer Center, New York, NY; with permission.*) (*B*) CT scan of the oral cavity shows spread of a right retromolar trigone tumor into the right buccal space involving the posterior aspect of the buccinator muscle.

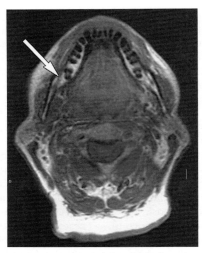

Fig. 15. Precontrast T1-weighted MR imaging shows diffuse enlargement of the right inferior alveolar nerve compatible with perineural spread of SCC. Because the inferior alveolar nerve is surrounded by fatty marrow, the enlarged nerve is easily seen on the precontrast T1-weighted sequence. The abnormal inferior alveolar nerve enhances postcontrast administration, which makes it blend in with the surrounding fatty marrow. Postcontrast T1-weighted sequence needs fat suppression for reliable identification of perineural spread.

recurrences are more easily detected on radiologic imaging (Fig. 21). Some radiographic features that may indicate locally recurrent disease include mass-like lesion with or without enhancement, abnormality along the margins of previous resection or reconstruction, bone invasion, and perineural spread. As on clinical examination, recurrence can be difficult to appreciate on diagnostic imaging

because of treatment-related changes, such as edema, fibrosis, and distortion of local anatomy after surgical manipulation. Unless otherwise indicated, it is advisable to wait approximately 12 weeks after completion of treatment before imaging to reduce false-positive results. In the appropriate circumstances, FDG PET scans can provide additional information and help direct the need for tissue diagnosis. Patients who have received radiation therapy as part of their treatment program may be at risk for developing osteoradionecrosis if the radiation portals include the mandible. Although the incidence of osteoradionecrosis is low in modern practice, its consequences, such as orocutaneous fistulas and pathologic fracture, can be devastating to the patient and treatment can be complicated. The differential diagnosis from recurrent tumor may be difficult, and unfortunately, PET scan is not specific in differentiating between these two entities.

The clinically node-negative neck in selected oral cancers can be managed safely by close surveillance. Clinical examination has been shown to be unreliable in detecting early nodal metastases compared with CT or MR imaging [11,12]. Although ultrasonography is not commonly used in the United States, it has become widely accepted in Europe [13]. Lymphatic metastases after treatment of the neck can be unpredictable because of distortion of normal lymphatic pathways. It is important to scrutinize the neck and upper mediastinum for unusual metastases, such as lateral retropharyngeal and paratracheal lymph nodes.

The lungs are the most common site for distant metastases from head and neck SCC. Routine screening for pulmonary metastases is generally limited to an annual chest radiograph, but CT of the chest may be appropriate for selected high-risk

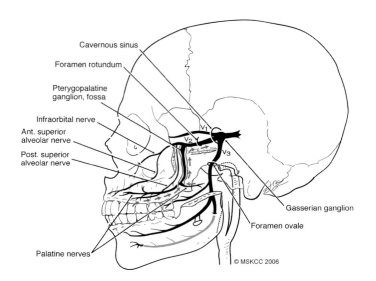

Cavernous sinus

Foramen rotundum

Pterygopalatine ganglion, fossa

Infraorbital nerve

Ant. superior alveolar nerve

Post. superior alveolar nerve

Palatine nerves

Gasserian ganglion

Foramen ovale

© MSKCC 2006

Fig. 16. The maxillary branch of the trigeminal nerve innervates the mucosa of the hard palate and upper alveolus. Perineural spread can occur along branches of these nerves in a retrograde fashion into the pterygopalatine fossa, where it can gain access to V2, or antegrade along any of the peripheral branches. (*Courtesy of* Memorial Sloan Kettering Cancer Center, New York, NY; with permission.)

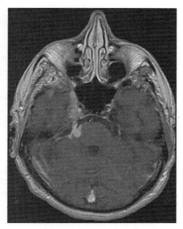

Fig. 17. Axial postcontrast T1-weighted MR imaging shows perineural spread involving V2 from the foramen rotundum, cavernous sinus, Meckel's cave, cisternal segment of the trigeminal nerve, and root entry zone in the pons.

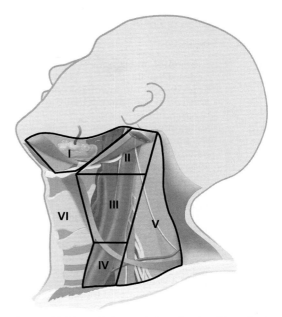

Fig. 18. Division of the neck into levels of lymphatic drainage. (*From* Shah JP, Patel SG. Head and neck surgery and oncology. 3rd edition. New York: Elsevier Science; 2003. p. 355; with permission.)

patients. No conclusive evidence supports the hypothesis that routine screening is cost-effective in improving overall outcome [14–16].

The risk for metachronous (subsequent) primary cancers increases progressively with time after successful treatment of the index primary oral cavity cancer [17]. Most of these tumors occur in locations that are easily accessible to the clinician, and there is no cost-effective role for imaging in screening for subsequent mucosal primary lesions of the head and neck. Patients who have oral cancers are also at risk for developing primary lung cancer, but the role for routine radiologic screening in this population remains undefined [17]. Annual chest radiographs have been recommended for early detection of subsequent primary lung cancer, but CT of the chest is a more sensitive examination that may be useful in selected high-risk patients [18].

The role of functional imaging (FDG-PET scan) has been investigated in screening after treatment of other head and neck cancers, such as laryngeal and hypopharyngeal [19]. The relatively lower risk for subsequent primary tumors and distant metastases in patients who have oral cancer makes it unlikely that this investigation will prove cost-effective.

Oropharynx

The oropharynx is the part of the upper aerodigestive tract that is immediately posterior to the oral cavity. It includes the base of tongue, tonsils, tonsillar pillars, posterior and lateral pharyngeal walls, and the inferior (anterior) surface of the soft palate. The oropharynx is separated from the oral cavity by the plane formed by the circumvalate papilla, anterior tonsillar pillars, and junction of the hard and soft palate. Superiorly, it extends to the level of the Passavant's ridge of the superior constrictor muscle, which is approximately at the plane of the hard palate. Inferiorly, the oropharynx ends at the level of pharyngoepiglottic folds.

This article focuses on SCC of the base of the tongue, tonsils/tonsillar pillars, and the soft palate subsites of the oropharynx. One should keep in mind that different subsites within the oropharynx contain a variable amount of lymphoid tissue. Lymphoma should be included in the differential diagnosis. Although less common, non–squamous cell malignancies, such as tumors that originate from the minor salivary glands, also can arise in the oropharynx.

Diagnosis

Base of the tongue carcinoma

The base of the tongue is the posterior third of the tongue or the part posterior to the circumvalate papilla. It extends inferiorly to end at the level of vallecula and houses the lingual tonsil [20]. SCC of the base of the tongue is often occult and asymptomatic; the lesions are often large by the time they cause symptoms, such as dysphagia or referred ear pain. Some patients present with nodal metastases without signs of a primary tumor [21]. These mucosal lesions can be invasive with deep

Table 3:	Levels of lymphatic drainage
Level	**Definition**
I	Submental and submandibular nodes. They lie above the hyoid bone, below the mylohyoid muscle, and anterior to the back of the submandibular gland.
IA	Submental nodes. They lie between the medial margins of the anterior bellies of the digastric muscles.
IB	Submandibular nodes. On each side, they lie lateral to the level IA nodes and anterior to the back of each submandibular gland.
II	Upper internal jugular nodes. They extend from the skull base to the level of the bottom of the body of the hyoid bone. They are posterior to the back of the submandibular gland and anterior to the back of the sternocleidomastoid muscle.
IIA	A level II node that lies either anterior, medial, lateral, or posterior to the internal jugular vein. If posterior to the vein, the node is inseparable from the vein.
IIB	A level II node that lies posterior to the internal jugular vein and has a fat plane separating it and the vein.
III	Middle jugular nodes. They extend from the level of the bottom of the body of the hyoid bone to the level of the bottom of the cricoid arch. They lie anterior to the back of the sternocleidomastoid muscle.
IV	Low jugular nodes. They extend from the level of the bottom of the cricoid arch to the level of the clavicle. They lie anterior to a line connecting the back of the sternocleidomastoid muscle and the posterolateral margin of the anterior scalene muscle. They are also lateral to the carotid arteries.
V	Nodes in the posterior triangle. They lie posterior to the back of the sternocleidomastoid muscle from the skull base to the level of the bottom of the cricoid arch and posterior to a line connecting the back of the sternocleidomastoid muscle and the posterolateral margin of the anterior scalene muscle from the level of the bottom of the cricoid arch to the level of the clavicle. They also lie anterior to the anterior edge of the trapezius muscle.

Table 3:	(continued)
Level	**Definition**
VA	Upper level V nodes extend from the skull base to the level of the bottom of the cricoid arch.
VB	Lower level V nodes extend from the level of the bottom of the cricoid arch to the level of the clavicle, as seen on each axial scan.

From Som PM, Curtin HD, Mancuso AA. An imaging-based classification for the cervical nodes designed as an adjunct to recent clinically based nodal classifications. Arch Otolaryngol Head Neck Surg 1999;125:388–96; with permission.

extension or can be exophytic and protrude into the airway (Fig. 22). Small lesions are difficult to detect on imaging because of lymphoid tissue at the base of the tongue, which normally enhances. The only finding on cross-sectional imaging when lesions are small may be subtle asymmetry at the base of the tongue. Unlike superficial spread of disease, deep plane infiltration is easily detected on imaging (Fig. 23). The extent of superficial spread is better appreciated clinically during endoscopic examination. On CT and MR imaging the tumors demonstrate mild to moderate enhancement. They are often isointense to muscle on T1-weighted images but are generally slightly hyperintense relative to muscle on T2-weighted images. The extent of the tumors is more easily appreciated on postcontrast images with fat saturation (Fig. 24).

In general, MR imaging is the preferred modality for evaluation of oropharyngeal tumors because of

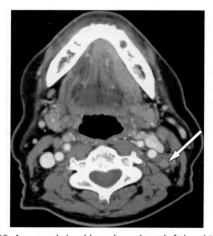

Fig. 19. A normal sized lymph node at left level II that has an eccentric focal metastatic deposit (*arrow*). This feature should be differentiated from a normal fatty hilum, which also would be eccentric but would be lower density and is seen in a reniform-shaped rather than round lymph node.

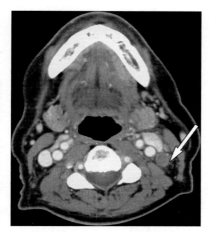

Fig. 20. Stranding of the soft tissue adjacent to a metastatic node indicates extracapsular nodal spread of disease. This feature is seen earlier on CT than MR imaging and portends a poorer prognosis for the patient.

superior soft tissue contrast and less amalgam artifact. Motion artifact can degrade image quality in patients who have bulky tumors, however. PET imaging, particularly when co-registered with CT, may localize the primary tumor in patients with unknown primaries.

Conservation therapy with chemotherapy and radiation has become the mainstay treatment of oropharyngeal cancers. Treatment is governed by tumor size, but tumor volume seems more important for therapy than T staging. Small-volume tumors can be treated with equivalent cure rates using surgery or radiation therapy, but definitive radiation therapy is the preferred treatment approach because surgical access via mandibulotomy is more invasive and has the potential for producing postoperative dysfunction [22]. Larger T-staged lesions are generally treated with concurrent chemotherapy and radiation therapy in an attempt to preserve function and the quality of life [23].

Tonsillar carcinoma

The anterior and posterior tonsillar pillars are mucosal folds over the palatoglossus and palatopharyngeal muscles, respectively. The faucial or palatine tonsils are located between the tonsillar pillars bilaterally. In this section, neoplasms that arise from the tonsillar fossa and the anterior and posterior pillars are grouped together. Carcinomas that arise at the tonsillar fossa are most common followed by lesions that arise from the anterior and the posterior pillars.

Small or early lesions are typically superficial and may be located within a tonsillar crypt so that they may be undetectable on CT/MR imaging. As the

Table 4: N staging for oral cavity and oropharyngeal tumors

Nx	Regional lymph nodes cannot be assessed
N0	No regional lymph node metastasis
N1	Metastasis in a single ipsilateral lymph node, 3 cm or less in greatest dimension
N2	Metastasis in a single ipsilateral lymph node, more than 3 cm but not more than 6 cm in greatest dimension; or in multiple ipsilateral lymph nodes, none more than 6 cm in greatest dimension; or in bilateral or contralateral lymph nodes, none more than 6 cm in greatest dimension
N2a	Metastasis in a single ipsilateral lymph node more than 3 cm but not more than 6 cm in greatest dimension
N2b	Metastasis in multiple ipsilateral lymph nodes, none more than 6 cm in greatest dimension
N2c	Metastasis in bilateral or contralateral lymph nodes, none more than 6 cm in greatest dimension
N3	Metastasis in a lymph more than 6 cm in greatest dimension

tumor grows it tends to create asymmetry of the tonsils, which can be indistinguishable from subtle tonsillar asymmetry that sometimes can be present in normal individuals (Fig. 25). The incidence of an asymmetric tonsil harboring cancer in a patient with an otherwise normal examination (ie, normal mucosa and no cervical adenopathy) is approximately 5% [24]. Tonsillar asymmetry should raise suspicion for tumor, particularly in a symptomatic patient. The larger or more advanced lesions may be exophytic or locally infiltrate the adjacent soft tissues of the neck (Fig. 26).

Similar to mucosal tumors at other sites, tonsillar carcinoma can present as a nonhealing, painless ulcer at first. As the tumor grows, however, the patient may develop painful swallowing, ipsilateral referred otalgia, and neck adenopathy. Advanced tonsillar fossa carcinomas can transgress the superior constrictor muscle to invade the parapharyngeal space. The tumors also can involve the anterior and posterior tonsillar pillars and grow along the palatoglossus and palatopharyngeal muscles, respectively. Lesions of the anterior tonsillar pillars can extend superiorly to the soft and hard palate and inferiorly to the tongue base [20]. Anteriorly, they can extend along the pharyngeal constrictor to the pterygomandibular raphe. When lesions involve the

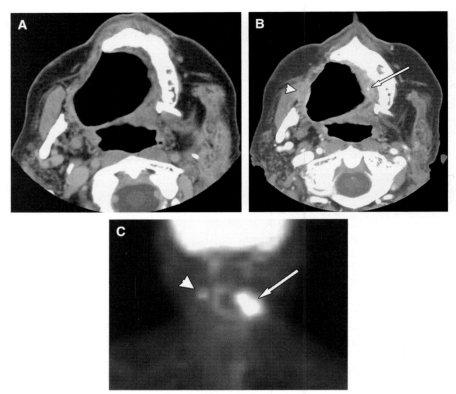

Fig. 21. CT scan of a patient with multiply recurrent SCC of the oral cavity. *(A)* Baseline posttreatment scan shows a right maxillectomy defect. *(B)* Recurrent tumor was easily seen on clinical examination *(arrow)*. Note the additional submucosal recurrence *(arrowhead)* that could not be appreciated on clinical examination. *(C)* Recurrent disease was FDG avid on PET scan, which was obtained for distant metastatic evaluation.

posterior tonsillar pillars they tend to grow along the palatopharyngeus muscle. They can extend superiorly to soft palate and inferiorly to involve the pharyngoepiglottic fold, middle constrictor, and even the upper thyroid cartilage [25]. The posterior oropharyngeal wall may get involved with posterior extension.

On CT the tumors can enhance similar to the tonsils. Invasion of the masticator and parapharyngeal space in advanced tumors is often readily detected on imaging (Fig. 27). On MR imaging the lesions are isointense to muscle on T1-weighted images but are slightly hyperintense relative to muscle on T2-weighted images. Fat-saturated postcontrast

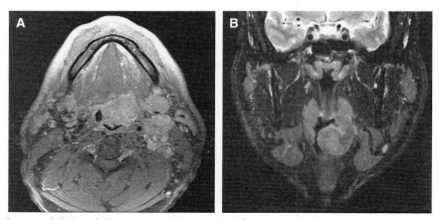

Fig. 22. Axial postgadolinium *(A)* and coronal T2-weighted fat saturated *(B)* images demonstrate an exophytic mass arising from the base of the tongue on the left side.

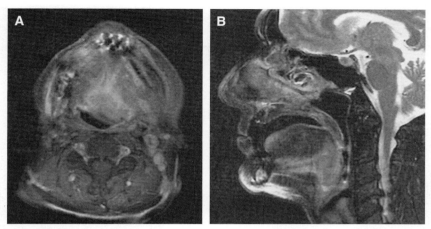

Fig. 23. Recurrent SCC of the tongue base involving the root of the tongue with extensive anterior extension is evident on the axial postcontrast (*A*) and sagittal T2-weighted image (*B*).

imaging helps in improving tumor delineation. PET CT can be helpful in localizing the primary tumor and guiding biopsy in patients who have "occult primaries" [26].

For early T1-T2 tonsillar lesions, definitive radiation therapy is the primary treatment of choice. Excellent locoregional control can be obtained. On the other hand, more advanced T3-T4 disease

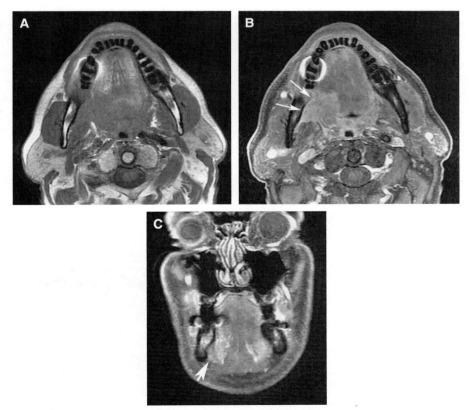

Fig. 24. Pre- (*A*) and postgadolinium with fat saturation (*B*) T1-weighted images. Advanced SCC of the tongue base extending to retromolar trigone abutting the mandible without mandibular invasion (*A, B*) (arrows). Coronal postcontrast image (*C*) demonstrates involvement of the posterior mylohyoid muscle with tumor extending into the submandibular space (*arrow*).

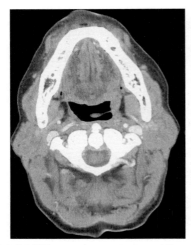

Fig. 25. Axial CT image demonstrates subtle asymmetric fullness of the left tonsil in a patient without prior tonsillectomy.

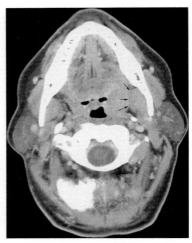

Fig. 27. Axial CT. Large left tonsillar mass extends into masticator space. The tumor abuts the medial pterygoid muscle without infiltrating the muscle (*arrows*).

is treated with concurrent chemotherapy and radiation therapy. Surgery is reserved for salvage [27].

Soft palate

The soft palate is a much less frequent subsite for SCC than the faucial tonsils or the base of the tongue. Carcinomas of the soft palate most commonly involve the oral aspect of the palate. As expected, SCC is the most common tumor of the soft palate, but minor salivary gland cancers are not infrequent [21].

When small, soft palate lesions may be undetectable on imaging and are best visualized during clinical evaluation. Early cancers appear as ulcerative mucosal lesions on direct visualization. Patients may have velopharyngeal insufficiency, hypernasal speech, difficulty swallowing, and

referred otalgia on presentation. Patients who have advanced lesions may have symptoms related to the sites of involvement by tumor, such as trismus and malocclusion—signs of pterygoid muscle invasion. These tumors commonly extend anteriorly to the hard palate or inferiorly to the tonsillar pillars (Fig. 28). They also can extend along the veli palatini muscles to involve even the skull base. The pterygopalatine fossa can become involved by tumor once the palatine nerves are diseased [21]. The tumors are best evaluated by MR imaging, particularly in the coronal plane.

Radiation therapy is the primary treatment modality for small tumors in many centers to preserve quality of life. More advanced T3 and T4 cancers are treated with radiation concurrent with chemotherapy. Surgery is reserved for salvage.

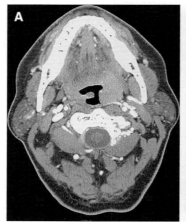
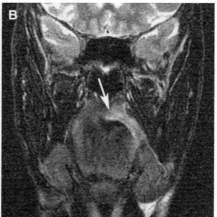

Fig. 26. Mildly enhancing left tonsillar mass on axial CT image (*A*). Coronal T2 fat-saturated image (*B*) of a different patient demonstrates superior extension of tonsillar SCC to left side of the soft palate (*arrow*).

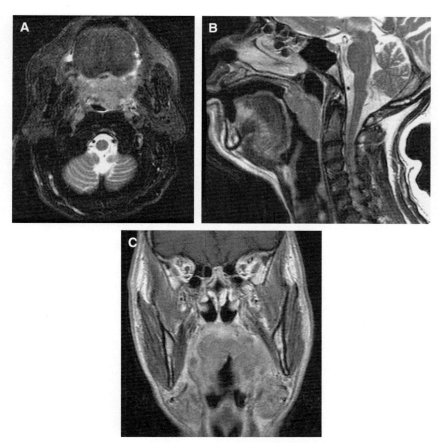

Fig. 28. Axial (*A*) and sagittal (*B*) T2-weighed images reveal a soft palate mass extending to the uvula. Postgadolinium image in the coronal plane (*C*) shows extension of tumor to the tonsillar fossae.

Staging

The TNM staging system is applicable to SCC and minor salivary gland carcinoma and not to nonepithelial tumors, such as those of mesenchymal origin. Although the surface extent of oropharyngeal cancer is best determined on clinical examination, cross-sectional imaging is invaluable in assessment of certain other features, such as deep tumor invasion and nodal staging.

Table 5: Tumor (T) staging for squamous cell carcinoma of the oropharynx

T1	Tumor ≤2 cm in maximal diameter
T2	Tumor 2–4 cm in maximal diameter
T3	Tumor >4 cm in maximal diameter
T4	4a Tumor invades the larynx, deep/extrinsic muscles of tongue, medial pterygoid, hard palate, or mandible
	4b Tumor invades lateral pterygoid muscle, pterygoid plates, lateral nasopharynx, or skull base or encases carotid artery

T stage

The primary tumor (T) staging depends mainly on tumor size (Table 5), and the treatment is determined by CT/MR features in addition to clinical findings [7]. The root of the tongue and the floor of the mouth should be inspected for possible anterior spread of a base of the tongue carcinoma. Base of the tongue carcinoma can spread posterolaterally to anterior tonsillar pillars and the faucial tonsils or inferiorly to pre-epiglottic fat or supraglottic larynx (Fig. 29) [25]. The third division of the trigeminal nerve should be inspected for signs of perineural spread.

Accurate staging of SCC arising from the palatine tonsils also depends on physical/endoscopic examinations and imaging. In advanced cases, numbness in the distribution of V3 and trismus indicate masticator space extension with involvement of V3. Numbness of the chin indicates mandibular extension and involvement of the inferior alveolar nerve. Fasciculation and atrophy of the hemitongue are signs of tumor in posterior sublingual space involving the twelfth nerve.

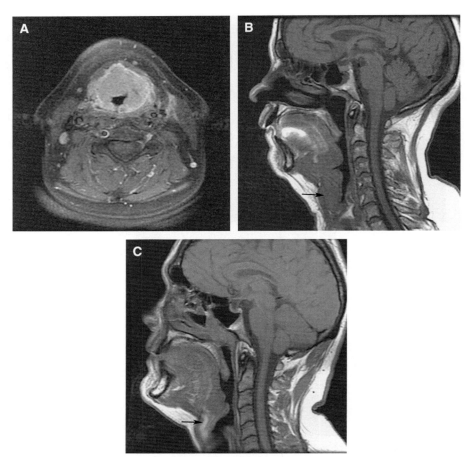

Fig. 29. Axial postgadolinium (*A*) and sagittal T1-weighted image (*B*) in a patient with base of the tongue SCC with involvement of the pre-epiglottic space and supraglottis. (*C*) Companion sagittal image of a different patient with base of the tongue SCC without involvement of the pre-epiglottic space. The pre-epiglottic fat and its replacement with tumor are marked with arrows (*B, C*).

N stage

Nodal staging of oropharyngeal carcinoma is the same as for cancers of the oral cavity (see Table 4). The oropharynx has the second highest incidence of nodal disease at presentation among other SCCs of the head and neck [28]. The lymph nodes in the upper jugular and spinal accessory chains and the retropharyngeal nodes are most commonly involved by oropharyngeal SCC. Nodal assessment is best performed on imaging at the time of primary tumor assessment. The oropharyngeal lymphatic metastases are mainly to level I-IV nodes, with level II being the most common site. The base of the tongue lymphatic drainage is mostly to level II-IV nodes. Nodal metastasis to both sides of the neck is common because of rich lymphatics and can be seen in up to 30% of patients who have tongue base carcinoma. Soft palatal carcinomas have a high incidence of nodal metastasis.

Approximately 60% of patients have nodal disease at the time of diagnosis [21].

Predominantly cystic SCC metastasis in the neck is most commonly seen with primary tumors of the palatine and lingual tonsils. Such cystic metastases should be differentiated from liquefaction necrosis that can occur in solid adenopathy [29]. These primary tumors arise in the tonsillar crypt epithelium and are of the transitional type instead of the usual SCC [30]. Cystic nodal metastases are not uncommonly confused for a branchiogenic cyst, and it is important to understand that the diagnosis of metastatic carcinoma must be ruled out, especially in adults. It is crucial to alert the clinician when cystic metastases are encountered in the neck on imaging because such primaries have a different behavior than the usual SCC. Such primary tumors can have different diagnostic/surgical implications when the primary site is

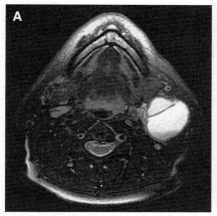 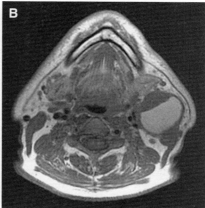

Fig. 30. Axial T2- (*A*) and T1-weighted (*B*) images of a patient with left tongue base SCC. Note lack of a significant mass at the tongue base and predominantly cystic metastasis on the left side containing hemorrhagic fluid.

not evident. The primary tumors of the oropharynx responsible for cystic metastases are often small and indolent and may be clinically occult. Patients are often younger and may not have history of risk factors, such as tobacco or alcohol use. Despite the typical small size of tumors of the tonsillar crypt epithelium, they metastasize early and lead to moderately large nodes (Fig. 30) [29]. In a patient who has cystic upper internal jugular chain nodal metastasis without a known primary, the ipsilateral faucial or lingual tonsil should be highly considered as a potential site for the occult tumor. The adenoidal pad of the Waldeyer's ring is a less frequent site responsible for cystic metastases. It should be noted that cystic metastases can be present in the setting of other tumors, such as papillary carcinoma of the thyroid [29,30].

M stage

The lungs are the most common site of distant metastases. Bony and hepatic metastases are less common in oropharyngeal SCC. Mediastinal node metastases are considered distant metastasis [7].

Disease-specific follow-up

Patients who have oropharyngeal cancer should be clinically followed with physical examinations every 6 to 8 weeks initially after treatment then every 2 months for the first 2 years, every 4 to 6 months the third and fourth years, and yearly in the fifth year. Posttreatment MR imaging should be obtained at least 3 months after completion of radiation therapy to minimize the confounding effect of posttreatment inflammatory changes. Close follow-up of high-risk patients or patients who are at high risk for tumor recurrence is encouraged, particularly during the 2 years after treatment [31]. Follow-up is important because most

recurrences occur during this time period. Imaging plays a crucial role during this period because it is not unusual for posttreatment changes to limit physical evaluation of the neck. FDG-PET has been shown to be a highly sensitive tool in detecting recurrent SCC of the head and neck [32,33].

In general, patients who have head and neck SCC have a 10% risk of developing a second aerodigestive tract primary malignancy. This number is even higher—approximately 15%—for tonsillar and base of the tongue cancers. It is important to be cognizant of this fact when following up patients who have a history of SCC.

Summary

In addition to familiarity with the locoregional anatomy, radiologists must have a solid understanding of the clinical behavior and spread patterns of oral cavity and oropharyngeal SCC to make a meaningful contribution to the treatment of patients.

References

[1] Jemal A, Siegel R, Ward E, et al. Cancer statistics, 2006. CA Cancer J Clin 2006;56(2):106–30.
[2] Davidson J, Gilbert R, Irish J, et al. The role of panendoscopy in the management of mucosal head and neck malignancy: a prospective evaluation. Head Neck 2000;22(5):449–54 [discussion: 454–5].
[3] Schwartz LH, Ozsahin M, Zhang GN, et al. Synchronous and metachronous head and neck carcinomas. Cancer 1994;74(7):1933–8.
[4] Shah JP, Medina JE, Shaha AR, et al. Cervical lymph node metastasis. Curr Probl Surg 1993; 30(3):273–344.

[5] Cooper JS, Pajak TF, Forastiere AA, et al. Postoperative concurrent radiotherapy and chemotherapy for high-risk squamous-cell carcinoma of the head and neck. N Engl J Med 2004;350(19):1937–44.

[6] Bernier J, Domenge C, Ozsahin M, et al. Postoperative irradiation with or without concomitant chemotherapy for locally advanced head and neck cancer. N Engl J Med 2004;350(19):1945–52.

[7] American Joint Committee on Cancer. AJCC cancer staging manual. 6th edition. New York: Springer; 2002.

[8] Spiro RH, Huvos AG, Wong GY, et al. Predictive value of tumor thickness in squamous carcinoma confined to the tongue and floor of the mouth. Am J Surg 1986;152(4):345–50.

[9] Spiro RH, Guillamondegui O Jr, Paulino AF, et al. Pattern of invasion and margin assessment in patients with oral tongue cancer. Head Neck 1999;21(5):408–13.

[10] Shah JP. Patterns of cervical lymph node metastasis from squamous carcinomas of the upper aerodigestive tract. Am J Surg 1990;160(4):405–9.

[11] Stevens MH, Harnsberger HR, Mancuso AA, et al. Computed tomography of cervical lymph nodes: staging and management of head and neck cancer. Arch Otolaryngol 1985;111(11):735–9.

[12] Merritt RM, Williams MF, James TH, et al. Detection of cervical metastasis: a meta-analysis comparing computed tomography with physical examination. Arch Otolaryngol Head Neck Surg 1997;123(2):149–52.

[13] van den Brekel MW, Castelijns JA, Stel HV, et al. Modern imaging techniques and ultrasound-guided aspiration cytology for the assessment of neck node metastases: a prospective comparative study. Eur Arch Otorhinolaryngol 1993;250(1):11–7.

[14] Merkx MA, Boustahji AH, Kaanders JH, et al. A half-yearly chest radiograph for early detection of lung cancer following oral cancer. Int J Oral Maxillofac Surg 2002;31(4):378–82.

[15] Stalpers LJ, van Vierzen PB, Brouns JJ, et al. The role of yearly chest radiography in the early detection of lung cancer following oral cancer. Int J Oral Maxillofac Surg 1989;18(2):99–103.

[16] Loh KS, Brown DH, Baker JT, et al. A rational approach to pulmonary screening in newly diagnosed head and neck cancer. Head Neck 2005;27(11):990–4.

[17] Lin K, Patel SG, Chu PY, et al. Second primary malignancy of the aerodigestive tract in patients treated for cancer of the oral cavity and larynx. Head Neck 2005;27(12):1042–8.

[18] Henschke CI, Shaham D, Yankelevitz DF, et al. CT screening for lung cancer: past and ongoing studies. Semin Thorac Cardiovasc Surg 2005;17(2):99–106.

[19] Ryan WR, Fee WE Jr, Le QT, et al. Positron-emission tomography for surveillance of head and neck cancer. Laryngoscope 2005;115(4):645–50.

[20] Mukherji SK, Pillsbury HR, Castillo M. Imaging squamous cell carcinomas of the upper aerodigestive tract: what clinicians need to know. Radiology 1997;205(3):629–46.

[21] Mukherji SK. Pharynx. In: Som PM, Curtin HD, editors. Head and neck imaging. St. Louis (MO): Mosby; 2003. p. 1485–9.

[22] Parsons JT, Mendenhall WM, Stringer SP, et al. Squamous cell carcinoma of the oropharynx: surgery, radiation therapy, or both. Cancer 2002;94(11):2967–80.

[23] Sessions DG, Lenox J, Spector GJ, et al. Analysis of treatment results for base of tongue cancer. Laryngoscope 2003;113(7):1252–61.

[24] Syms MJ, Birkmire-Peters DP, Holtel MR. Incidence of carcinoma in incidental tonsil asymmetry. Laryngoscope 2000;110(11):1807–10.

[25] Million RR, Cassisi NJ, Mancuso AA. The oropharynx. In: Million RR, Cassisi NJ, editors. Management of head and neck cancer: a multidisciplinary approach. Philadelphia: JB Lippincott; 1994. p. 402–31.

[26] Braams JW, Pruim J, Kole AC, et al. Detection of unknown primary head and neck tumors by positron emission tomography. Int J Oral Maxillofac Surg 1997;26(2):112–5.

[27] Chao KS, Ozyigit G, Blanco AI, et al. Intensity-modulated radiation therapy for oropharyngeal carcinoma: impact of tumor volume. Int J Radiat Oncol Biol Phys 2004;59(1):43–50.

[28] Som PM. Lymph nodes of the neck. Radiology 1987;165(3):593–600.

[29] Goldenberg D, Sciubba J, Koch WM. Cystic metastasis from head and neck squamous cell cancer: a distinct disease variant? Head Neck 2006;28(7):633–8.

[30] Thompson LD, Heffner DK. The clinical importance of cystic squamous cell carcinomas in the neck: a study of 136 cases. Cancer 1998;82(5):944–56.

[31] Harnsberger HR. Handbook of head and neck imaging. St. Louis (MO): Mosby; 1995. p. 272–3.

[32] Wong RJ, Lin DT, Schoder H, et al. Diagnostic and prognostic value of [(18)F]fluorodeoxyglucose positron emission tomography for recurrent head and neck squamous cell carcinoma. J Clin Oncol 2002;20(20):4199–208.

[33] Goerres GW, Schmid DT, Bandhauer F, et al. Positron emission tomography in the early follow-up of advanced head and neck cancer. Arch Otolaryngol Head Neck Surg 2004;130(1):105–9 [discussion: 120–1].

ELSEVIER
SAUNDERS

RADIOLOGIC
CLINICS
OF NORTH AMERICA

Radiol Clin N Am 45 (2007) 21–43

Lung Cancer

Michelle S. Ginsberg, MD[a,b,*], Ravinder K. Grewal, MD[a,b],
Robert T. Heelan, MD[a,b]

Lung cancer is the most frequently occurring cancer in the world, and in the United States it is the second most common cancer diagnosed. Accurate staging by imaging can have a significant impact on appropriate treatment and surgical options. Familiarity with the different histologic subtypes of lung cancer and the typical and atypical appearances of lung cancer is vital. Radiologists serve a critical role in the diagnosis, staging, and follow-up of patients with lung cancer.

Incidence

Lung cancer is the most frequently occurring cancer in the world; 1.2 million new cases or 12.3% of the world's total cancer incidence were diagnosed in the year 2000. In the United States, lung cancer is the second most common cancer diagnosed in men and women. An estimated 174,470 new cases of lung cancer will be diagnosed in 2006, accounting for 13% of cancer diagnoses of which 92,700 cases will be in men and 81,770 cases among women [1]. The incidence is declining significantly in men, from a high of 102.1 per 100,000 in 1984 to 79.8 in 2000. In the 1990s, the increasing trend previously noted among women leveled off with an incidence at 52.8 per 100,000. The long-term trends in the age-adjusted incidence among men and women are consistent with the historic pattern of tobacco use, which reflects a 30-year lag time between increasing prevalence of smoking in women and development of lung cancer as compared with men. The lifetime probability of developing lung cancer in men in the United States is 1 in 13; for women the probability is 1 in 17. This is based on data from 1998 to 2000 [2].

Incidence rates of lung cancer also differ by ethnicity. African Americans and Native Hawaiians

a Department of Radiology, Memorial Sloan-Kettering Cancer Center, 1275 York Avenue, New York, NY
10021, USA
b Weill Medical College of Cornell University, New York, NY, USA
* Corresponding author. Memorial Sloan-Kettering Cancer Center, 1275 York Avenue, New York, NY 10021,
USA
E-mail address: ginsberm@mskcc.org (M.S. Ginsberg).

doi:10.1016/j.rcl.2006.10.004

are at a significantly greater risk of lung cancer than whites, Japanese Americans, and Latinos among those who smoked no more than 20 cigarettes per day. At levels exceeding 30 cigarettes per day, however, these differences were not significant [3]. African Americans have the highest rate of smoking (29%) but smoke the fewest number of cigarettes per day and have higher nicotine levels after same number of cigarettes smoked. This may represent variation in metabolism of nicotine and differences in smoking behavior (ie, depth and frequency of inhalation) that may underlie exposure to carcinogens.

Mortality

Lung cancer is the leading cause of death in smokers and the leading cause of cancer mortality in men and women in the United States. There will be an estimated 160,460 deaths from lung cancer in the United States in 2006. An estimated 90,330 deaths among men and 72,130 deaths among women will account for about 29.8% of all cancer deaths in the United States [1]. In 2006, the American Cancer Society described a historic drop in cancer death from lung cancer by 369 total cancer deaths. Death rates have continued to decrease significantly in men since 1991 by 1.8% per year. The rate of increase in women, which had continued to increase, has slowed since the early 1990s. Mortality rates remain closely related to smoking patterns and lung cancer incidence rates. The decrease in smoking rates observed have reflected the decline in smoking observed over the past 30 years, although smoking patterns among women lag behind those of men. Overall, lung cancer mortality rates and trends are similar to those observed for incidence, because survival for lung cancer is poor.

Histologic types

Non–small cell lung cancer

Adenocarcinoma is the most common cell type representing 50% of all cases and is the most common cell type in nonsmokers. CT usually demonstrates a solitary peripheral pulmonary nodule or mass, which can be spiculated or lobulated. It is often subpleural and asymptomatic because of its peripheral location (Fig. 1). It may be associated with concomitant lung disease, such as focal and diffuse fibrosis. It is a slower-growing tumor; however, it can metastasize early. Subclassification is very difficult, with mixed subtype as the most common subtype. This is a glandular epithelial tumor with acinar, papillary, or solid growth patterns. In the 1981 World Health Organization classification, four subtypes of lung

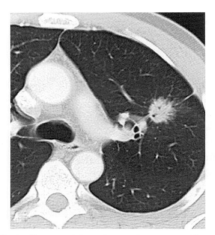

Fig. 1. A 41-year-old male smoker presenting with spiculated left upper lobe nodule with linear extension to the pleura. Histologically proved to be poorly differentiated adenocarcinoma.

adenocarcinoma were recognized including acinar, papillary, bronchioloalveolar (BAC), and solid carcinoma with mucus production.

BAC subtype of adenocarcinoma represents 3% of lung cancers. According to the 2004 World Health Organization classification the strict definition of BAC is that of a noninvasive tumor with no stromal, vascular, or pleural invasion and mantling of pre-existing airspaces "lepidic growth" along alveolar walls [4]. There are three radiologic patterns. A solitary nodule is the most common appearance, similar to adenocarcinoma. It represents 60% to 90% of presentations of this histologic subtype. Ground glass density can be seen especially peripherally within the lesion, representing the classic lepidic growth (along the alveolar walls) that is associated with this tumor. The second most common appearance is the pneumonic process, which is dense consolidation that can have air bronchograms similar to pneumonia. This presentation is seen in up to 20% of cases. Nodules can also be seen in association with this appearance, which can be bilateral because it is spread by the tracheobronchial tree and can disseminate throughout both lungs. A large dominant mass with satellite nodules within the same lobe or multiple nodules in more than one lobe can also be seen. The least common appearance is multiple small subcentimeter irregularly marginated nodules.

There are three histologic subtypes that have important clinical associations. The nonmucinous subtype is associated with a solitary nodule and a better clinical outcome. The mucinous subtype presents as a pseudopneumonic or multifocal-multinodular appearance and has a worse clinical outcome. Histologically, this type shows mucin production with mucin pooling in alveolar spaces. The third subtype is a mixed mucinous and nonmucinous type. These different appearances have different clinical implications. Diffuse or multicentric growth patterns can be seen with both nonmucinous and mucinous BAC, but this is more characteristic of mucinous tumors.

Most lung adenocarcinomas with a BAC pattern are not pure BAC, however, but rather adenocarcinomas, mixed subtype with invasive patterns. This applies to tumors presenting with a diffuse-multinodular and solitary nodule pattern. The percent of BAC versus invasive components in lung adenocarcinoma seems to be prognostically important [4].

Atypical adenomatous alveolar hyperplasia is a premalignant lesion thought to be a precursor to BAC and found in lung adjacent to areas of invasive adenocarcinoma. Small BAC can be indistinguishable, however, from atypical adenomatous alveolar hyperplasia both histologically and radiologically.

Squamous cell carcinoma represents approximately 30% of all lung cancers. It is associated with the best prognosis. Although it generally grows locally rapidly, distant metastases occur at a later phase. There is a strong association with smoking.

Most tumors are between 3 and 5 cm when detected and centrally located, resulting in postobstructive atelectasis or pneumonia (Fig. 2). Patients may also present with signs and symptoms related to invasion of adjacent central structures, such as involvement of the recurrent laryngeal nerve. Hemoptysis, which is associated with central tumors, can also be a presenting symptom with squamous cell carcinoma. When these lesions occur peripherally they may be large before presentation and can lead to chest wall invasion and Pancoast's syndrome. Pancoast's syndrome refers to involvement of the brachial plexus and cervical sympathetic nerves associated with severe pain in the shoulder region radiating toward the axilla and scapula; atrophy of hand and arm muscles; Horner

syndrome (constellation of signs produced because of interruption of the sympathetic innervation); and compression of blood vessels with edema. Pancoast's tumors can occur with any histology but are more common with both squamous cell and adenocarcinoma. The term "superior sulcus" tumor refers to its location in the superior pulmonary sulcus at the lung apex, from which it can invade locally the chest wall and brachial plexus.

Undifferentiated large cell carcinoma represents up to 5% of lung cancers. It generally presents as a large peripheral mass (>70% tumors are >4 cm on presentation) with rapid growth and early metastases, especially to mediastinum and brain. This histology generally has a poor prognosis and has a strong association with smoking (Fig. 3). There are several histologic subtypes of this tumor. Giant cell has a more aggressive behavior. Large cell neuroendocrine carcinoma also is more aggressive and can have a similar prognosis to small cell carcinoma. It differs histologically from small cell neuroendocrine tumors in appearance and response to chemotherapy, which is generally poorer. For the poorly-differentiated high-grade tumors, electron microscopy or immunohistochemistry may be needed to confirm endocrine features and diagnose this subtype.

The histologic distinction between these categories may not always be clear and different portions of a tumor may have different histologies. Poorly differentiated squamous cell carcinoma can be difficult to distinguish from a high-grade adenocarcinoma or undifferentiated large cell carcinoma.

Small cell lung cancer

Small cell lung cancer (SCLC), previously called "oat cell carcinoma" for the small, round cell shape of the cancer cells, is an aggressive tumor often presenting with generalized symptoms and distant metastases. Although these tumors respond initially to chemotherapy, most patients develop drug resistance. SCLC represents approximately 20% all lung

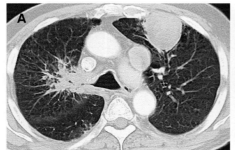 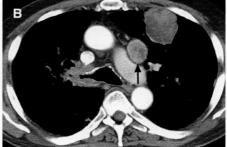

Fig. 2. A 75-year-old smoker with metastatic squamous cell carcinoma. (*A*) Note spiculated right central mass with encasement of the right main stem bronchus. A contralateral metastasis is seen in the left upper lobe. (*B*) Mediastinal lymphadenopathy (*arrow*).

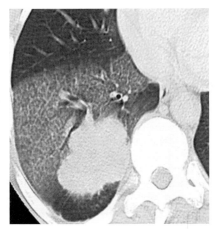

Fig. 3. Large right lower lobe mass with adjacent ground glass density consistent with hemorrhage. Patient presented with hemoptysis.

cancer cases. It has the greatest association with tobacco use, with almost 98% of patients with SCLC having a history of smoking [5]. The proportion of patients with SCLC has decreased over the last decade. SCLC is of a high-grade morphology and pathologic diagnosis is usually made on light microscopic findings, although electron microscopy or immunohistochemistry can be helpful.

Multiple primary carcinomas

Synchronous lesions are defined as the presence of two tumors at the same time or closely following initial diagnosis. The incidence of synchronous multiple primary tumors is less than 3.5% of all lung cancers [6]. This number may even be higher depending on the cell type and how carefully further primary tumors are sought and the rigidity of

the criteria used to define the tumors as primary lesions. Difference in cell type is an accepted criterion; however, tumors of the same histologic type must be physically quite separate and separated by noncancerous lung tissue (Fig. 4) [7]. Metachronous lesions are defined as the second cancers appearing after a time interval, usually 12 months or more. The peak incidence is between the third and eighth postoperative years. These lesions comprise at least two thirds of multiple pulmonary neoplasms. Ten percent to 32% of patients surviving resection for lung cancer may develop a second primary tumor. The reported incidence has increased presumably because second primary lung cancer can be distinguished from recurrence and satellite disease. These lesions are regarded as multiple primary lesions only if they show unique histologic features. Adenocarcinoma has replaced squamous cell cancer as the most common histologic type of multiple carcinoma [8,9].

Screening

Surveillance and early detection

Lung cancer has a poor prognosis because it is typically diagnosed at an advanced stage as a result of a patient's symptoms, by which time it is incurable. The possibility of detection of early stage lung cancer, and which if treated aggressively by surgery could result in a high cure rate, has long been of interest.

Efforts using induced bronchial sputum cytology to detect early lung cancer did not prove successful [10–12]. The use of chest radiograph to detect early lung cancer had decidedly mixed results, with some centers detecting stage I lung cancer in

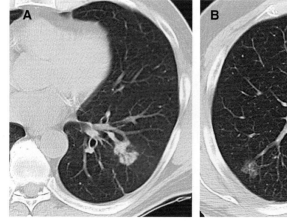
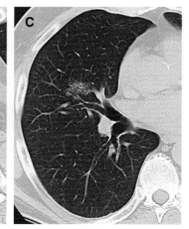

Fig. 4. A 68-year-old smoker with synchronous adenocarcinoma of the lung. (*A*) Left lower lobe nodule with air bronchograms. (*B*) Right upper lobe ground glass nodule. (*C*) Right middle lobe ground glass nodule. All were of slightly different histologies.

approximately 40% of patients. This was accompanied by the failure of these efforts to impact on mortality from lung cancer [13], resulting in a long pause in attempts at screening high-risk asymptomatic patients, lasting through the 1980s and most of the 1990s.

Those supporting imaging screening claimed that the study group and observation groups, particularly in the Mayo Clinic study, which compared a randomized study group receiving quarterly chest radiographs with an observation group for which only periodic clinical follow-up was recommended, were contaminated by noncompliance in the study group, and by the tendency of the observation patients to get tested [13,14]. The numbers of patients entered was claimed to be insufficient to answer the screening efficacy mortality question (ie, the study was "underpowered") [13]. Those opposing imaging screening claimed that there were various kinds of statistical bias introduced which caused a spurious increase in the diagnosis of small or early stage lung cancers accompanied by no decrease in late stage diagnosed lung cancers with any decrease in lung cancer mortality in the study group. These most notably included lead time bias [15] (screening diagnosis does not lead to a real increase in life span); length bias [15] (screening misses tumors that progress rapidly); and overdiagnosis bias [16] (diagnosis of pseudodisease [ie, nodules or "tumors" that would not have resulted in the patient's death because of an extremely slow rate of growth]).

The issue of lung cancer screening resurfaced in the early 1990s with the development of more advanced CT technology allowing faster breathhold scanning of the chest. During the 1990s Japanese investigators established the feasibility of CT screening to detect early lung cancer, and noting an increase in the number of early stage cancers diagnosed [17,18]. In 1999, Henschke and coworkers [19] published a prevalence study of CT scanning of 1000 high-risk patients. Twenty seven lung cancers were diagnosed and treated, of which 23 were stage I (85%). This paper was controversial because it proposed universal screening. A methodologic dispute followed as to whether follow-up studies of screening CT should be single arm or a randomized controlled trial (ie, whether all patients should receive the low-dose CT screening alone or whether they should be randomly assigned either to receive the test or not receive the test, or to receive another screening test, such as chest radiograph, with the results being compared between the two groups). This latter method was considered to be definitive for eliminating the possibility of significant bias and for detecting real differences in mortality from lung cancer between the two groups.

Henschke and coworkers [20] embarked on an international single-armed study that enrolled more than 25,000 participants: lung cancer continued to be detected on initial screening and on follow-up at stage I in 80% of patients. Moreover, this group claimed to have devised an imaging method for accurately differentiating benign non-calcified nodules from small lung cancers, involving careful follow-up and evaluation of size, both on measurement and by three-dimensional volumetric study, and use of sophisticated percutaneous biopsy procedures [21].

Swensen and coworkers [22], in a single-armed study of 1500 patients, demonstrated an apparent increase in diagnosis of small, early stage tumors. In comparing mortality from the CT study with their prior chest radiograph study from the 1980s, however, no difference in mortality between these two groups could be confirmed. In addition, the Mayo Clinic study found a significant incidence of work-up (including invasive procedures) of non-cancerous masses to eliminate false-positive diagnoses.

It is thought that a large randomized trial of low-dose CT versus chest radiograph will be able to answer the issues raised by the overdiagnosis claim [23] and to this end a large randomized study sponsored by the National Cancer Institute and the American College of Radiology Imaging Network [24] has enrolled, with initial examination, 53,000 individuals into a randomized study involving comparison of CT and chest radiograph screening. Initial accrual has been completed and results, including early mortality results, should be available in the next several years.

Asymptomatic patients

With the increasing awareness of the relationship between smoking and lung cancer, individuals at risk are requesting low-dose CT screening outside of a clinical research study. Low-dose CT scans (40 mA, compared with conventional 200–300 mA CT dose) have the advantage of offering a diagnostic procedure at a radiologic dose that is comparable with plain posteroanterior and lateral chest radiographs. The potential reward is the diagnosis of lung cancer in a high-risk patient when it is both smaller and at an earlier stage. The downside of screening is the diagnosis of false-positives, with consequent morbidity and potential mortality associated with invasive diagnostic procedures [22]. At this time, screening has not shown a decrease in lung cancer mortality. Experience with diagnosing early lung cancer in a screening setting in asymptomatic patients has resulted in some guidelines in the evaluation of small pulmonary nodules [20–25].

- Nodules <5 mm are seldom caused by lung cancer.
- Growth of nodules is ominous and should be aggressively evaluated, including by percutaneous biopsy. Growth is the screening gold standard for lung cancer diagnosis. There are, however, instances of growth of benign nodules.
- Lack of growth over time of 5- to 10-mm nodules should be confirmed over a 2-year time period.
- Small foci of clustered nodules are usually inflammatory or postinflammatory in origin.
- Randomly distributed nodules are nonspecific. They have a large differential diagnosis including inflammatory, inhalational, and neoplastic processes, both metastatic and primary in the lung.

Symptomatic patients

Symptomatic patients with lung cancer frequently present on chest radiograph or CT with pleural effusions, mediastinal lymphadenopathy, or distant metastasis, all hallmarks of advanced disease. Patients with advanced lung cancer may present with fever and cough, blood-tinged sputum, brain or bone symptoms, weakness, weight loss, or other clinical indications of advanced disease. Whether the patient is symptomatic or asymptomatic, histologic confirmation is crucial, usually obtained either by percutaneous lung biopsy; bronchoscopy with biopsy (or alveolar lavage); or surgical exploration by open thoracotomy or video-assisted thoracoscopic surgery procedures.

Diagnosis

Imaging diagnosis of lung cancer frequently occurs in the context of screening or detection of nodules on a routine CT scan or chest radiograph in asymptomatic patients. These tumors tend to be smaller at diagnosis and not to have spread beyond their local confines. Diagnosis of lung cancer in patients whose work-up is precipitated by the development of symptoms, however, usually results in diagnosis of later-stage lung cancer, which is generally larger in size and may have spread regionally or distantly.

The location of these lesions can be described as central or peripheral. The shape of the borders of these lesions can be suggestive, but is not diagnostic of malignancy. In particular the presence of spiculation (Fig. 5) is thought to indicate a higher likelihood of malignancy [26]. Clearly defined edges [27] may indicate an inflammatory process. Cavitation, frequently an indication of long-standing or advanced lung cancer, is most commonly seen with squamous cell lung cancer (Fig. 6) [28].

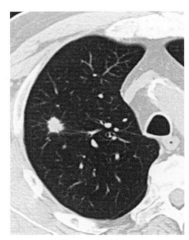

Fig. 5. A 68-year-old man with squamous cell carcinoma, moderately differentiated, of right upper lobe. Peripheral spiculated nodule with corona radiata. The spiculation suggests a malignant lesion with aggressive behavior.

In recent years, particularly with the development of surveillance programs, which tend to detect tumors at a smaller size, debate continues to occur as to whether detection and treatment of these small tumors, which seem to be earlier-stage lung cancers, translates into improved mortality. Yabuuchi and coworkers [29] correlated CT characteristics of small peripheral lung tumors with well-differentiated and poorly differentiated adenocarcinoma. Smoothness of tumor margin and a solid tumor appearance without air-bronchograms were more commonly found in poorly differentiated adenocarcinoma (all patients in this study had

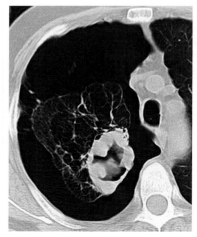

Fig. 6. A 60-year-old man with a cavitated mass that represents squamous cell cancer. Note the large pneumothorax.

lung cancer). The presence of air-bronchograms was associated with well-differentiated adenocarcinoma. Henschke and coworkers [30] in analyzing their data from the Early Lung Cancer Action Project divided their group of 233 noncalcified nodules into three groups: (1) solid (Fig. 7), (2) part solid (Fig. 8), and (3) nonsolid–ground glass opacity (Fig. 9). Nodules detected at screening that were part solid (ie, containing a solid and ground glass [nonsolid] component) had the greatest chance of being malignant (63%). Nonsolid nodules, composed of ground glass material, had an 18% chance of being malignant, whereas purely solid nodules had only a 7% chance of being malignant.

Lee and coworkers [31] in evaluating T1 stage non–SCLC (NSCLC), including imaging and histopathologic findings, found that T1 lung cancers with a large ground glass attenuation component (50% or more of tumor volume) had a better prognosis and less likelihood of mediastinal nodal or extrathoracic metastasis. Solid T1 lesions with a spiculated margin or with bronchovascular bundle thickening in the surrounding lung more frequently demonstrated local vessel invasion, regional lymph node metastasis, and distant metastatic disease. They suggest that patients with these morphologic features should have a work-up for extrathoracic metastases, including positron emission tomography scan, brain MR imaging, or mediastinoscopy. Li and coworkers [32] described three morphologic characteristics of screening detected or small peripheral lung nodules: nodules with pure ground glass opacity and that had a round shape were found more often to be malignant. These pure ground glass opacity lesions, especially when small, may represent premalignant atypical adenomatous hyperplasia. Mixed ground glass opacities (ie, with ground glass opacity at the periphery and a high attenuation zone at the center) were more often seen

in malignant lesions than in benign, which agreed with Henschke's observation. Among solid nodules a polygonal shape or a smooth or somewhat smooth margin was present less frequently in malignant than in benign lesions. They concluded that certain morphologic characteristics at thin-section CT can be helpful in differentiating small malignant nodules from benign ones. These characteristics of screening-detected small nodules may reflect radiographic characteristics of the very early development of lung cancers rather than the well-described appearance of more advanced lung cancers.

Up to one half of patients with central tumors exhibit signs of locally advanced tumor with peripheral lung collapse or obstructing pneumonia [33]. The central location of these tumors results in early involvement of adjacent structures (vessels, lymph nodes, and bronchi) resulting, in the latter instance, in peripheral lung collapse or obstructive pneumonia (Fig. 10). In some instances, the peripheral consolidation or collapse of the lung may be distinguished from central tumor on contrast-enhanced CT scans, allowing visualization of the normal enhanced peripheral anatomy distinct from the central inhomogeneously enhanced or necrotic tumor (Fig. 11) [34]. The role of MR imaging in this area is questionable [35]. The presence of a persistent segmental or lobar pneumonia or an incompletely healed infiltrate, despite appropriate antibiotic therapy, should precipitate a careful search for a central obstructing pulmonary neoplasm. Rate of growth is measured by volume-doubling times and is not, in general, reliable for distinguishing tumor from a benign process. Recent CT volumetric analysis indicates a wide range of doubling times with more than 20% exhibiting markedly slow growth (doubling time greater that 465 days) [36].

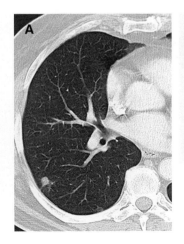
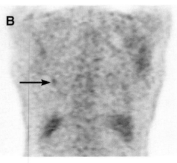

Fig. 7. (*A*) Small solid nodule detected in an asymptomatic 69-year-old man. In Henschke's data, this has a 7% chance of being malignant. (*B*) The positron emission tomography scan was weakly positive (*arrow*). This increases the likelihood of malignancy, but remains a nonspecific finding. Following resection, pathology revealed histoplasma granuloma.

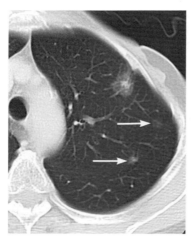

Fig. 8. A 65-year-old woman with a left upper lobe nodule with a solid core and large nonsolid periphery. At histology this was adenocarcinoma with bronchioalveolar features. Note two smaller lesions adjacent (*arrows*).

Common cell types of lung cancer as described previously have certain typical radiographic appearances; however, recognizing unusual presentations and suggesting the correct diagnosis is also of primary importance. Adenocarcinoma when located peripherally may directly invade the pleura and grow circumferentially around the lung and mimic diffuse malignant mesothelioma [37], pleural metastases, or metastatic involvement of the pleura by thymoma. Centrally located tumors may directly invade mediastinal structures or extend by the pulmonary veins into the left atrium. BAC most commonly presents as a solitary nodule with surrounding ground glass opacity. Although less common, consolidation and multiple small pulmonary nodules are other forms of

presentations (Fig. 12). Unusual radiographic appearances include lobar atelectasis, expansile consolidation without air bronchograms, or elongated lobulated opacity resembling mucoid impaction [38,39].

Squamous cell carcinoma less commonly may present as a solitary peripheral nodule with or without cavitation. When the tumor cavitates, the inner wall is typically thick and irregular, and if secondarily infected may develop an air-fluid level. The unusual appearance of undifferentiated large cell carcinoma is a centrally located mass.

Fluorodeoxyglucose positron emission tomography scanning

Malignant tumors have a higher rate of metabolism because of the higher glucose use. Glucose and fluorodeoxyglucose (FDG) uptake by malignant cells is higher compared with surrounding tissues. After intravenous administration FDG is taken up by cells in a similar fashion to unlabeled D-glucose, which is then converted to FDG-6-phosphatase after being phosphorylated by hexokinase. FDG-6-phosphatase cannot then be further dephosphorylated or degraded by the glycolytic pathway [40]. FDG is ultimately filtered by kidneys and resorbed by glucose transporters.

The standardized uptake value (SUV) or standardized uptake ratio is used to provide an objective measurement of positron activity in the region of interest. SUV is calculated as maximum activity concentration detected in the lesion divided by injected activity and corrected for body weight.

It has been shown that FDG uptake in untreated primary NSCLC is related to the expression of glucose transporter-1 expression [41]. There is correlation between the degree of differentiation of lung adenocarcinoma and both Glut-1 expression and

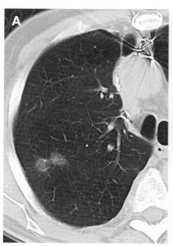
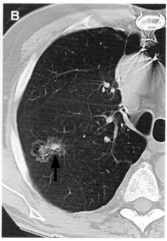

Fig. 9. An 81-year-old man with non–small cell lung cancer. (*A*) CT scans with two separate foci of ground glass density (nonsolid) in the right lung. This nonsolid appearance is frequently seen in bronchioloalveolar carcinoma. (*B*) Same levels in the right lung 1 year later. The tumor densities have increased in size and have developed small central solid cores (*arrow*), suggesting evolution to more aggressive adenocarcinoma in the central region.

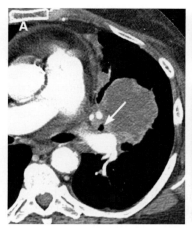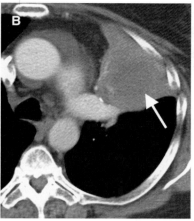

Fig. 10. (*A*) Largely central necrotic mass encasing the left upper lobe bronchus (*arrow*) and left hilar vessels. (*B*) More superiorly the mass extends into the left upper lobe, again demonstrating central necrosis (*arrow*) with some associated peripheral collapse.

FDG uptake. That is likely why FDG uptake has been shown to be significantly lower in BACs [42].

FDG-PET has a sensitivity ranging from 90% to 100% and specificity ranging from 69% to 95% [43–45] in detecting malignancy in a solitary nodule (**Fig. 13**). Small nodules (<7 mm) may not be detected by FDG-PET imaging because the amount of FDG uptake in these lesions cannot be reliably resolved [44] and may be below the threshold of resolution of current PET-CT scanners. An FDG-PET scan is indicated when the appearance of a nodule on CT is discordant with the pretest probability of cancer [46]. An SUV value >2.5 in a pulmonary lesion is highly suggestive of a malignant process [47] or active infection or inflammation. It has been observed that an SUV <2.5 has a 100% specificity for benign lesions >1.2 cm [48]. Similar findings have been reported, however, in the evaluation of lung lesions as small as 7 mm [44].

False-positive results on a PET scan can be caused by metabolically active infectious or inflammatory lesions. Granulomatous diseases like sarcoidosis, tuberculosis, or fungal infections can commonly produce significant FDG accumulation [49]. In geographic locations where prevalence of pulmonary fungal infections is high, there is low specificity and negative predictive value of FDG-PET in the evaluation of pulmonary lesions [50].Occasionally, adenocarcinoma <1 cm can have relatively less FDG accumulation and can result in a high false-negative rate of cancer detection [51,52]. A recent retrospective study evaluating the role of FDG-PET in indeterminate lesions <1 cm reported a sensitivity of 93%, specificity of 77%, positive predictive value of 72%, and negative predictive value of 94%. In this series, the prevalence of malignancy was found to be 39% [43].

Note that focal or pure BAC can result in a false-negative FDG-PET scan [53,54]. Similarly, in carcinoid tumors, an FDG-PET scan can yield false-negative results [55]. In about 5% of T1 indolent cancers, such as a focal nodular pure BAC or a carcinoid tumor, there is no significant FDG uptake [31].

Staging of non–small cell lung cancer

The process of staging, although separate from diagnosis, usually takes place in tandem with diagnostic procedures. The International System for Staging Lung Cancer, which follows the standard TNM

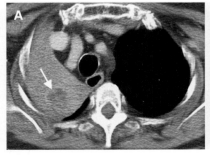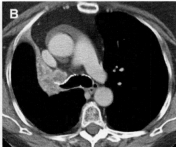

Fig. 11. A 79-year-old woman with non–small cell carcinoma. Patient with advanced, symptomatic lung cancer. (*A*) CT scan demonstrates a 3-cm right lung tumor within right upper lobe collapse (*arrow*). (*B*) Central hilar adenopathy (N2) with occlusion of the right upper lobe bronchus. MR image of brain (not shown) also detected a metastasis (M1 disease).

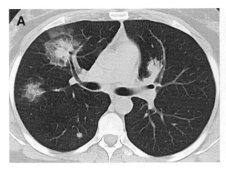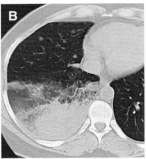

Fig. 12. A 35-year-old nonsmoking woman with multifocal bronchioalveolar carcinoma. (*A*) CT image demonstrates bilateral masses with ground glass and solid components. (*B*) Dense consolidation in the right lower lobe and smaller nodules in the right middle lobe.

format (Fig. 14) [56], is universally accepted and provides a useful framework for NSCLC staging. Small cell cancer is staged and treated differently (see later).

In the past there have been two competing systems for mapping mediastinal lymph nodes, but in 1996 the two systems were unified and adapted by the American Joint Committee on Cancer (Fig. 15) [57,58]. The new unified system provided for a numbered and a descriptive classification for lymph node staging, resulting in a standardized and easily understood system of reproducible lymph node mapping. The staging for NSCLC is not perfect, however, reflecting some intrinsic problems with the system and the complex anatomy in the thorax and the consequent variety of possibilities of regional and distant spread of disease. It is frequently difficult or impossible to determine the extent of tumor because of the presence of other abnormalities (eg, the true size of a tumor mass may be obscured by

surrounding lung infiltrate or consolidation or a large pleural effusion). There are several descriptive ambiguities associated with this staging system, of which three examples are given below:

- N2 tumor, which invades mediastinal structures (Fig. 16). Is this considered a meaningful N2 or is it more advanced disease?
- Recurrence of tumor following surgery: in lung, brain, bone, and so forth. There is no staging for this situation. It is designated recurrent disease.
- Two synchronous lung cancers are staged separately and independently. Prognosis is determined by the most advanced-stage tumor (Fig. 17).

Pathologic staging more accurately reflects the patient's true extent of disease than clinical staging, because of the fact that it is performed during the actual surgical removal of tumor and

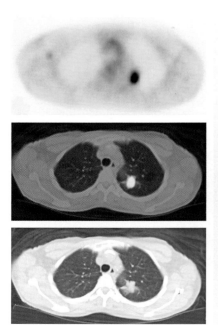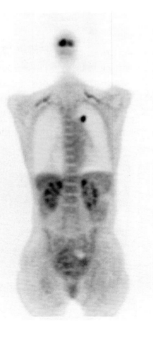

Fig. 13. A 65-year-old woman with lung nodule for evaluation. FDG-PET scan showed increased uptake in a nodule in the left upper lobe consistent with malignancy. Biopsy demonstrated poorly differentiated adenocarcinoma.

TNM	Stage	Percent surviving 5 years after treatment	
		Clinical stage (% with 95% CI)	Pathological stage (% with 95% CI)
CIS	0		
T1N0M0	IA	61	67
T2N0M0	IB	38	57
T1N1M0	IIA	34	55
T2N1M0	IIB	24	39
T3N0M0	IIB	22	38
T3N1M0	IIIA	9	25
T1-3N2MO	IIIA	13	23
T4N0-2M0	IIIB	7	–
Tany N3M0	IIIB	3	–
Tany Nany M1	IV	1	–

Primary tumor (T)
TX   Malignant cells in Sputum or bronchial washings but primary not visualized.
T0   No Primary tumor
Tis   Carcinoma in *situ*
T1   Tumor ≤ 3 cm in greatest dimension, surrounded by lung ir visceral pleura.
T2   Tumor with any of the following features of size or extent: > 3 cm in greatest dimension.
      Involves main bronchus ≥ 2 cm distal to the carina. Invades the visceral pleura. Associated with
      atelectasis or obstructive pneumonitis that extends to the hilar region but does not involve the entire lung.
T3   Tumor of ant size that directly invades any of the following: chest wall (including superior sulcus tumors),
      diaphragm, mediastinal pleura, parietal pericardium; or tumor in the main bronchus < 2 cm distal to the carina,
      but without involvement of the carina; or associated atelectasis or obstructive pneumonitis of the entire lung.
T4   Tumor of any size that invades any of the following: mediastinum, heart, great vessels, trachea, esophagus,
      vertebral body, carina; or tumor with malignant pleural or pericardial effusion, [a](see below) or with satellite
      tumor nodule(s) within the ipsilateral primary-tumor lobe of the lung.
Regional lymph nodes (N)
NX   Regional lymph nodes cannot be assessed.
N0   No regional lymph node metastasis.
N1   Ipsilateral peribronchial and/or hilar lymph nodes, and intra pulmonary nodes involved by direct extension.
N2   Metastasis to ipsilateral mediastinal and/or subcranial lymph node(s).
N3   Metastasis to contralateral mediastinal or hilar lymph node(s), any scalene or supraclavicular lymph node(s).
Distant metastasis (M)
MX   Presence of metastasis cannot be assessed.
M0   No distant metastasis.
M1   Distant metastasis; separate metastatic tumor nodule(s) in the ipsilateral
      non primary-tumor lobe(s) of the lung.

[a]Most pleural effusions are due to tumor. However, there are a few patients in whom
  multiple cytopathologic examinations of pleural fluid show no tumor. In these cases, the fluid is
  non bloody and is not an exudate. When these elements and clinical judgment
  dictate that the effusion is not related to the tumor, the effusion should be excluded as a staging
  element and disease should be staged T1, T2, or T3. Pericardial effusion is classified according
  to the same rules.

Fig. 14. International system for Staging Lung Cancer and Lung Cancer Survival by Stage. (*Data from* Mountain CF. Revisions in the International System for Staging Lung Cancer. Chest 1997;111:1710–7.)

the anatomic relationship of the tumor to surrounding structures may be ascertained (eg, adjacent to or invading a particular structure). Also, other foci of tumor may be found that were not seen on presurgical procedures (satellite nodules or regional lymph nodes containing tumor). Once diagnosis is achieved, detailed clinical staging must be performed, which is defined as staging procedures that occur before the definitive therapeutic intervention. Surgical staging comprises all staging information from the therapeutic surgical procedure, including findings at surgery and confirmatory pathologic findings, representing a further refinement of clinical staging. In patients who undergo operation, the clinical preoperative staging is subject to verification by the surgical and pathologic findings, which not infrequently uncover more advanced disease than the clinical staging. Surgical staging frequently results in an upgrade of the clinical stage. This may be fairly simple in cases of early or small lung cancer. A CT scan alone in the presence of a small nodule <7 mm demonstrating growth over time, if negative for regional abnormality, may suffice as the sole preoperative diagnostic procedure, although some clinicians advocate extensive preoperative work-up for all patients diagnosed with cancer, including small T1 lesions. If, however, there are equivocal or abnormal findings (eg, borderline-size nodes or an adrenal

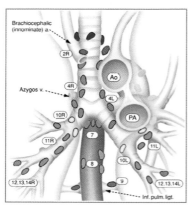

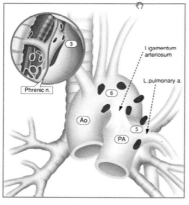

Superior Mediastinal Nodes

● 1 Highest Mediastinal

● 2 Upper Paratracheal

● 3 Pre-vascular and Retrotracheal

◐ 4 Lower Paratracheal
     (including Azygos Nodes)

N₂ = single digit, ipsilateral
N₃ = single digit, contralateral or supraclavicular

Aortic Nodes

● 5 Subaortic (A-P window)

● 6 Para-aortic (ascending
     aorta or phrenic)

Inferior Mediastinal Nodes

◐ 7 Subcarinal

◐ 8 Paraesophageal
     (below carina)

◐ 9 Pulmonary Ligament

N₁ Nodes

○ 10 Hilar

◐ 11 Interlobar

◐ 12 Lobar

◐ 13 Segmental

◐ 14 Subsegmental

(Mountain/Dresler modifications from Naruke/ATS-LCSG Map)   © 1997 Reprints are permissible for educational use only

Fig. 15. Mediastinal lymph node mapping figure. (*From* Mountain CF, Dresler CM. Regional lymph node classification for lung cancer staging. Chest 1997;111:1718–23; with permission.)

mass), further work-up may be indicated. FDG-PET scan (discussed later) may be considered in these situations. In cases of advanced lung cancer at presentation (eg, regional lymph nodes, pleural effusion), when the efficacy of surgery may be questioned, a complete staging work-up should be performed. This should include CT of the chest, FDG-PET scan, brain MR imaging, and other procedures as may be clinically warranted, including MR imaging of other organs, as indicated by the patient's symptoms, to determine if the patient is truly a candidate for useful surgical intervention.

In advanced lung cancer (stage III B/IV) surgery is contraindicated because it represents incurable disease. There is no surgical-pathologic staging because surgery is not performed. Surgery is contraindicated in these patients with advanced tumor, including those patients with T4 tumor (ie, with invasion of central mediastinal structures [including spine] or malignant pleural effusion or satellite tumor nodules within the primary-tumor lobe of lung). Some surgeons resect satellite tumor nodules if they are in the same lobe as the primary tumor, reasoning that they are part of the local-regional process and are potentially completely resectable. Patients with stage III B by virtue of positive contralateral mediastinal or hilar nodes, or either contralateral or ipsilateral scalene or supraclavicular nodes, are not considered resectable. Any M1 (distant metastasis) is unresectable.

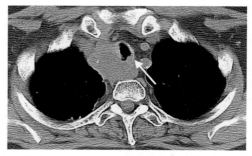

Fig. 16. Extensive mediastinal adenopathy invading the trachea (arrow). This N2 disease is more extensive (involving or invading mediastinal structures in a manner described for T4 primary lung masses) than standard enlarged mediastinal metastatic disease contained within a lymph node capsule.

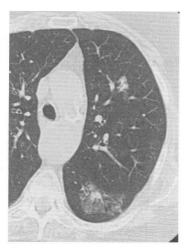

Fig. 17. Left upper lobe solid nodule with an irregular shape. A mass in the superior segment of the left lower lobe is of ground glass opacity with a central core. Although both were adenocarcinomas, they differed significantly in their morphology and immunohistologic staining properties, causing the pathologist to designate them as two separate primary lung cancers.

By its nature, pathologic staging uncovers equal or more advanced neoplasm than clinical staging and is more accurate. It seldom results in downstaging of a neoplasm; occasionally, it may diagnose benign disease in a lesion previously thought malignant. This delineation of more advanced tumor by surgical intervention explains the improved 5-year survival seen in Fig. 8 in patients who are staged pathologically for each stage: clinical staging discovers less advanced disease; pathologic staging uncovers tumor involvement not seen on clinical staging. This more accurate pathologic appraisal results in a greater percentage of patients in each staging group actually belonging to that group, and not having more advanced disease, as in the clinical staging group, accounting for the apparent superior 5-year survivals with pathologic staging.

CT and positron emission tomography in staging of mediastinal lymphadenopathy

In the era before CT, plain chest radiography was the most commonly used noninvasive method for preoperative evaluation of lung cancer. Earlier reports of CT scanning in patients with lung cancer aroused great optimism in the radiologic community concerning the ability of this modality accurately to stage lung cancer. Indeed, early reports, which were poorly controlled and not correlated with surgical-pathologic findings, indicated high accuracy for CT in detecting regional, mediastinal, and distant metastases. A standard morphologic criterion for abnormality of lymph nodes was a short axis measurement of 10 mm or more. It seems clear now that this somewhat simplistic approach to lung cancer staging was flawed. Eventually, larger series of patients undergoing pretreatment CT were analyzed with more rigorous criteria for truth testing, including thoracotomy, mediastinoscopy, and other invasive procedures designed accurately to determine the ability of CT to evaluate mediastinal and hilar lymph nodes, raising serious doubts concerning exaggerated claims for CT's accuracy in this regard [59,60]. The cooperative Radiology Diagnostic Oncology Group, in comparing the accuracy of CT and MR imaging in staging lung cancer in the mediastinum, found that the two procedures were equally inaccurate, with sensitivity for CT and MR imaging at 52% and 48%, respectively, and specificity for CT and MR imaging at 69% and 64%, respectively [36]. McLoud and coworkers [60] in a study of CT accuracy in diagnosing mediastinal involvement with excellent surgical-pathologic correlation reported a sensitivity and specificity of CT on a per patient basis of 64% and 62%. The sensitivity for CT in individual nodal stations involved with tumor was 44%. A significant number of false-positives (benign enlarged lymph nodes) and false-negatives (normal-sized lymph nodes containing tumor) were encountered. Other carefully performed studies placed the overall percent accuracy of CT in detecting mediastinal lymph node metastasis in the upper 60s to low 70s.

Initially, MR imaging with its ability to scan in any plane was proposed as a replacement for CT in staging lung cancer, justified by its claimed intrinsic diagnostic superiority related to its ability to scan in all planes. The Radiology Diagnostic Oncology Group study, however, demonstrated no advantage for MR imaging over CT in staging lung cancer. In addition, MR imaging was considerably more xpensive and time consuming to perform. There does seem to be some advantage for MR imaging in evaluating extent of invasion of superior sulcus tumors through the lung apex into the lower neck [61].

CT, although clearly useful in describing the properties of the primary tumor (T stage) and in detecting distant metastatic disease (frequently in patients who are symptomatic), was demonstrated to be a flawed modality in the evaluation of mediastinal lymphadenopathy. Some observers in the surgical community suggested a return to more invasive staging procedures as a routine, such as cervical mediastinoscopy [62].

Dales and coworkers [63] reviewed all available studies of CT in the detection of mediastinal metastasis between January 1980 and 1988. A total of 42 studies were pooled and a meta-analysis was performed, indicating a sensitivity, specificity, and accuracy of 79%. This was considered unreliable as a truth test because of the unacceptable number of false-positive and false-negative examinations, potentially resulting in unnecessary surgery in patients with advanced disease or depriving patients of potentially curative surgery in the mistaken belief that they had advanced disease. At the end of the article the author stated "we believe that no clinically important advances (in detection of mediastinal lymph node tumor involvement) will be made until lymph node size is replaced by a fundamentally different indicator of lymph node pathology."

FDG-PET is useful in the evaluation and staging of lung cancer and assessment of prognosis and treatment response [64]. It has been shown that FDG-PET can be more accurate than CT for staging of NSCLC. In patients with potentially resectable disease it can help in reducing the rate of unnecessary surgical procedures [65,66] because an FDG-PET scan can identify involved lymph nodes, although they may be normal sized. M and N staging is better assessed with FDG-PET than with CT imaging. Additionally, FDG-PET scanning can be more accurate than CT scanning or endoscopic ultrasound for the detection of mediastinal metastases [67]. FDG-PET can be particularly helpful and more accurate than CT for the detection of N1 and N2-N3 disease (Fig. 18).

In patients with suspected or proved NSCLC considered resectable by standard staging procedures, FDG-PET can prevent unnecessary thoracotomy in one out of five patients [68]. In a multicenter randomized trial involving 188 patients with NSCLC, conventional staging work-up as compared with conventional work-up plus FDG-PET was evaluated and it was concluded that unnecessary surgery in one of five patients was prevented by the addition of FDG-PET to the conventional work-up. Additionally, 27% of patients were upstaged based on the FDG-PET findings [69].

In a prospective study of 102 patients with NSCLC, the sensitivity and specificity of FDG-PET in detecting mediastinal lymph node metastasis were 91% and 86%, respectively, and the investigators concluded that invasive procedures, such as mediastinoscopy, are probably not necessary in patients with negative mediastinal findings on FDG-PET scan. Detection of local and distant metastases in patients with NSCLC can improve with a FDG-PET scan (Fig. 19) [70].

The prognostic value of FDG-PET has been investigated by several groups. In a study of a group of 155 patients with NSCLC median survival was compared with the SUV of the primary tumor. As the mean SUV increased, the median survival decreased [71]. A retrospective study of 100 patients demonstrated that

in a group with an SUV >9, the 2-year survival rate was 68%, whereas with those in the group with an SUV <9, the survival rate increased to 96% [72]. Another study that included 162 patients with stage I to IIIB NSCLC of which 93 patients were treated with surgery and 69 patients were treated with radiotherapy concluded that the SUV for the primary tumor was the most significant prognostic factor among that group of patients. Patients with a low SUV ≤5 showed significantly better disease-free survival than those with a high SUV >5 [73].

In patients with stage I NSCLC, the FDG-PET uptake had a significant independent postoperative prognostic value for recurrence. The incidence of metastases was high if the SUV was high [74]. The SUV values, however, had a wide range from 5 to 20 [75].

A recent multicenter trial evaluating 465 patients with NSCLC noted that obtaining an FDG-PET study initially after first presentation does not decrease the overall number of diagnostic tests, although invasive procedures, such as mediastinoscopies, were performed significantly less often if a PET-CT scan was obtained. There were limitations with this study, however, such as different levels of clinical experience with FDG-PET interpretation, which varied among institutions, and also the fact that the PET scans were not read in conjunction with the CT scan [76].

For small, peripherally located T1 or T2 tumors, however, FDG-PET has no demonstrable benefit in the diagnosis, staging, or determination of prognosis of these patients. Only 55% of these tumors were FDG-PET avid after the exclusion of BAC [77]. Another study involving patients with stage I-II NSCLC found that PET provides potential for more appropriate stage-specific treatment but may not lead to a significant decrease in the actual number of thoracotomies avoided [78]. In locally advanced NSCL patients, FDG-PET was found to have additional value over CT in monitoring response to induction chemotherapy. It may be feasible to predict response and patient outcome even after one course of induction chemotherapy [79]. It has been shown that in patients with known or suspected lung cancer evaluated with FDG-PET, the results had major impact on staging and management of their lung cancer [80]. PET-CT is also more accurate than PET and CT alone for staging NSCLC [81].

Staging of small cell lung cancer

SCLC is not staged according to the TNM system. It is described as either limited-stage disease or extensive-stage disease. Standard staging procedures for SCLC include CT scans of the chest and abdomen, bone scan, and CT scan or MR

A   B

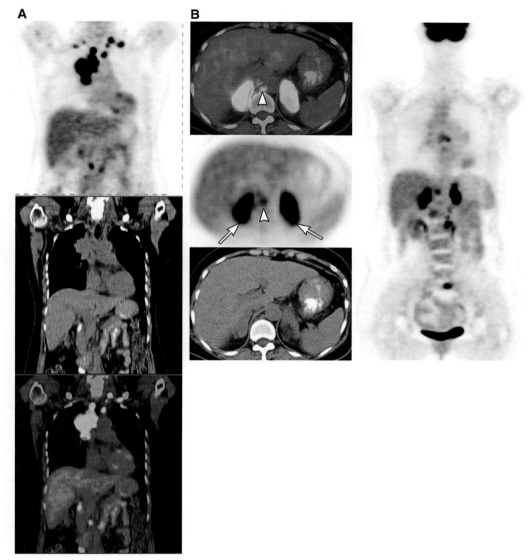

Fig. 18. A 56-year-old woman with non–small cell lung carcinoma. (*A*) FDG-PET scan demonstrates increased uptake in the right upper lung in a paramediastinal mass with lymph node metastases bilaterally in the lower neck, paratracheal region, and the para-aortic region in the upper abdomen. (*B*) There is also increased activity in the adrenal glands (*arrows*) and in a retrocrural lymph node (*arrowhead*) consistent with metastases.

imaging of the brain. Patients with limited-stage disease have involvement restricted to the ipsilateral hemithorax within a single radiation port (Fig. 20). Extensive-stage disease is defined as the presence of metastatic disease. Limited-stage disease is treated with curative intent with chemotherapy and radiation therapy. The median survival time for patients with limited-stage disease is approximately 18 months. A small subset of these patients present with a single solitary nodule that can be resected. These cases are considered very early stage limited disease and have a better prognosis. Extensive-stage disease is treated primarily with chemotherapy, with a median survival time of approximately 9 months [82]. These tumors are usually centrally located and present as a hilar or perihilar mass associated with extensive bilateral mediastinal lymphadenopathy [83]. The primary tumor may be obscured by adenopathy and which may lead to associated lobar collapse. It is the most common cause of superior vena cava syndrome. Less commonly seen are peripheral lesions with associated hilar adenopathy.

There are limited data regarding the role of FDG-PET in the work-up of patients with SCLC [84]. Some preliminary data with a small number of

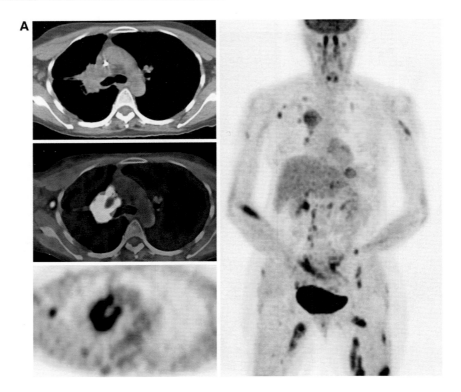

Fig. 19. A 54-year-old woman with adenocarcinoma of the right lung. (*A*) FDG-PET showed increased uptake in the right hilar mass. Whole body maximum intensity projection image demonstrates extensive nodal metastases in the chest and abdomen. (*B*) Note musculoskeletal metastases in the legs.

patients provided a potential use of FDG-PET for the staging of patients with SCLC (Fig. 21) [85]. FDG-PET influences staging and can help in improving management of patients with SCLC. A study by Brink and coworkers [86] evaluated the clinical impact of FDG-PET on primary staging of patients with newly detected SCLC. In this study, FDG-PET showed 100% sensitivity in the detection of the primary tumor. The sensitivity of FDG-PET was significantly better than that of CT in the detection of extrathoracic lymph node involvement and distant metastases, with exception of brain where a brain MR image or CT is more sensitive than an FDG-PET scan.

Follow-up imaging

Immediate postoperative period

In the immediate postoperative period, chest radiography is performed to assess for lobar collapse, tension pneumothorax, pulmonary edema, or other acute processes. In the weeks and months after surgery, postoperative pneumothorax decrease in size and are replaced by fluid or compensatory expansion of the remaining lung. Patients with pneumonectomy usually have complete opacification of the hemithorax with shift of the mediastinum into the surgical side. Occasionally, air fluid levels may persist; however, if it is stable or the patient is asymptomatic, it is not clinically significant. An increase in the air component of the postoperative hydropneumothorax should raise concern, however, for a bronchopleural fistula.

The radiologic follow-up of patients after the immediate postoperative period varies according to the referring surgeon. Follow-up examinations generally include chest radiography and chest CT. Extrathoracic imaging is not usually ordered unless there are clinical symptoms that are suggestive of potential metastatic disease. Assessing for recurrent disease and for metastatic disease is vital for the radiologist interpreting the CT scan or radiograph.

Long-term follow-up

The standard treatment of choice for localized stage I through IIIA remains surgical resection with and without chemoradiation therapy. Unfortunately, the 5-year survival for all stages of lung cancer remains at 15% [1]. Careful follow-up may lead to earlier detection of recurrences or earlier detection of a second primary bronchogenic carcinoma. The risk of developing a second lung cancer in patients

B

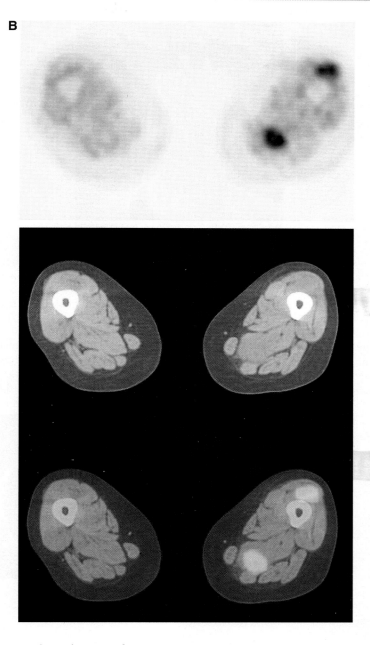

Fig. 19 (continued)

who survived resection of a NSCLC is approximately 1% to 2% per patient per year and for SCLC survivors it is approximately 6%. Ten years after the initial treatment in those who survived SCLC, the risk increases to greater than 10% per patient per year. This risk of developing a second primary lung cancer can translate into an important cumulative risk [87]. This cumulative risk can make death from a second lung cancer a common cause of death in lung cancer survivors.

The current recommendations for routine follow-up after complete resection of NSCLC at the authors' institution are as follows: for 2 years following surgery a contrast-enhanced chest CT scan every 6 months and then yearly noncontrast chest CT scans. Recurrence on CT is the primary goal in the initial years and a contrast-enhanced scan should be obtained optimally to evaluate the mediastinum. Because identifying an early second primary lung cancer becomes of more clinical

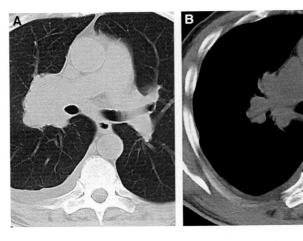

Fig. 20. A 56-year-old man presenting with limited stage small cell lung cancer. Note larger right hilar mass (*A*) and mediastinal lymphadenopathy (*B*) that can be contained in a single radiation port.

importance in the subsequent years a noncontrast scan suffices to evaluate the lung parenchyma.

Posttreatment imaging

Radiation therapy changes

All references should be related to the end of the radiation therapy treatment period. Imaging performed within 3 months of the conclusion of therapy may show ground glass opacities, which may indicate radiation pneumonitis. This may occasionally appear nodular but is within the lung that was treated with radiation. At follow-up imaging, the nodules are seen to coalesce into areas of consolidation and eventually become a component of the radiation fibrosis. Radiation fibrosis consists of a well-defined area of consolidation associated with volume loss and bronchiectasis. Fibrosis can progress slowly over 3 to 12 months after radiation therapy ends but stabilize within 2 years (Fig. 22). Most fibrosis occurs within the first 12 months

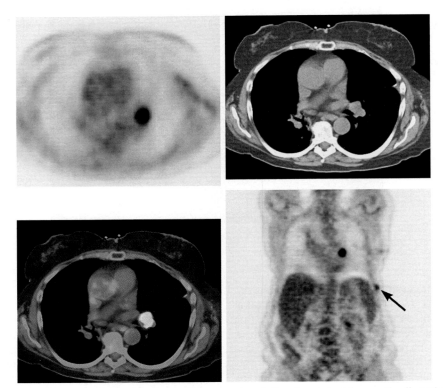

Fig. 21. A 64-year-old woman following chemotherapy and radiation treatment for small cell carcinoma of the right lung developed a left hilar mass, which had increased uptake on an FDG-PET scan consistent with tumor recurrence. Focus of uptake in a left lower rib (*arrow*) is consistent with a new rib metastasis.

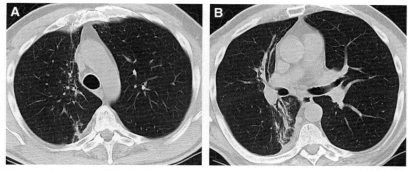

Fig. 22. (A) Right paramediastinal fibrotic changes within the radiation port. (B) Three years later after treatment with radiation and chemotherapy demonstrates typical postradiation changes of right paramediastinal consolidation and traction bronchiectasis.

and has a well-defined border [88]. Changes occurring within radiation fibrosis that had previously been confirmed to have stabilized could represent recurrent tumor or infection. Recurrent tumor may manifest as a convex bulge in the border of the radiation fibrosis or as a tumor extending into adjacent structures, such as the mediastinum or chest wall. Filling in of the bronchiectasis within the fibrosis is also an indication of recurrent tumor and may occur without any other evidence of recurrence [89]. Infection within the radiation fibrosis can have a similar manifestation, however, with opacities filling the bronchiectasis.

Thermal ablation

The use of imaging-guided thermal ablation, which includes radiofrequency, microwave and cryoablation, is a relatively new application in the treatment of lung neoplasms. It may be used in those patients who may not be surgical candidates or in those patients who are not candidates for conventional radiation (external beam or brachytherapy) and chemotherapy because of coexisting morbidities or of the higher stage of their inoperable tumor that may respond poorly to conventional treatment. On the immediate post–radiofrequency ablation CT, the most common imaging finding is ground glass opacity adjacent to the treated tumor. Between 1 and 3 months after radiofrequency ablation most patients have resolution of this ground-glass opacity and can develop cavitation within the treated tumor (Fig. 23). This is more common if a lesion is located in the inner two thirds of the lung or in close proximity to a segmental bronchus. Pleural thickening and scar formation in the region of pleura traversed by the radiofrequency electrode is often seen. Tumor size can be variable in the first 6 months after radiofrequency ablation. If there is growth of the lesion beyond 6 months it is usually consistent with residual or recurrent disease [90].

Future directions

Despite "better treatment for lung cancer," survival remains poor. Treatment up until recently was focused on surgery, radiation therapy, and chemotherapy. New molecular and genetic understanding of tumor biology has led to research involving targeted therapies. There may be genes that may make certain individuals susceptible to lung cancer. More recently, research has been centered on identifying patients who respond and may have mutated forms of an epidermal growth factor receptor on their tumors and may respond to a drug that targets epidermal growth factor receptors. Drugs that take advantage of those molecular differences and thereby block the activity of molecules necessary for cancer cells to survive are being developed. Such dugs as gefitinib and erlotinib have led to unexpected insight that mutations are found in a substantial number of NSCLCs, particularly in never-smokers with adenocarcinoma. These discoveries promise to alter the approach toward lung cancer [91,92]. Molecular imaging of lung cancer may in the future aid in earlier diagnosis of lung cancer.

Computer-aided diagnosis

The goal of lung cancer screening with CT is to detect small cancers. Computer-aided diagnosis has been reported to be effective in facilitating detection of small pulmonary nodules at CT. Most computer-aided diagnosis schemes that are used to facilitate detection of focal lung lesions are designed and optimized for solid nodules. It has been postulated that a program can be developed by combining the texture and pixel attenuation features of localized ground glass opacity with an artificial neural network classification to facilitate detection of localized ground glass opacity in the lung at CT [93]. Lung cancers missed at low-dose CT screening have been studied with the use of computer-aided diagnosis. Li and coworkers

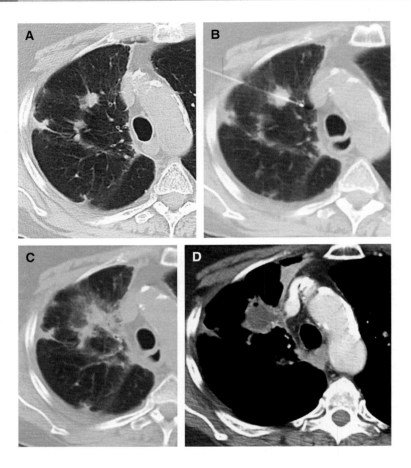

Fig. 23. A 72-year-old man with small cell lung cancer. (*A*) Nodule seen in the right upper lobe. (*B*) Radiofrequency probe within the nodule. (*C*) Nodule immediately postradiofrequency treatment demonstrates peripheral ground glass density representing adequate treatment. (*D*) Three months after treatment lesion is low in density consistent with necrotic tumor.

[94] evaluated whether a computer-aided diagnosis scheme can help radiologists detect missed lesions at least 6 mm. They included lesions with pure ground glass opacity, mixed ground glass opacity, and solid opacity. Lung cancers missed at low-dose CT were very difficult to detect, even in an observer study. The use of computer-aided diagnosis, however, did improve radiologists' performance in the detection of these subtle cancers. Future development may improve the radiologists' performance in the detection of these subtle cancers. Growth of lung nodules in the future will likely be assessed by automated three-dimensional volumetric measurements. This may lead to the more accurate measurement of growth of a nodule and also possibly may help discriminate malignant versus benign disease based on growth patterns and rates.

Summary

Lung cancer prevention by smoking cessation is an important aspect in discussions on lung cancer. Survival for lung cancer is clearly better for earlier-stage tumors, and whereas it sounds reasonable that early detection in an asymptomatic population is beneficial, there are no definitive data that screening for lung cancer leads to a decrease in mortality.

Accurate staging by imaging can have a significant impact on appropriate treatment and surgical options. Staging of newly diagnosed NSCLC is performed according to the International System for Staging Lung Cancer using the TNM system. Because the extent of the disease determines whether the patient is treated by means of surgical resection, radiation therapy, chemotherapy, or a combination of these modalities, radiologic imaging plays an important role in the staging evaluation [90]. SCLC is not staged according to the TNM system but rather as limited-stage disease or extensive-stage disease. Accurate staging by imaging of SCLC is also extremely important. Staging by combined modalities, such as CT and FDG-PET, has been shown to be more accurate than CT or PET alone.

Radiologists need to be aware of entire spectrum of manifestations of lung cancer. Familiarity with the different histologic subtypes of lung cancer and the typical and atypical appearances of lung cancer is vital. Radiologists serve a critical role in the diagnosis, staging, and follow-up of patients with NSCLC. This includes suggesting the possibility of synchronous and metachronous lung cancers because it has serious implications in the staging and prognosis of these patients.

References

[1] American Cancer Society. Cancer facts and figures 2006. Atlanta (GA): American Cancer Society; 2006.

[2] Probability of Developing or Dying of Cancer Software, Version 5.1 Statistical Research and Applications Branch, NCI, 2003. Available at: http://srab.cancer.gov/devcan. Accessed February 20, 2004.

[3] Haiman CA, Stram DO, Wilkens LR, et al. Ethnic and racial differences in the smoking-related risk of lung cancer. N Engl J Med 2006;354:333–42.

[4] Travis WD, Garg K, Franklin WA, et al. Evolving concepts in the pathology and computed tomography imaging of lung adenocarcinoma and bronchioloalveolar carcinoma. J Clin Oncol 2005;23:3279–87.

[5] Khuder SA. Effect of cigarette smoking on major histological types of lung cancer: a meta-analysis. Lung Cancer 2001;31:139–48.

[6] Bower SL, Choplin RH, Muss HB. Multiple primary bronchogenic carcinomas of the lung. AJR Am J Roentgenol Am J Roentgenol 1983;140:253–8.

[7] Martini N, Melamed M. Multiple primary lung cancers. J Thorac Cardiovasc Surg 1975;70:606–12.

[8] Asaph JW, Keppel JF, Handy JR Jr, et al. Surgery for second lung cancers. Chest 2000;118:1621–5.

[9] Antakli T, Schaefer RF, Rutherford JE, et al. Second primary lung cancer. Ann Thorac Surg 1995;59:863–7.

[10] Kubik A, Polak J. Lung cancer detection: results of a randomized prospective study in Czechoslovakia. Cancer 1986;57:2427–37.

[11] Melamed MR, Flehinger BJ, Zaman MB, et al. Screening for early lung cancer: results of the Memorial Sloan-Kettering Study in New York. Chest 1984;86:44–53.

[12] Tockman M. Survival and mortality from lung cancer in a screened population: the Johns Hopkins Study. Chest 1986;89:325S.

[13] Fontana RS. The Mayo Lung Project. Presented at the International Conference on Prevention and Early Diagnosis of Lung Cancer. Varese, Italy, December 9–10, 1988.

[14] Fontana RS, Sanderson DR, Woolner LB, et al. Screening for lung cancer: a critique of the Mayo Lung Project. Cancer 1991;67(Suppl4):1155–64.

[15] Flehinger BJ, Kimmel M, Melamed MR. The effect of surgical treatment on survival from early lung cancer: implications for screening. Chest 1992;101:1013–8.

[16] Swensen SJ, Jett JR, Midthun DE, et al. Computed tomographic screening for lung cancer: home run or foul ball? Mayo Clin Proc 2003;78:1187–8.

[17] Kaneko M, Eguchi K, Ohmatsu H, et al. Peripheral lung cancer: screening and detection with low-dose spiral CT versus radiography. Radiology 1996;201:798–802.

[18] Sone S, Takashima S, Li F, et al. Mass screening for lung cancer with mobile spiral computed tomography scanner. Lancet 1998;351:1242–5.

[19] Henschke CI, McCauley DI, Yankelevitz DF, et al. Early lung cancer action project: overall design and findings from baseline screening. Lancet 1999;354:99–105.

[20] Henschke CI, Yankelevitz DF, Miettinen OS, et al. Computed tomographic screening for lung cancer: the relationship of disease to tumor size. Arch Intern Med 2006;166:321–5.

[21] Yankelevitz DF, Vazquez M, Henschke CI. Special techniques in transthoracic needle biopsy of pulmonary nodules. Radiol Clin North Am 2000;38:267–79.

[22] Swensen SJ, Jett JR, Hartman TE, et al. CT screening for lung cancer: five-year prospective experience. Radiology 2005;235:259–65.

[23] Bach PB, Kelley MJ, Tate RC, et al. Screening for lung cancer: a review of the current literature. Chest 2003;123:72S–82.

[24] Hillman BJ, Schnall MD. American College of Radiology Imaging Network: future clinical trials. Radiology 2003;227:631–2.

[25] Henschke CI, Yankelevitz DF, Naidich DP, et al. CT screening for lung cancer: suspiciousness of nodules according to size on baseline scans. Radiology 2004;231:164–8.

[26] Kuriyama K, Tateishi R, Doi O, et al. CT-pathologic correlation in small peripheral lung cancers. AJR Am J Roentgenol 1987;149:1139–43.

[27] Theros EG. Varying manifestations of peripheral pulmonary neoplasms: a radiologic-pathologic correlative study. AJR Am J Roentgenol 1977;128:893–914.

[28] Chaudhuri MR. Primary pulmonary cavitating carcinomas. Thorax 1973;28:354–66.

[29] Yabuuchi H, Murayama S, Murakami J, et al. High-resolution CT characteristics of poorly differentiated adenocarcinoma of the peripheral lung: comparison with well differentiated adenocarcinoma. Radiat Med 2000;18:343–7.

[30] Henschke CI, Yankelevitz DF, Mirtcheva R, et al. CT screening for lung cancer: frequency and significance of part-solid and nonsolid nodules. AJR Am J Roentgenol 2002;178:1053–7.

[31] Lee KS, Jeong YJ, Han J, et al. T1 non-small cell lung cancer: imaging and histopathologic findings and their prognostic implications. Radiographics 2004;24:1617–36.

[32] Li F, Sone S, Abe H, et al. Malignant versus benign nodules at CT screening for lung cancer: comparison of thin-section CT findings. Radiology 2004;233:793–8.

[33] Byrd RB, Miller WE, Carr DT, et al. The roentgenographic appearance of squamous cell carcinoma of the bronchus. Mayo Clin Proc 1968;168:327–32.

[34] Onitsuka H, Tsukuda M, Araki A, et al. Differentiation of central lung tumor from postobstructive lobar collapse by rapid sequence computed tomography. J Thorac Imaging 1991;6:28–31.

[35] Tobler J, Levitt RG, Glazer HS, et al. Differentiation of proximal bronchogenic carcinoma from postobstructive lobar collapse by magnetic resonance imaging: comparison with computed tomography. Invest Radiol 1987;22:538–43.

[36] Winer-Muram HT, Jennings SG, Tarver RD, et al. Volumetric growth rate of stage I lung cancer prior to treatment: serial CT scanning. Radiology 2002;223:798–805.

[37] Rosado-de-Christenson ML, Templeton PA, Moran CA. Bronchogenic carcinoma: radiologic-pathologic correlation. Radiographics 1994;14: 429–46.

[38] Wiesbrod GL, Towers MJ, Chaimberlin DW, et al. Thin-walled cystic lesions in bronchioalveolar carcinoma. Radiology 1992;185:401–5.

[39] Huang D, Wiesbrod GL, Chaimberlin DW. Unusual radiologic presentations of bronchioalveolar carcinoma. J Can Assoc Radiol 1986;37: 94–9.

[40] Langen KJ, Braun U, Rota Kops E, et al. The influence of plasma glucose levels on fluorine-18-fluorodeoxyglucose uptake in bronchial carcinomas. J Nucl Med 1993;34:355–9.

[41] Brown RS, Leung JY, Kison PV, et al. Glucose transporters and FDG uptake in untreated primary human non-small cell lung cancer. J Nucl Med 1999;40:556–65.

[42] Higashi K, Ueda Y, Sakurai A, et al. Correlation of Glut-1 glucose transporter expression with (18F) FDG uptake in non-small cell cancer. Eur J Nucl Med 2000;27:1778–85.

[43] Herder GJ, Golding RP, Hoekstra OS, et al. The performance of (18F)-fluorodeoxyglucose positron emission tomography in small solitary pulmonary nodules. Eur J Nucl Med Mol Imaging 2004;31:1231–6.

[44] Lowe VJ, Fletcher JW, Gobar L, et al. Prospective investigation of positron emission tomography in lung nodules. J Clin Oncol 1998;16:1075–84.

[45] Gould MK, Maclean CC, Kuschner WG, et al. Accuracy of positron emission tomography for diagnosis of pulmonary nodules and mass lesions: a meta-analysis. JAMA 2001;285:914–24.

[46] Ost D, Fein A. Management strategies for the solitary pulmonary nodule. Curr Opin Pulm Med 2004;10:272–8.

[47] Duhaylongsod FG, Lowe VJ, Patz EF Jr, et al. Detection of primary and recurrent lung cancer by means of F-18 fluorodeoxyglucose positron emission tomography (FDG PET). J Thorac Cardiovasc Surg 1995;110:130–9.

[48] Patz EF Jr, Lowe VJ, Hoffman JM, et al. Focal pulmonary abnormalities: evaluation with F-18 fluorodeoxyglucose PET scanning. Radiology 1993; 188:487–90.

[49] Roberts PF, Follette DM, von Haag D, et al. Factors associated with false-positive staging of lung cancer by positron emission tomography. Ann Thorac Surg 2000;70:1154–9 [discussion: 1159–60].

[50] Croft DR, Trapp J, Kernstine K, et al. FDG-PET imaging and the diagnosis of non-small cell lung cancer in a region of high histoplasmosis prevalence. Lung Cancer 2002;36:297–301.

[51] Ost D, Fein AM, Feinsilver SH. Clinical practice: the solitary pulmonary nodule. N Engl J Med 2003;348:2535–42.

[52] Shankar LK, Sullivan DC. Functional imaging in lung cancer. J Clin Oncol 2005;23:3203–11.

[53] Kim BT, Kim Y, Lee KS, et al. Localized form of bronchioloalveolar carcinoma: FDG PET findings. AJR Am J Roentgenol 1998;170:935–9.

[54] Marom EM, Sarvis S, Herdon JE, et al. T1 lung cancers: sensitivity of diagnosis with fluorodeoxyglucose PET. Radiology 2002;223:453–9.

[55] Erasmus JJ, McAdams HP, Patz EF Jr, et al. Evaluation of primary pulmonary carcinoid tumors using positron emission tomography with 18-F-fluorodeoxyglucose. AJR Am J Roentgenol 1998; 170:1369–73.

[56] Mountain CF, Dresler CM. Regional lymph node classification for lung cancer staging. Chest 1997;111:1718–23.

[57] Mountain CF. Revisions in the international system for staging lung cancer. Chest 1997;111:1710–7.

[58] Cymbalista M, Waysberg A, Zacharias C, et al. CT demonstration of the 1996 AJCC-UICC regional lymph node classification for lung cancer staging. Radiographics 1999;9:899–900.

[59] Webb WR, Gatsonis C, Zerhouni EA, et al. CT and MR imaging in staging non-small cell bronchogenic carcinoma: report of the Radiologic Diagnostic Oncology Group. Radiology 1991;178:705–13.

[60] McLoud TC, Bourgouin PM, Greenberg RW, et al. Bronchogenic carcinoma: analysis of staging in the mediastinum with CT by correlative lymph node mapping and sampling. Radiology 1992;182:319–23.

[61] Heelan RT, Demas BE, Caravelli JF, et al. Superior sulcus tumors: CT and MR imaging. Radiology 1989;170:637–41.

[62] Gdeedo A, Van Schil P, Corthouts B, et al. Prospective evaluation of computed tomography and mediastinoscopy in mediastinal lymph node staging. Eur Respir J 1997;10:1547–51.

[63] Dales RE, Stark RM, Raman S. Computed tomography to stage lung cancer: approaching a controversy using meta-analysis. Am Rev Respir Dis 1990;141:1096–101.

[64] Erasmus JJ, McAdams HP, Patz EF Jr, et al. Thoracic FDG PET: state of the art. Radiographics 1998;18:5–20.

[65] Kelly RF, Tran T, Holmstrom A, et al. Accuracy and cost-effectiveness of (18F)-2-fluoro-deoxy-D-glucose-positron emission tomography scan in potentially resectable non-small cell lung cancer. Chest 2004;125:1413–23.

[66] Hoekstra CJ, Stroobants SG, Hoekstra OS, et al. The value of (18F) fluoro-2-deoxy-D-glucose

positron emission tomography in the selection of patients with stage IIIA-N2 non-small cell lung cancer for combined modality treatment. Lung Cancer 2003;39:151–7.

[67] Toloza EM, Harpole L, McCrory DC. Noninvasive staging of non-small cell lung cancer: a review of the current evidence. Chest 2003;123(1 Suppl):137S–1346S.

[68] Reed CE, Harpole DH, Posther KE, et al. Results of the American College of Surgeons Oncology Group Z0050 trial: the utility of positron emission tomography in staging potentially operable non-small cell lung cancer. J Thorac Cardiovasc Surg 2003;126:1943–51.

[69] van Tinteren H, Hoekstra OS, Smith EF, et al. Effectiveness of positron emission tomography in the preoperative assessment of patients with suspected non-small-cell lung cancer: the PLUS multicentre randomized trial. Lancet 2002;359:1388–93.

[70] Pieterman RM, van Putten JWG, Meuzelaar JJ, et al. Preoperative staging of non-small-cell lung cancer with positron-emission tomography. N Engl J Med 2000;343:254–61.

[71] Ahuja V, Coleman RE, Herndon J, et al. The prognostic significance of fluorodeoxyglucose positron emission tomography imaging for patients with non-small cell lung carcinoma. Cancer 1998;83:918–24.

[72] Downey RJ, Akhurst T, Gonen M, et al. Preoperative F-18 fluorodeoxyglucose–positron emission tomography maximal standardized uptake value predicts survival after lung cancer resection. J Clin Oncol 2004;22:3255–60.

[73] Sasaki R, Komaki R, Macapinlac H, et al. (18F) fluorodeoxyglucose uptake by positron emission tomography predicts outcome of non-small-cell lung cancer. J Clin Oncol 2005;23:1136–43.

[74] Higashi K, Ueda Y, Arisaka Y, et al. 18 F- FDG uptake as a biologic prognostic factor for recurrence in patients with surgically resected non–small cell lung cancer. J Nucl Med 2002;43:39–45.

[75] Prevost S, Boucher L, Larivee P, et al. Bone marrow hypermetabolism on 18F-FDG PET as a survival prognostic factor in non-small cell lung cancer. J Nucl Med 2006;47:559–65.

[76] Herder GJ, Kramer H, Hoekstra OS, et al. POORT study group. Traditional versus up-front (18F) fluorodeoxyglucose- positron emission tomography staging of non-small-cell lung cancer: a Dutch cooperative randomized study. J Clin Oncol 2006;24:1800–6.

[77] Port JL, Andrade RS, Levin MA, et al. Positron emission tomographic scanning in the diagnosis and staging of non-small cell lung cancer 2 cm in size or less. J Thorac Cardiovasc Surg 2005;130:1611–5.

[78] Viney RC, Boyer MJ, King MT, et al. Randomized controlled trial of the role of positron emission tomography in the management of stage I and II non-small-cell lung cancer. J Clin Oncol 2004;22:2357–62.

[79] Hoekstra CJ, Stroobants SG, Smit EF, et al. Prognostic relevance of response evaluation using (18F)-2-fluoro-2-deoxy-D-glucose positron emission tomography in patients with locally advanced non-small-cell lung cancer. J Clin Oncol 2005;23:8362–70.

[80] Seltzer MA, Yap CS, Silverman DH, et al. The impact of PET on the management of lung cancer: the referring physician's perspective. J Nucl Med 2002;43:752–6.

[81] Lardinois D, Weder W, Hany TF, et al. Staging of non-small-cell lung cancer with integrated positron-emission tomography and computed tomography. N Engl J Med 2003;348:2500–7.

[82] Simon GR, Wagner H. Small cell lung cancer. Chest 2003;123:259S–71S.

[83] Pearlberg JL, Sandler MA, Lewis JW Jr, et al. Small-cell bronchogenic carcinoma: CT evaluation. AJR Am J Roentgenol 1988;150:265–8.

[84] Schumacher T, Brink I, Mix M, et al. FDG-PET imaging for the staging and follow-up of small cell lung cancer. Eur J Nucl Med 2001;28:483–8.

[85] Pandit N, Gonen M, Krug L, et al. Prognostic value of (18 F) FDG-PET imaging in small cell lung cancer. Eur J Nucl Med Mol Imaging 2003;30:78–84.

[86] Brink I, Schumacher T, Mix M, et al. Impact of (18F) FDG-PET on the primary staging of small-cell lung cancer. Eur J Nucl Med Mol Imaging 2004;31:1614–20.

[87] Johnson BE. Second lung cancers in patients after treatment for an initial lung cancer. J Natl Cancer Inst 1998;90:1335–45.

[88] Munden RF, Swisher SS, Stevens CW, et al. Imaging of the patient with non–small cell lung cancer. Radiology 2005;237:803.

[89] Libshitz HI, Sheppard DG. Filling in of radiation therapy–induced bronchiectatic change: a reliable sign of locally recurrent lung cancer. Radiology 1999;210:25–7.

[90] Bojarski JD, Dupuy DE, Mayo-Smith WW. CT imaging findings of pulmonary neoplasms after treatment with radiofrequency ablation: results in 32 tumors. AJR Am J Roentgenol 2005;185:466–71.

[91] Pao W, Miller VA. Epidermal growth factor receptor mutations, small-molecule kinase inhibitors, and non-small-cell lung cancer: current knowledge and future directions. J Clin Oncol 2005;10:2556–68.

[92] Lynch TJ, Bell DW, Sordella R, et al. Activating mutations in the epidermal growth factor receptor underlying responsiveness of non-small-cell lung cancer to gefitinib. N Engl J Med 2004;350:2129–39.

[93] Kim KG, Goo JM, Kim JH, et al. Computer-aided diagnosis of localized ground-glass opacity in the lung at CT: initial experience. Radiology 2005;237:657–61.

[94] Li F, Arimura H, Suzuki K, et al. Computer-aided detection of peripheral lung cancers missed at CT: ROC analyses without and with localization. Radiology 2005;237:684–90.

RADIOLOGIC
CLINICS
OF NORTH AMERICA

Radiol Clin N Am 45 (2007) 45–67

Imaging Breast Cancer

Lia Bartella, MD, FRCR[a,b],*, Clare S. Smith, MB, BCh, BAO, FRCR[a],
D. David Dershaw, MD[a,b], Laura Liberman, MD[a,b]

Breast cancer is now the most common nonskin cancer in women in the United States. Women have an average risk of one in eight of being diagnosed with breast cancer at some time in their lives. Although the breast cancer diagnosis rate has increased, there has been a steady drop in the overall breast cancer death rate since the early 1990s [1], most likely due to a combination of screening, improved treatments, and better awareness.

Invasive ductal carcinoma is the most common breast cancer histologic type, accounting for 70%

to 80% of all cases. Invasive lobular carcinoma is the second most common histologic type (5% to 10% of all breast cancers). It is associated with a high rate of multifocality and bilaterality and can be difficult to diagnose clinically and mammographically because of its tendency to spread diffusely through breast tissue instead of forming a mass and causing architectural distortion. Other less common cancers include tubular, medullary, mucinous, and papillary cancers. Cystosarcoma, phyllodes, angiosarcoma, and lymphoma also occur in the breast but are not considered typical breast

[a] Department of Radiology, Breast Imaging Section H-118, Memorial Sloan-Kettering Cancer Center, 1275 York Avenue, New York, NY 10021, USA
[b] Weill Medical College of Comell University, New York, NY, USA
* Corresponding author. Memorial Sloan-Kettering Cancer Center, 1275 York Avenue, New York, NY 10021.
E-mail address: bartelll@mskcc.org (L. Bartella).

0033-8389/07/$ – see front matter © 2006 Elsevier Inc. All rights reserved.
radiologic.theclinics.com

doi:10.1016/j.rcl.2006.10.007

cancers. Inflammatory cancer is diagnosed clinically based on the association with edema, erythema, and skin dimpling. Paget's disease is a relatively rare disease, affecting the nipple–areolar complex. It accounts for 1% of all breast cancer cases.

In situ carcinoma is contained within the duct, and the basement membrane surrounding the duct is not breached. Ductal carcinoma in situ (DCIS) originates from the major lactiferous ducts. Approximately 30% to 50% of patients who have DCIS will develop invasive ductal carcinoma over a 10-year period [2]. Lobular carcinoma in situ (LCIS) arises from the terminal duct lobule and can be distributed diffusely throughout the breast. In contrast to DCIS, women who have LCIS have up to 30% risk of developing invasive carcinoma, mostly of the ductal type and with equal frequency in both breasts [3]. Therefore, LCIS is considered a marker of increased risk rather than a precursor of breast cancer.

Controversy exists around the diagnosis and treatment of DCIS, particularly in relation to screening and the phenomenon of overdiagnosis (finding early neoplasms, of which many would not become clinically evident if screening had not occurred). It has been estimated that 1 in 3 in situ tumors are overdiagnosed at the first screen and 1 in 25 are overdiagnosed at subsequent screens [4]. It is not yet possible to say which patients who have DCIS will go on to develop invasive cancers and whether survival rates would be the same if surgery were undertaken only after early invasive cancer had been diagnosed (Tables 1–3). The diagnosis and management of breast cancer has undergone tremendous changes over the years. The mammogram has taken over from clinical examination in the diagnosis of breast cancer. Ultrasound and stereotactic biopsy have replaced many surgical biopsies, and early detection of breast cancer has resulted in breast conservation and sentinel lymph node biopsy, replacing the radical mastectomy and axillary lymph node dissection. Mammography remains the traditional first-line radiologic test of choice in the detection and diagnosis of breast cancer; however, mammography is not perfect. About 10% of cancers are mammographically occult even after they are palpable and, in women who have dense breasts, the sensitivity of mammography can be as low as 68% [5]. This low sensitivity has led to the expansion of breast imaging to include sonography and MR imaging and the development of newer imaging techniques such as positron emission tomography (PET), lymphoscintigraphy, scintimammography, breast tomosynthesis, and contrast-enhanced mammography to aid in the detection and staging of breast cancer and to monitor response to therapy.

Mammography is used for diagnostic and screening purposes. Diagnostic mammography is commonly used to identify possible breast cancers in women who present with signs or symptoms and it has higher sensitivities (85%–93%) compared with screening mammography [6,7]. Tumors detected by diagnostic mammography are larger and more likely to be node positive than those detected by screening mammography [8]. The last decade has seen the development of full-field digital mammography. Digital mammography devices are similar to film-screen units except that the film-screen cassette used to record the image is replaced by a digital detector. Digital mammography has a number of advantages over traditional film-screen mammography. It has a higher contrast resolution yet maintains a good dynamic range. It allows for digital transmission and storage of images, eliminating the need for the film library. The images can be manipulated to enhance visualization of subtle structures and calcifications, and the procedure is quicker for the patient because there are no wait times for the films to be processed. It also eliminates film artifacts such as dust and uses a lower dose of radiation [9]. The major disadvantage of digital mammography is cost, with digital systems currently costing approximately one to four times as much as film-screen systems. The results of the largest trial to date comparing digital versus film mammography for breast cancer screening, the Digital Mammographic Imaging Screening Trial [10], were recently published. In this multicenter trial, the investigators found that digital mammography was better than conventional film mammography at detecting breast cancer in young, premenopausal, and perimenopausal women and in women who have dense breasts; however, there was no significant difference in diagnostic accuracy between digital and film mammography in the population as a whole or in the other predefined subgroups.

Breast sonography is well established as a valuable imaging technique. The current indications for performing breast ultrasound, as listed in the "ACR Practice Guideline for the Performance of Breast Ultrasound Examination," include identification and characterization of palpable and nonpalpable abnormalities, evaluation of clinical and mammographic findings, guidance of interventional procedures, evaluation of breast implants, and treatment planning for radiation therapy [11]. It is also the imaging technique of choice to evaluate palpable masses in women younger than age 30 years and in lactating and pregnant women. Its advantage lies in the fact that it is easily accessible, relatively low in cost, and does not involve the use of ionizing radiation. Its main disadvantage is that its performance

Table 1: TNM staging system

Primary tumor – T	
TX	Primary tumor cannot be assessed
T0	No evidence of primary tumor
Tis	Carcinoma in situ
Tis (DCIS)	Ductal carcinoma in situ
Tis (LCIS)	Lobular carcinoma in situ
Tis (Paget's)	Paget's disease of the nipple with no tumor (note: Paget's disease associated with a tumor is classified according to the size of the tumor)
T1	Tumor ≤2.0 cm in greatest dimension
T1mic	Microinvasion ≤0.1 cm in greatest dimension
T1a	Tumor >0.1 cm but ≤0.5 cm in greatest dimension
T1b	Tumor >0.5 cm but ≤1.0 cm in greatest dimension
T1c	Tumor >1.0 cm but ≤2.0 cm in greatest dimension
T2	Tumor >2.0 cm but ≤5.0 cm in greatest dimension
T3	Tumor >5.0 cm in greatest dimension
T4	Tumor of any size with direct extension to (a) chest wall or (b) skin, only as described below
T4a	Extension to chest wall, not including pectoralis muscle
T4b	Edema (including peau d'orange) or ulceration of the skin of the breast, or satellite skin nodules confined to the same breast
T4c	Both T4a and T4b
T4d	Inflammatory carcinoma
Regional lymph nodes – N	
NX	Regional lymph nodes cannot be assessed (eg, previously removed)
N0	No regional lymph node metastasis
N1	Metastasis to movable ipsilateral axillary lymph node(s)
N2	Metastasis to ipsilateral axillary lymph node(s) fixed or matted, or in clinically apparent ipsilateral internal mammary nodes in the absence of clinically evident axillary lymph node metastasis
N2a	Metastasis in ipsilateral axillary lymph nodes fixed to one another (matted) or to other structures
N2b	Metastasis only in clinically apparent* ipsilateral internal mammary nodes and in the absence of clinically evident axillary lymph node metastasis
N3	Metastasis in ipsilateral infraclavicular lymph node(s) with or without axillary lymph node involvement, or in clinically apparent* ipsilateral internal mammary lymph node(s) and in the presence of clinically evident axillary lymph node metastasis; or, metastasis in ipsilateral supraclavicular lymph node(s) with or without axillary or internal mammary lymph node involvement
N3a	Metastasis in ipsilateral infraclavicular lymph node(s)
N3b	Metastasis in ipsilateral internal mammary lymph node(s) and axillary lymph node(s)
N3c	Metastasis in ipsilateral supraclavicular lymph node(s)
Distant metastasis – M	
MX	Distant metastasis cannot be assessed
M0	No distant metastasis
M1	Distant metastasis
Histologic grade – G	
GX	Grade cannot be assessed
G1	Low combined histologic grade (favorable)
G2	Intermediate combined histologic grade (moderately favorable)
G3	High combined histologic grade (unfavorable)

is operator dependent and it can be time-consuming.

Several studies have shown that breast sonography can help distinguish benign from malignant solid nodules [12] and that the use of ultrasound as an adjunct to mammography has led to an overall increase in diagnostic accuracy [13]. Studies on the impact of ultrasound have also shown that its use can affect management in 64% of patients and prevent unnecessary biopsies in 22% [14]. Ultrasound is also useful in the assessment of the axilla in a patient who has newly diagnosed breast

Table 2: Stage grouping

Stage	Tumor	Node	Metastasis
0	Tis	N0	M0
I	T1	N0	M0
IIA	T0	N1	M0
	T1	N1	M0
	T2	N0	M0
IIB	T2	N1	M0
	T3	N0	M0
IIIA	T0	N2	M0
	T1	N2	M0
	T2	N2	M0
	T3	N1	M0
	T3	N2	M0
IIIB	T4	N0	M0
	T4	N1	M0
	T4	N2	M0
IIIC	Any T	N3	M0
IV	Any T	Any N	M1

cancer. If lymph nodes are seen to have cortical contour bulges or masses, then ultrasound-guided percutaneous needle biopsy can confirm metastatic involvement, obviating the need for sentinel lymph node biopsy [15].

An American College of Radiology Imaging Network trial (Protocol 6666) is now underway to assess the efficacy of screening breast sonography. The primary aim of this multicenter protocol is to determine whether screening whole-breast sonography can identify mammographically occult cancers and whether such results can be generalized across multiple centers.

Breast cancer screening

Abundant evidence has accumulated over the past 4 decades to support the ability of mammographic screening to decrease breast cancer mortality. Seven prospective randomized trials have been conducted. Study designs of these trials have differed, with variable intervals between mammographic screenings, variable ages at invitation to screening and cessation of screening, and even with varying mammographic techniques. (Table 4) [16].

Table 3: Stage and 5-year survival rate

Stage	Rate (%)
0	100
I	100
IIA	92
IIB	81
IIIA	67
IIIB	54
IV	20

Because of these differences, the conclusions of these studies have varied from trial to trial. Based on these trials, however, there is little doubt that mammographic screening has efficacy. A recent meta-analysis of data from these seven trials shows a 24% mortality reduction in women invited to screening.

The estimation of mortality reduction with mammographic screening is generally considered to be underestimated by these trials because of noncompliance of those invited to screening and contamination of the control groups (the women included in these studies who were not invited to be screened). The percentage of women invited to screening who actually underwent screening was as low as 67%. Although they underwent some screening, many women did not undergo all the screening mammography to which they were invited. This lack of compliance degrades the impact of screening on breast cancer mortality in all studies. In addition, of the women not invited to screening, some underwent mammographic screening outside of the study situation, further decreasing the study's estimate of the impact of mammography.

Results of prospective randomized trials have now been augmented by experience with population-based screening. In the Uppsala region of Sweden, a comparison of breast cancer mortality before and after the introduction of mammographic screening has estimated a 39% mortality reduction due to screening [17]. In Italy, the rate of fatal breast cancer cases has been reduced by 50% with the introduction of mammographic screening [18]. These data suggest that the impact of screening may be greater than that estimated by prospective randomized trials.

Although the benefit of mammographic screening is widely accepted, limitations and adverse effects from screening are also generally acknowledged and include biopsies to diagnose benign lesions, anxiety about mammography and biopsy results, scarring from biopsies, and time lost from work to undergo screening and follow-up. Of biopsies done on the basis of mammographic abnormalities, only 25% to 45% result in a diagnosis of carcinoma.

The failure of mammography to detect all breast cancers is also widely acknowledged, with the false-negative rate of screening mammography usually in the 20% to 30% range. Tumors without associated calcifications and subtle masses are particularly difficult to diagnose. Invasive lobular carcinoma and uncalcified DCIS are especially difficult to detect with mammography.

Despite these limitations, mammography has been incorporated in the routine medical care of

Table 4: Results of prospective randomized trials of mortality reduction by mammographic screening

Study	Year begun	Age of women (y)	Mammography interval (mo)	% Participation of invited women	% Mortality reduction (95% CI)
HIP	1963	40–64	12	67	24 (7–38)
Two county, Sweden	1977	40–74	24	89	32 (20–41)
Malmo	1976	45–69	18–24	74	19 (−8–39)
Stockholm	1981	40–64	24	81	26 (−10–50)
Gothenburg	1982	39–59	18	84	16 (−39–49)
Canada NBSS1	1980	40–49	12	100	−3 (−26–27)
Canada NBSS2	1980	50–59	12	100	−2 (−33–22)
All trials combined					24 (18–30)

Abbreviations: CI, confidence interval; HIP, health insurance plan of greater NY; NBSS, National Breast Cancer Screening study.
Data from Smith RA, Saslow D, Sawyer KA, et al. American Cancer Society guidelines for breast cancer screening: update 2003. CA Cancer J Clin 2003;53:141–69; and Heywang-Koebrunner SH, Dershaw DD, Schreer I. Diagnostic breast imaging. 2nd edition. New York: Thieme; 2001.

women. The usual recommendation for mammographic screening in the United States is currently annual mammography starting at age 40 years [19]. No upper age limit has been applied to the screening recommendation in the United States.

In women at higher risk than the general population, screening for the development of breast cancer may be more aggressive. Women at highest risk are those who are gene positive on testing for *BRCA* genes or who have a very strong family history. These histories include multiple first- and second-degree relatives who have had breast or ovarian carcinoma, a first-degree relative who has had breast cancer before age 50 years, male relatives who have had breast cancer, and Ashkenazi Jewish women who have a family history of breast or ovarian cancer. In some families, gene-positive women have been calculated to have up to an 85% lifetime risk of developing breast cancer. In families in which premenopausal breast cancer develops, it has been recommended that women should start screening 10 years earlier than the youngest age at which breast cancer was diagnosed, starting as early as age 25 years. Because breast cancers in younger women may grow more quickly and because familial breast cancers may grow more quickly than sporadic cancers, it has been suggested that screening may be useful more frequently than every 12 months in this population. Although 6-month mammographic screening has been suggested for these women, there are no data to indicate whether it is of any advantage over annual examinations.

Other women at significantly higher risk include those who have a personal history of breast cancer or prior biopsy diagnosis of atypical ductal hyperplasia (ADH) or LCIS. Screening for these women should commence at the time of diagnosis. Women treated for Hodgkin's disease with mantle radiation are at risk for developing radiation-induced breast cancer and should commence screening as early as 8 years after their cure [20].

The addition of other imaging modalities to mammography in the screening algorithm for high-risk women has undergone some study, but screening with nonmammographic imaging remains controversial. It should be remembered that mammography is the cornerstone of breast cancer screening, and there are no recommendations that it be abandoned for other screening modalities. The ability of mammography to detect subcentimeter carcinomas based on easily identified microcalcifications has not been replaced by any other screening tool [21].

When used in a high-risk population, there are data to suggest that sonography and MR imaging can detect early, curable cancers not found by mammography. In a study of Dutch women who had a genetic predisposition to develop breast cancer, MR imaging was able to find more cancers than mammography at initial and follow-up screenings. Cancers found by both modalities had a similar prognosis, and the positive predictive values of mammography and MR imaging were comparable [22]. Other studies from the United States and Europe support these results. Data for sonographic screening are less compelling, suggesting a sensitivity that is inferior to MR imaging and an inability to detect most in situ disease. There may also be a lower positive predictive value for sonographically recommended biopsies than those based on mammographic or MR imaging findings. The wider availability and lesser cost of sonography compared with MR imaging, however, may make it the study of choice in some situations when a second modality is desired.

Percutaneous image-guided biopsy

Percutaneous image-guided biopsy is increasingly used as an alternative to surgical biopsy for the histologic assessment of breast lesions [23]. Guidance for percutaneous biopsy may be provided by stereotaxis, ultrasound, or MR imaging. Most often, stereotactic guidance is used for biopsy of calcifications; ultrasound guidance for biopsy of masses; and MR imaging guidance for lesions identified only with breast MR imaging. Tissue acquisition for percutaneous biopsy is usually accomplished with automated core needles or vacuum-assisted biopsy probes. Vacuum-assisted probes are preferable for stereotactic-guided or MR imaging–guided biopsies; for ultrasound-guided biopsies, automated core needles and vacuum-assisted probes are useful. For small imaging lesions in which the imaging target is removed at percutaneous biopsy, placement of a localizing marker is helpful.

Percutaneous image-guided biopsy, compared with surgical biopsy, is faster, less invasive, has fewer complications, and causes minimal to no scarring. Percutaneous biopsy spares the need for surgical biopsy in approximately 80% of patients, often obviating surgery in women who have benign disease and decreasing the number of operations necessary in women who have breast cancer [24]. Finally, percutaneous biopsy, compared with surgical biopsy, has a lower cost of diagnosis. At the authors' facility, the cost of diagnosis was decreased by 20% by using stereotactic 11-gauge vacuum-assisted biopsy and by more than 50% with ultrasound-guided 14-gauge automated core biopsy [25,26].

Guidance

Stereotaxis

Stereotactic biopsy is based on the principle that the three-dimensional location of a lesion can be assessed based on its apparent positional change on two angled (stereotactic) images. Validation studies of stereotactic 14-gauge automated core biopsy demonstrated 87% to 96% concordance between results of stereotactic and surgical biopsies; obtaining multiple specimens with a long excursion gun and a dedicated table yielded the best results [27]. Although prone tables provide more working room, decrease the likelihood of patient motion or vasovagal reaction, and provide a physical and psychologic barrier between the patient and the procedure than upright units, they are more expensive and require more space. Digital imaging is

valuable in stereotactic biopsy because it enables image processing that improves lesion conspicuity and shortens procedure times.

Stereotactic biopsy is most often used for lesions evident as calcifications. Vacuum-assisted biopsy probes are preferable to automated core biopsy needles for tissue acquisition of calcifications at stereotactic biopsy because they provide better retrieval of calcifications [28] and better characterization of complex lesions such as ADH and DCIS, lesions that are often evident as calcifications at mammography [29,30]. "Underestimation" is defined as the diagnosis of cancer at surgery in a lesion that yielded ADH at percutaneous biopsy or the diagnosis of invasive cancer at surgery in a lesion that yielded DCIS at percutaneous biopsy. The likelihood of underestimation is significantly lower among lesions that undergo stereotactic 11-gauge vacuum-assisted biopsy compared with 14-gauge automated core biopsy [31,32]. There is a learning curve for stereotactic biopsy, with better results obtained after the first 5 to 20 cases for 14-gauge automated core biopsy and after the first 5 to 15 cases for 11-gauge vacuum-assisted biopsy [33]. In a validation study of stereotactic 11-gauge vacuum-assisted biopsy, false-negative cases were encountered in 3% of all cancers; the false-negative rate was significantly higher among radiologists who had previously performed fewer than 15 cases rather than 15 or more cases (10% versus 0.6%, $P < .01$) [32].

Ultrasound

Ultrasound-guided biopsy, first performed with 14-gauge automated core needles, is a fast, safe, and accurate procedure. Ultrasound guidance has numerous advantages over stereotactic guidance, including speed, multipurpose equipment, lack of ionizing radiation, accessibility of all areas of the breast and axilla, real-time needle visualization, multidirectional sampling, and lower cost. The main disadvantage of ultrasound guidance is that sonographically inapparent lesions (eg, specific lesions evident as calcifications or masses that are not visualized on ultrasound) may not be amenable to ultrasound-guided biopsy. Ultrasound-guided biopsy can also be performed with vacuum-assisted devices [33]. The vacuum-assisted biopsy devices are faster and more often achieve complete excision of the imaging target but have no other significant benefit compared with 14-gauge automated core needles for ultrasound-guided biopsy [34].

Ultrasound-guided biopsy is generally performed for sonographically evident masses initially identified by imaging or palpation. A mass identified at mammography and ultrasound could potentially undergo biopsy under stereotactic or ultrasound guidance; however, ultrasound guidance is often preferable due to shorter procedure time, lack of ionizing radiation, and lower cost. Soo and colleagues [35] found that a subset (23%) of calcific lesions had a sonographic correlate and were therefore amenable to percutaneous biopsy under ultrasound guidance [35]. A sonographic correlate was more likely in calcific lesions categorized as Breast Imaging Reporting and Data System (BI-RADS) 5, highly suggestive of malignancy, compared with calcific lesions classified as BI-RADS 4, suspicious of malignancy (89% versus 17%, *P* < .001). Targeting the sonographic mass (if present) associated with the calcifications may facilitate diagnosis of the invasive component of a lesion containing invasive cancer and DCIS, thereby decreasing the frequency of underestimation. If screening breast ultrasound proves to be efficacious, then ultrasound-guided biopsy will be the method of choice for diagnosis of lesions identified at screening sonography [36].

MR imaging

MR imaging can demonstrate breast cancers that are not identified by mammography, sonography, or physical examination. The specificity of breast MR imaging, however, is limited, ranging from 37% to 97%. Furthermore, among lesions identified at MR imaging that warrant biopsy, ultrasound fails to reveal a sonographic correlate in up to 77% [37]. To benefit from breast MR imaging, it is necessary to have the capability to perform biopsy of lesions identified with MR imaging only. MR imaging–guided percutaneous breast biopsy poses several challenges, including the necessity to remove the patient from the closed magnet to perform the biopsy, limited access to the medial breast tissue, the transient nature of contrast enhancement, and the difficulty in confirming lesion retrieval [38]. Dedicated MR imaging–guided biopsy equipment has been developed to overcome some of these challenges, including coils, breast immobilization and compression devices, needle guides, localizing markers, and nonferromagnetic needles with minimal artifact.

MR imaging–guided biopsy is more expensive than biopsies done under stereotactic or ultrasound guidance and is generally reserved for lesions identified only at MR imaging. Pioneered in Europe [39], MR imaging–guided vacuum-assisted biopsy has been further refined in the United States [40–43]. For MR imaging–guided percutaneous biopsy, vacuum-assisted biopsy probes have several advantages over automated core needles for tissue acquisition: they are faster, acquire a larger volume of tissue, and provide more accurate characterization of lesions such as ADH and DCIS, lesions that are

encountered more frequently among the high-risk patients undergoing breast MR imaging examination than among the general population. In published experience from the authors' institution, the median time to perform MR imaging–guided biopsy of a single lesion was 33 minutes; MR imaging–guided biopsy histology yielded cancer in 25% (Fig. 1), with more than half of the cancers being DCIS [41].

Percutaneous biopsy: future directions

Percutaneous biopsy provides an excellent alternative to surgery for histologic diagnosis. Further work is necessary to optimize lesion selection for biopsy, to refine the equipment and techniques for performing percutaneous biopsy, to develop evidence-based criteria to optimize the biopsy method for specific clinical scenario, to evaluate cost-effectiveness of different biopsy procedures, and to assess long-term outcomes. These studies will allow more women to benefit from the use of minimally invasive techniques to diagnose benign and malignant lesions of the breast.

Staging breast cancer

Preoperative staging

Traditional preoperative planning for breast cancer involves clinical examination and mammogram. It was shown from a study of 282 mastectomy specimens [44] (performed for unifocal breast cancer) assessed clinically and mammographically that most breasts (63%) had additional sites of cancer that were undetected by clinical examination or mammography. Additional foci of cancer were found pathologically within 2 cm of the index cancer in 20% and greater than 2 cm away from the index cancer in 43%. Seven percent had additional foci of carcinoma more than 4 cm away from the index cancer, which likely represent cancer within a separate breast quadrant. The presence of undetected residual disease that is not removed entirely at surgery is the rational for performing postoperative radiation therapy in patients who are treated with breast conservation therapy.

It is known that disease may or may not be left behind in the breast; however, it has not been possible without the addition of MR imaging to reliably identify which patients have additional multifocal or multicentric cancer. Many studies have shown that MR imaging is able to detect additional foci of cancer in the breast that has been overlooked by conventional techniques. Several investigators have shown that MR imaging is able to detect additional foci of disease in up to one third of patients [45,46], which may possibly result

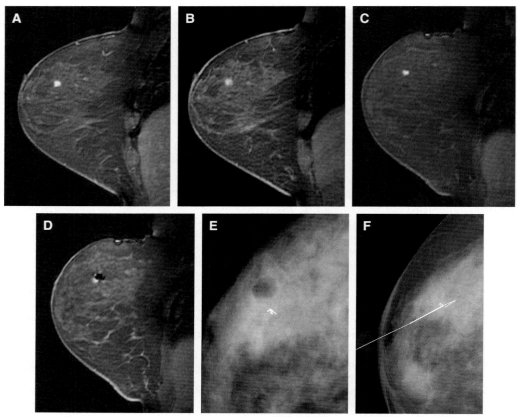

Fig. 1. A 62-year-old asymptomatic woman who has a strong family history of breast cancer (sister at ages 53 and 69 years, daughter at age 33 years) and moderately dense breasts without suspicious findings at mammography (not shown). (A) Sagittal, fat-suppressed, T1-weighted MR image of the right breast obtained within 2 minutes after injection of intravenous gadolinium at high-risk screening MR imaging examination shows an intensely enhancing 0.7-cm mass in the right breast upper inner quadrant. (B) Sagittal, T1-weighted, fat-suppressed, delayed image of the right breast after contrast injection during the high-risk screening MR imaging examination shows washout of contrast from the right breast upper inner quadrant mass. This lesion, which had no mammographic or sonographic correlate, was interpreted as suspicious for carcinoma, and biopsy was recommended. (C) On the day of MR imaging–guided vacuum-assisted biopsy, a sagittal, T1-weighted, fat-suppressed scout image demonstrates that the lesion is still present. (D) Images obtained after tissue acquisition and clip placement show low signal artifact from air and clip at the biopsy site. The lesion has been sampled. (E) Collimated mammographic image of the right breast after biopsy and clip placement demonstrates air and the clip that has deployed in the breast. Histologic analysis yielded invasive ductal carcinoma. (F) Mediolateral mammographic image of the right breast on the day of breast conserving surgery demonstrates preoperative localization of the clip under mammographic guidance. Surgery yielded invasive ductal carcinoma, 0.5 cm, adjacent to the needle biopsy site. The sentinel nodes were free of tumor.

in a treatment change [47]. MR imaging can potentially provide valuable information for preoperative planning in the single-stage resection of breast cancer [48,49]. By using breast MR imaging as a complementary test to the conventional imaging techniques, more precise information can be obtained about the extent of breast cancer, ultimately improving patient care.

Patient selection for preoperative breast MR imaging may include the young patient, the patient who has dense or moderately dense breasts, and the patient who has difficult tumor histology, such as infiltrating lobular carcinoma and tumors with extensive intraductal component (EIC) in which tumor size assessment is difficult [50]. Infiltrating lobular carcinoma is known to be difficult to detect on mammography; for this neoplasm, MR imaging has been shown to assess the extent of disease more accurately than mammography [51,52]. MR imaging has also been shown to demonstrate unsuspected DCIS, which can be helpful when assessing extent of disease in preoperative testing [53,54]. EIC is associated with a known invasive carcinoma when greater than 25% of the tumor is DCIS. EIC can also be associated with residual carcinoma and positive margins after lumpectomy, and there is some evidence that the presence of EIC may indicate an increased risk of local recurrence.

MR imaging defines the anatomic extent of disease more accurately than mammography, particularly in tumors with difficult histologies, as discussed previously. Breast MR imaging can give helpful information for staging on tumor size, presence or absence of multifocal or multicentric disease, and whether the chest wall or pectoralis muscle is invaded [55]. Chest wall involvement is an important consideration for the surgeon before surgical planning. Mammography does not image the ribs, intercostal muscles, and serratus anterior muscle that compose the chest wall. Tumor involvement of the chest wall changes the patient's stage to IIIB, indicating that the patient may benefit from neoadjuvant chemotherapy before surgery. Tumor involvement of the pectoralis muscle does not alter staging, and surgery can usually proceed. Knowledge that the muscle is involved, however, may alter the surgeon's plan; for example, when the full thickness of the pectoralis major muscle is involved with tumor, the surgeon may be more inclined to perform a radical instead of a modified radical mastectomy (Fig. 2).

Controversy exists regarding the use of MR imaging to stage breast cancer. MR imaging may identify cancer, especially additional DCIS that is currently treated with adjuvant chemotherapy and radiation therapy. It is being argued that staging with MR imaging results in surgical overtreatment of the patient's breast cancer. For example, many women who may be candidates for breast conservation therapy may be overtreated with mastectomy based on the MR imaging results that additional disease was found elsewhere. The challenge is in knowing what is and what is not clinically significant disease on MR imaging. At this time, identification of significant disease that will not be treated with radiation therapy is not possible and all additional disease is treated surgically. In a recent study by Liberman [56], 666 nonpalpable, mammographically occult MR imaging–detected lesions were reviewed; the frequency of malignancy was found to increase significantly with lesion size ($P<.001$), and only 3% of lesions smaller than 0.5 cm were found to be malignant. Trials that involve radiologists in addition to radiation oncologists and surgeons are needed to answer these perplexing questions.

Sentinel lymph node biopsy

For patients who have invasive breast cancer, lymph node status is one of the most important prognostic factors [57]. Traditionally, lymph node status has been assessed with axillary dissection. Advances in breast cancer screening and increased public awareness have meant that many women are now diagnosed at an earlier stage when the axillary lymph nodes are free of metastasis. For many of these patients, axillary dissection, with its complications such as lymphedema, has no benefit. Sentinel lymph node biopsy has emerged as a minimally invasive alternative to axillary dissection, where a negative sentinel node obviates the need for the latter.

The sentinel node is the node in the tumor bed that is most likely to harbor tumor cells because it is the first to receive lymphatic drainage from the

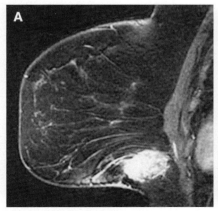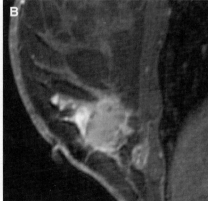

Fig. 2. (A) Posteriorly located breast cancer. Sagittal, fat-suppressed, T1-weighted image demonstrates the chest wall to be free of tumor. The patient went on to have successful surgical excision and conservation treatment for this invasive ductal cancer. (B) Posteriorly located irregular heterogeneously enhancing breast carcinoma. An enhancing mass is noted involving the chest wall. Appearances demonstrate extension of the tumor into the intercostal muscles, which would make the patient IIIB. Primary management now is chemotherapy, rather than surgical. This tumor was not detected on the patient's mammogram.

tumor. A number of studies have shown that the findings in the sentinel node accurately predict the status of the other axillary nodes [58,59]. The technique that is used varies between institutions. A radiotracer that is taken up by macrophages and allows visualization of the lymphatics is injected into the breast. In the United States, technetium 99m sulfur colloid (filtered or unfiltered) is used. In Europe and Australia, other tracers such as technetium 99m nanocolloid are widely available. The site of injection also varies between institutions. Most investigators favor peritumoral or sub/intradermal injections or a combination of these. Lymphoscintigraphy is performed the afternoon before or the morning of surgery, depending on the size of the colloid particle injected and whether it is filtered. Images are acquired in two planes, usually anterior and oblique, using a high-resolution camera, and the site of the sentinel node should be marked on the patient's skin, making sure the arm is abducted in the same position as in the operating room, allowing the surgeon to focus attention on the correct spot in the axilla (Figs. 3 and 4).

At surgery, localization of the sentinel node is performed by external counting with a gamma probe. Intraoperative lymphatic mapping using isosulfur dye, injected intradermally, peritumorally, subdermally, or in the periareolar region is also often performed to locate the sentinel node. Using a combined technique of blue dye and radioisotope mapping, success rates of 97% in identifying the sentinel lymph node have been reported [60]. With increasing experience in the radioisotope technique, the blue dye technique only marginally improves radio-guided identification of the sentinel node. After the sentinel nodes have been removed, a thorough histopathologic examination of the nodes, including multisectioning and immunohistochemistry analysis, is performed. Completion axillary node dissection is then performed if the sentinel node is positive.

Overall, the sensitivity of sentinel node biopsy (SNB) for node involvement ranges from 71% to 100% and the average false-negative rate is 8.4% [61]. The American Society of Breast Surgeons recommends that a sentinel lymph node identification sensitivity of 85% with a false-negative rate of 5% or less is required to abandon axillary dissection.

More recently, investigators have been evaluating other imaging techniques to assess the axilla. PET is a noninvasive imaging modality that can detect lymph nodes. A number of studies have compared fludeoxyglucose F 18 (FDG)-PET to SNB or axillary lymph node dissection and have found that although the sensitivity is relatively low, the specificity is greater than 94% [62,63], suggesting that FDG-PET cannot replace histologic staging in early breast cancer but may be able to identify women who can forego SNB, requiring axillary node dissection instead. The use of MR imaging in evaluating the axilla has also been assessed [64]. Presently, there is no imaging modality able to detect microscopic nodal metastasis detected at SNB.

Breast MR imaging

Breast MR imaging has become an important and powerful tool in breast imaging. The performance and clinical uses of breast MR imaging are more standardized and defined than they were several

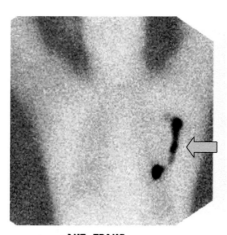
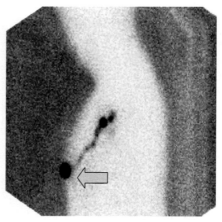

ANT TRANS   LT LAT TRANS

Fig. 3. Lymphoscintigraphy performed in a 47-year-old woman who subsequently underwent left breast conservation therapy and sentinel lymph node biopsy for a 1.3-cm moderately to poorly differentiated invasive ductal carcinoma. The images demonstrate a chain of draining nodes in the left axilla (*arrow in left image*). Radiotracer is also demonstrated at the intradermal injection site overlying the primary tumor (*arrow in right image*). Seven lymph nodes removed at surgery were negative for metastasis.

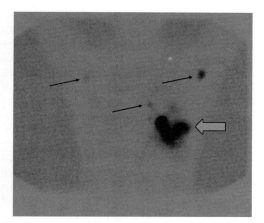

Fig. 4. Lymphoscintigraphy performed in a 40-year-old woman, pre left mastectomy for recurrent ductal carcinoma. She previously had left breast conservation therapy and sentinel lymph node biopsy for a node-negative invasive ductal carcinoma. The images demonstrate radiotracer activity at the intradermal injection site overlying the primary tumor (*white arrow*) and tracer activity in draining nodes in the left axilla, in the left intramammary lymph nodes, and in a contralateral draining right axillary node (*black arrows*). The left axillary sentinel node was removed at surgery and yielded metastatic disease.

decades ago. In the past few years, great strides have been made in the realm of breast intervention, with new coils and needles now available. More sequences that have an increase in image quality and speed of acquisition are available from manufacturers. The use of breast MR imaging for cancer detection is changing the current algorithms in the detection and treatment of breast cancer. By being able to detect cancer that is occult on conventional imaging such as mammography and sonography, MR imaging can provide valuable information about breast cancer that was, up to this point, unimaginable [65,66]. This section addresses current and evolving trends in breast MR imaging for cancer detection. Preoperative staging and screening are addressed in respective sections in this article.

Indications for the use of breast MR imaging

Many studies have shown that breast MR imaging is best used in situations in which there is a known cancer, a suspected cancer, or a high probability of finding cancer. For example, in the preoperative evaluation of the patient with a known cancer, the ability of MR imaging to detect multifocal (within the same quadrant of the breast) and multicentric (within different quadrants) disease that was previously unsuspected facilitates accurate staging [45–48,50,67,68]. Incidental synchronous contralateral carcinomas have also been detected when screening

the contralateral breast in patients who have known cancer [46,49,69]. In the patient who has positive margins following an initial attempt at breast conservation, MR imaging can detect residual disease [69–71] and, in the patient who has inoperable locally advanced breast cancer, MR imaging can assess response to neoadjuvant chemotherapy [72–75]. Suspected recurrence can be confirmed with MR imaging in the previously treated breast [76,77], and breast MR imaging is absolutely indicated in the patient who has axillary node metastases with unknown primary [78–82]. Another indication that is promising is the use of MR imaging for high-risk screening [83–87].

During the past few decades, as breast MR imaging has been incorporated into the clinical evaluation of the breast, it has become apparent that standardization of image acquisition and terminology is important. The American College of Radiology committee on standards and guidelines has published a document for the performance of breast MR imaging [88], and the recent publication of the BI-RADS lexicon [89] includes a section about breast MR imaging so that standardized terminology can be used when describing findings on breast MR imaging. The existence of standardized guidelines in image acquisition and interpretation may help disseminate this technology from academic centers to the community.

Neoadjuvant chemotherapy response

Response to neoadjuvant chemotherapy for locally advanced breast cancer can be assessed with MR imaging. A complete pathologic response (elimination of tumor) following neoadjuvant therapy is strongly predictive of excellent long-term survival. Minimal response suggests a poor long-term survival regardless of postoperative therapy. MR imaging may find a role in being able to predict at an earlier time, perhaps after several cycles of chemotherapy, which patients are responding to neoadjuvant chemotherapy. Early knowledge of suboptimal response may allow switching to alternative treatment regimens earlier rather than later. Unless the response is dramatic, it currently takes longer to predict response because the mammogram and physical examination may be compromised due to fibrosis. Studies have shown MR imaging to be superior to mammography, sonography, and clinical examination in measuring residual disease after neoadjuvant chemotherapy [90–92]. MR imaging showed 89% to 97% correlation with pathology, whereas clinical examination demonstrated 55% correlation and mammography demonstrated 52% correlation. There are limitations with MR imaging in assessing early treatment response. A recent study has shown that although early changes of tumor measurements were observed with MR imaging after one cycle of chemotherapy (2 weeks), these changes were not statistically significant. It has been shown, however, that the final change in MR imaging volume was a significant predictor of recurrence-free survival. A multicenter trial (American College of Radiology Imaging Network Protocol 6657) is under way to further assess the predictive value of early changes in tumor volume and changes in tumor vascularity, as measured by MR imaging [93].

Assessment of residual disease

For patients who have undergone lumpectomy with positive margins, MR imaging can be helpful in the assessment of residual tumor load. Postoperative mammography is able to detect residual calcifications, although it is limited in the evaluation of residual uncalcified DCIS or residual mass. MR imaging is able to detect bulky residual disease at the lumpectomy site and residual disease in the same quadrant (multifocal) or a different quadrant (multicentric). MR imaging can be helpful in the determination of whether the patient would best be served with directed re-excision (residual disease at the lumpectomy site or multifocal disease) or whether the patient warrants mastectomy (multicentric disease) (Fig. 5). Evaluation for microscopic residual disease directly at the lumpectomy site is not the role of MR imaging because the surgeon will perform re-excision based on pathologic margins and not based on MR imaging results. If multicentric disease is identified on MR imaging before mastectomy, then it is important to sample and verify this impression. A study [70] has shown that MR imaging was able to detect residual disease in 23 of 33 cases (70%) and alone identified multifocal or multicentric disease in 9 of 33 cases (27%). The authors looked at 100 women who underwent MR imaging for positive margins [94]. Fifty-eight patients had residual disease at surgery: 20 multicentric, 15 multifocal, and 23 unifocal. MR identified 18 of 20 cases (90%) of multicentric, 14 of 15 cases (93%) of multifocal, and 18 of 23 cases (78%) of unifocal residual disease. Eight false-negative findings included 2 cases of multicentric DCIS occult to MR imaging and 6 cases of residual disease (4 subcentimeter invasive and 2 microscopic DCIS) directly at the lumpectomy site. Overall sensitivity for detection of residual cancer was 86% (50/58) and specificity was 68% (28/41).

Tumor recurrence at the lumpectomy site

Tumor recurrence after breast conservation occurs at an overall rate of 1% to 2% per year. Recurrence directly at the lumpectomy site occurs earlier than elsewhere in the breast and usually peaks several years following conservation therapy. Evaluation of the lumpectomy site by mammography is extremely limited due to postoperative scarring, and physical examination may have greater sensitivity than mammography in the detection of recurrence. Mammography is able to detect 25% to 45% of recurrences and is more likely to detect recurrent tumors associated with calcifications than recurrences without calcifications. In one study [76], all recurrences of invasive carcinoma (enhanced with nodular enhancement and linear enhancement) were observed in the cases of DCIS recurrence. Most scars showed no enhancement.

Knowing when to image for potential recurrence is problematic because scar tissue can enhance for years following surgery. Because recurrence peaks in the first few years following surgery and the most likely site of recurrence is the lumpectomy site, the usefulness of the information obtained from a costly MR imaging study needs to be weighed against the benefit obtained from a potentially less expensive needle biopsy of the area.

Occult primary breast cancer

Patients presenting with axillary metastases suspicious for breast primary and a negative physical examination and negative mammogram should undergo breast MR imaging [81,82]. In patients

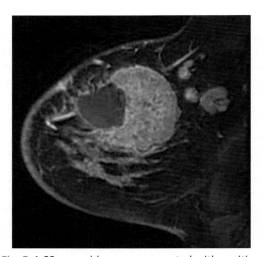

Fig. 5. A 33-year-old woman presented with positive-margins status post lumpectomy for a palpable mass that was mammographically occult. The MR image demonstrated a large residual mass surrounding the lumpectomy bed, in addition to enhancing skin nodules and thickening and enlarged axillary nodes; the patient had advanced local disease and was therefore treated with chemotherapy.

who have this rare clinical presentation, MR imaging has been able to detect cancer in 90% to 100% of cases when a tumor is present. The tumors are generally small (under 2 cm); thus, they may evade detection by conventional imaging and physical examination.

The identification of the site of malignancy is important therapeutically. Patients traditionally undergo mastectomy because the site of malignancy is unknown. Whole-breast radiation can be given, although it is generally not recommended because survival is equal but the recurrence rate is higher (up to 23%). Thus, when a site of malignancy can be identified, the patient can be spared mastectomy and offered breast conservation therapy, thereby having a significant impact on patient management (Fig. 6). In one study, the results of the MR examination changed therapy in approximately one half of cases, usually allowing conservation in lieu of mastectomy [78]. If a site of malignancy is not identified on MR imaging, it may be reasonable for the patient to receive full breast radiation with careful follow-up with MR imaging examination rather than mastectomy.

Proton MR spectroscopy of the breast

Proton MR spectroscopy (1H MRS) provides biochemical information about the tissue under investigation. The diagnostic value of 1H MRS in cancer is typically based on the detection of elevated levels of choline compounds, which is a marker of active tumor [95]; these compounds include choline, phosphocholine, glycerophosphocholine, and taurine. At the field strengths used for in vivo work (1.5–4 T), these multiple resonances cannot be spectrally resolved and thus appear as a single peak, termed "total choline-containing compounds" (tCho). For the brain and prostate, 1H

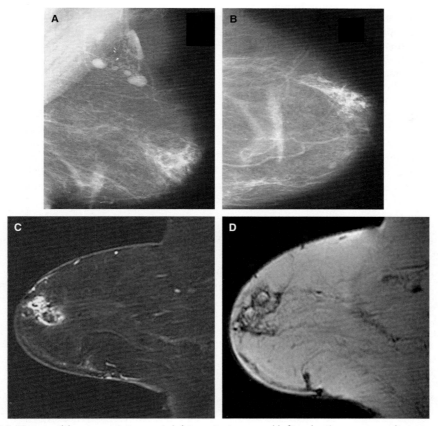

Fig. 6. (*A*, *B*) A 60-year-old woman status post right mastectomy and left reduction mammoplasty presented with a palpable mass in the left breast. Postreduction changes were seen on the mammogram. The patient refused biopsy for the palpable mass, so MR imaging was performed. (*C*) T1-weighted, fat-suppressed sagittal image through the left breast demonstrated a peripherally enhancing lesion at the site of the palpable abnormality. (*D*) The non–fat-suppressed image confirmed the presence of fat in the lesion, consistent with fat necrosis.

MRS is approved by the US Food and Drug Administration (FDA) and is widely used.

The use of proton MR spectroscopy in the breast

1H MRS has been suggested as an adjunct to breast MR imaging [96]. Studies performed on 1.5-T MR scanners have reported sensitivities of 70% to 100% and specificities of 67% to 100% for breast 1H MRS. Fewer studies performed on 4-T scanners have reported sensitivities of 46% to 61% and specificities of 83% to 94% [97,98]. The use of 1H MRS in the breast has predominantly been performed using a single-voxel technique (SVS), but the use of MR spectroscopy has also been tried [99]. One disadvantage is that the voxel size has been a limiting factor in SVS. It has been shown that voxels less than 1 cm^3 yield large errors in tCho measurements, even at 4 T [98]. MR spectroscopy provides information about the spatial distribution of metabolites, which is useful for studying multiple lesions. This method is technically more challenging than SVS, encountering more problems in the quantification of metabolite levels. Qualitative and quantitative approaches have been used in choline measurements. Scanning at 4 T allows detection of tCho in benign lesions and normal subjects, therefore magnifying the need for a quantitative method for choline detection. Quantification has been performed in studies at 1.5 T [100] and at 4 T [98], with similar absolute choline levels (0.4–5.8 mmol/L and 0.4–10 mmol/L, respectively) being reported. Higher signal-to-noise ratio has been reported on previous MR spectroscopy studies at 4 T, enabling the detection of tCho in smaller lesions and the occasional detection of other metabolites such as taurine, creatine, and glycine [98].

Differentiating benign from malignant breast lesions

Multiple in vivo 1H MRS studies aimed at improving the discrimination between benign and malignant breast lesions have been done at several centers (Table 5) [98–107]. In a group of patients studied at the Memorial Sloan-Kettering Cancer Center (MSKCC) [96], the sensitivity of 1H MRS was 100% and the specificity was 88%, which compared favorably to prior reports of breast 1H MRS. The use of 1H MRS as an adjunct to breast MR imaging would have significantly (P<.01) increased the positive predictive value of biopsy from 35% to 82%. If 1H MRS had been used as an adjunct to MR imaging in the 40 lesions with unknown histology, then biopsy may have been spared in 58% of the lesions and none of the cancers would have gone undetected. These data suggest that 1H MRS may be a useful supplement to breast MR imaging, thereby reducing the number of benign biopsy samples without compromising the diagnosis of breast cancer (Fig. 7).

All cancers in the study reported by Bartella and colleagues [96] were identified by 1H MRS (Fig. 8); there were no false-negative cases. A choline peak was identified at 1H MRS in a variety of cancer histologies, including 16 invasive cancers (infiltrating ductal, infiltrating lobular, and infiltrating mixed ductal and lobular) and 1 DCIS. Three false-positive cases are included in this report: a fibroadenoma, a chronic inflammatory lesion with atypia (Fig. 9), and ADH with columnar cell alteration. A false-positive choline peak has previously been reported with a fibroadenoma [101,102]. To the authors' knowledge, which is limited by the small number of published series on breast single-voxel 1H MRS, the other two lesions

Table 5: **In vivo 1H MRS studies performed on 1.5-T magnets in order to differentiate benign from malignant lesions**

Study	Malignant lesions	Benign lesions	Sens (%)	Spec (%)	TP	TN	FN	FP	PPV (%)
Roebuck et al, 1998 [100]	10	7	70	86	7	6	3	1	88
Kvistad et al, 1999 [102]	11	11	82	82	9	9	2	2	82
Cecil et al, 2001 [103]	23	15	83	87	19	13	4	2	90
Yeung et al, 2001 [101]	24	6	92	83	22	5	2	1	97
Jagannathan et al, 2001 [110]	32	14	81	86	26	12	6	2	93
Tse et al, 2003 [106]	19	21	89	100	17	21	2	0	100
Huang et al, 2004 [107]	18	12	100	67	18	8	0	4	82
Bartella et al, 2006 [96]	31	26	100	88	31	23	0	3	91
Sum	168	112	87	85	149	97	19	15	90

Abbreviations: FN, false-negative cases; FP, false-positive cases; PPV, positive predictive value; Sens, sensitivity; Spec, specificity; TN, true-negative cases; TP, true-positive cases.
Adapted from Bartella L, Morris EA, Dershaw DD, et al. Proton MR spectroscopy with choline peak as malignancy marker improves positive predictive value for breast cancer diagnosis: preliminary study. Radiology 2006;239(3):691; with permission.

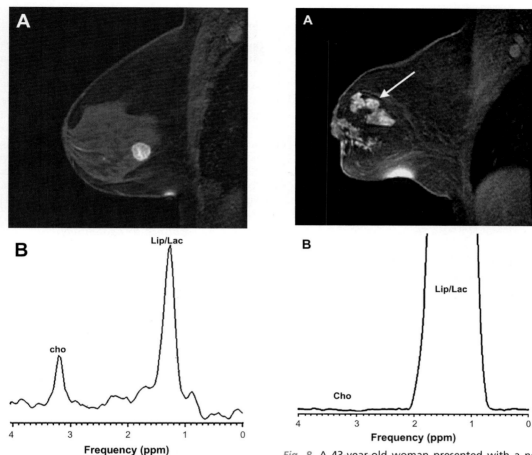

Fig. 7. A 52-year-old woman with a mammographically detected, biopsy-proven invasive ductal carcinoma in the left breast. (A) Sagittal, T1-weighted, MR image of left breast immediately after injection of intravenous gadolinium shows a 1.5-cm rim-enhancing mass. (B) MR spectroscopy of this lesion demonstrated a positive choline peak at a frequency of 3.2 ppm, with a signal-to-noise ratio greater than 2; this is a true positive finding. Cho, choline; Lac, lactate; Lip, lipid. (From Bartella L, Morris EA, Dershaw DD, et al. Proton MR spectroscopy with choline peak as malignancy marker improves positive predictive value for breast cancer diagnosis: preliminary study. Radiology 2006;239(3):689; with permission.)

Fig. 8. A 43-year-old woman presented with a new palpable mass in the right breast. MR imaging–guided biopsy followed by surgical excision yielded benign fibrosis and ductal hyperplasia. (A) Postcontrast sagittal, T1-weighted MR image of the right breast demonstrates an irregular 4.2-cm mass (arrow). (B) Spectrum obtained from MR spectroscopy did not demonstrate a positive choline resonance peak, and there was only noise level at a frequency of 3.2 ppm; this is a true negative finding. Cho, choline; Lac, lactate; Lip, lipid. (From Bartella L, Morris EA, Dershaw DD, et al. Proton MR spectroscopy with choline peak as malignancy marker improves positive predictive value for breast cancer diagnosis: preliminary study. Radiology 2006;239(3):690; with permission.)

have not previously been reported. In view of the presence of atypia in these two lesions, excision would have been the standard of care. Further work is necessary to evaluate the frequency and characteristics of false-positive findings on 1H MRS.

Characterization of histopathologic subtypes

MRS has been shown to be highly sensitive for all invasive breast cancers, regardless of histology

[98,108]. Based on preliminary results from an ongoing study at MSKCC, 1H MRS at 1.5 T was performed on 30 invasive breast cancers [108]. Significantly, a choline peak was detected in one case of DCIS [96]. This lesion is of interest, in light of prior reports, and suggests that DCIS may not manifest a choline peak [100,104]. Further study with additional DCIS lesions is essential. At 4 T, the tCho levels did not appear to be related to different histologic subtypes [98].

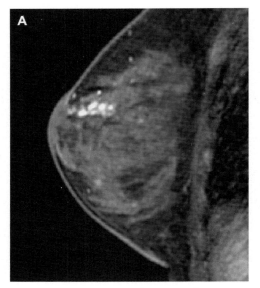

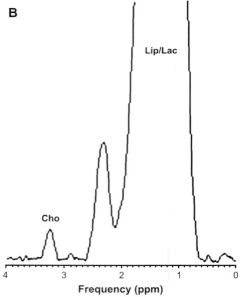

Fig. 9. A 51-year-old woman who had a positive family history for breast cancer presented with a suspicious lesion detected on a high-risk screening breast MR imaging examination. (*A*) Postcontrast sagittal, T1-weighted MR image of the left breast shows ductal clumped enhancement in the retroareolar region. (*B*) A magnified spectrum of this lesion demonstrated a positive choline resonance peak, with a signal to noise ratio greater than 2. Excision of this lesion yielded an atypical chronic inflammatory lesion; this is a false-positive finding. Cho, choline; Lac, lactate; Lip, lipid. (*From* Bartella L, Morris EA, Dershaw DD, et al. Proton MR spectroscopy with choline peak as malignancy marker improves positive predictive value for breast cancer diagnosis: preliminary study. Radiology 2006;239(3):689; with permission.)

Evaluation of normal and lactating breast parenchyma

In a small series performed at MSKCC, normal breast glandular parenchyma had no choline signal detected at 1.5 T, regardless of menstrual status or stage in the menstrual cycle [109]. Yet, choline signal can be detected in normal breast tissue at higher field strengths [98]. Choline signal has also been documented in the lactating breast [102,110]. Despite the limited existing data, this detection suggests the increasing need for the quantification of choline concentrations [97,98]. A recent study performed at 7 T on normal volunteers detected tCho and taurine in normal glandular parenchyma [111].

Predicting response to neoadjuvant chemotherapy

An early pilot study has shown that using a 1.5-T magnet, a change in tCho was observed after the completion of treatment, which was confirmed with pathology [110]. In a more recent pilot study performed on a 4-T system, 1H MRS was able to predict clinical response in patients who had locally advanced breast cancer within 24 hours of receiving the first dose of neoadjuvant chemotherapy. These results suggest that the addition of 1H MRS may offer a substantial advantage over MR imaging alone in the prediction of response to neoadjuvant chemotherapy [112].

MR spectroscopy of axillary lymph nodes in breast cancer patients

Yeung and colleagues [113] reported the role of in vivo MR spectroscopy in the evaluation of axillary nodes using choline as a marker for metastases. This study was performed on a 1.5-T magnet using a 14-cm circular receive-only surface coil that was placed against the affected breast to improve the signal-to-noise ratio. They detected axillary nodal metastases with a sensitivity of 82% and a specificity of 100%. In vitro MR spectroscopy was used to characterize the metabolic profile of axillary nodes and distinguish metastatic lymph nodes from noninvolved ones [114,115]. Over 40 metabolites were identified. The specificity of in vitro MR spectroscopy in detecting axillary node metastases using the glycerophosphocholine-phosphocholine/threonine ratio was 80%, and the specificity was 91%.

High-resolution magic angle spinning MR spectroscopy of breast tissue

Studies have been performed looking at ex vivo MR spectroscopic imaging of breast tissue to establish the metabolic profile of breast tumor and noninvolved breast tissue [116]. Metabolite composition has been investigated in perchloric acid extracts from tissue and in intact tissue using high-resolution magic angle spinning MR spectroscopy using nuclear MR spectrometers (DRX-400/DRX-600 BRUKER, Rheinsteiten, Germany). More than 30 different metabolites were detected and assigned [116]. The total amount of choline on average was found to be more than 10 times higher in tumor tissue than in noninvolved tissue [116]. The relative intensities of the resonances of these compounds were also found to be different in cancerous and in noninvolved tissue.

Positron emission tomography and breast cancer

PET is different than other imaging modalities in that it gives metabolic information in addition to anatomic detail. FDG-PET has outperformed conventional imaging modalities in determining extent of disease and in evaluating disease recurrence (Fig. 10) [117,118]. Currently, this modality is used for treatment monitoring and is approved by the FDA as an adjunct to conventional imaging modalities. Studies have also suggested that FDG-PET

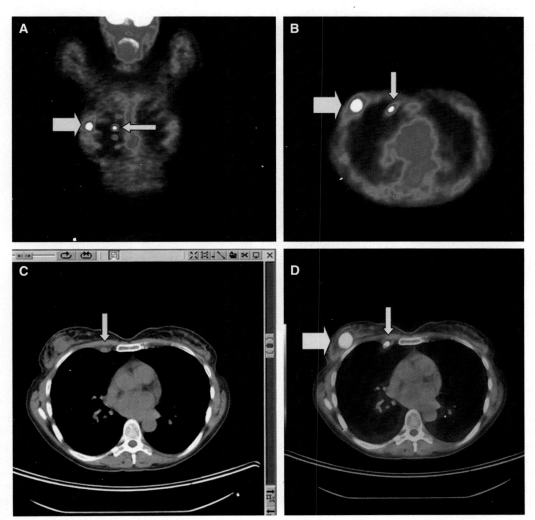

Fig. 10. FDG PET/CT performed on a 50 year old woman with newly diagnosed invasive ductal carcinoma of the right breast with palpable right axillary nodes. Coronal PET (*A*), axial PET (*B*), axial CT (*C*), and fusion PET/CT (*D*) demonstrate hypermetabolic activity in the primary tumor (*thick arrow*, SUV 12.2), within right axillary nodes and right intramammary lymph nodes (*thin arrow*, SUV 4.2). Sagittal PET (*E*), axial PET (*F*), axial CT (*G*), and fusion axial PET/CT (*H*) demonstrate hypermetabolic activity in L1 vertebral body (*thick arrow*, SUV 5). A biopsy of the L1 lesion confirmed mestatic disease. Of note, a bone scan performed at the same time demonstrated no abnormality. The patient underwent chemotherapy and bisphosphonates therapy and a PET/CT performed 3 months later showed a marked decrease in metabolic activity in all the lesions.

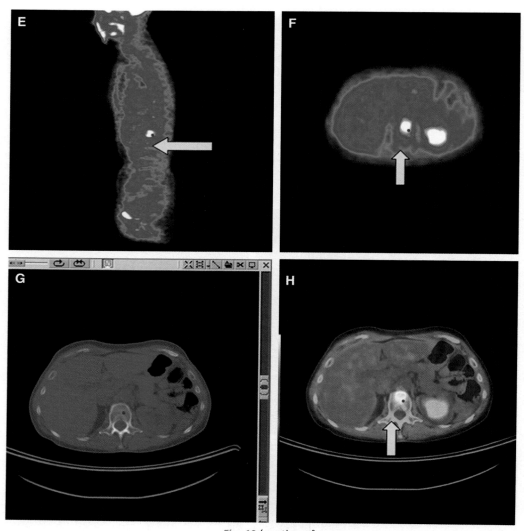

Fig. 10 (continued)

enables early assessment of treatment response in patients undergoing chemotherapy [119,120]. Investigators have also looked at the role of PET in the evaluation of suspicious breast lesions [121]. It seems that presently, PET is inadequate for the detection of small primary tumors; however, the high positive predictive value may be helpful in cases in which conventional imaging is inconclusive.

Dedicated PET mammography units have been developed with a higher spatial resolution to try to detect smaller breast cancers [122,123]. New tracers are also being investigated for use in breast cancer. The use of antibodies as potential tracers for specific cell receptors has also been increasing. For example, 68-Ga-Dota-F(ab')2-Herceptin allows sequential PET imaging of HER 2 expression and may be useful in predicting early tumor response [124].

Other new techniques

Other new imaging modalities being assessed for their ability to detect breast cancer include scintimammography, tomosynthesis, and contrast-enhanced mammography. Previously, scintimammography was performed with a general-purpose gamma camera. Recently, however, investigators have begun to use high-resolution, small field-of-view cameras specific to breast imaging, with encouraging results [125,126]. Tomosynthesis of the breast involves the mathematic processing of a set of planar images of the breast acquired at different angles. It is hoped that this method of evaluating the breast will reduce the number of false-positive and false-negative mammograms due to overlapping tissue.

The use of contrast agents has also been used in MR imaging to improve the sensitivity of mammography. Two small studies using nonionic iodinated contrast with temporal subtraction [127] and dual energy subtraction [128] have performed well, demonstrating cancers with few false positives.

Summary

Advances in breast imaging have revolutionized breast cancer management. Screening mammography remains the "gold standard" for breast cancer detection. Modalities such as digital mammography, breast ultrasound, and breast MR imaging play increasingly important roles in breast imaging. Percutaneous needle biopsy provides a faster, less invasive, and less expensive method than surgery for breast diagnosis. SNB provides a less invasive method than axillary dissection for staging the axilla. MR spectroscopy may improve specificity of breast cancer diagnosis. New modalities such as PET, breast tomosynthesis, and contrast-enhanced mammography may also contribute to the breast imaging evaluation. Further work is necessary to refine and evaluate these newer modalities so that women can be offered the most accurate and least invasive techniques for breast cancer diagnosis, staging, monitoring, and treatment.

References

[1] Edwards BK, Brown ML, Wingo PA, et al. Annual report to the nation on the status of cancer, 1975–2002, featuring population-based trends in cancer treatment. J Natl Cancer Inst 2005; 97(19):1407–27.

[2] Page DL, Dupont WD, Rogers LW, et al. Intraductal carcinoma of the breast: follow-up after biopsy only. Cancer 1982;49(4):751–8.

[3] Rosen PP, Kosloff C, Lieberman PH, et al. Lobular carcinoma in situ of the breast. Detailed analysis of 99 patients with average follow-up of 24 years. Am J Surg Pathol 1978;2(3):225–51.

[4] Yen MF, Tabar L, Vitak B, et al. Quantifying the potential problem of overdiagnosis of ductal carcinoma in situ in breast cancer screening. Eur J Cancer 2003;39(12):1746–54.

[5] Rosenberg RD, Hunt WC, Williamson MR, et al. Effects of age, breast density, ethnicity, and estrogen replacement therapy on screening mammographic sensitivity and cancer stage at diagnosis: review of 183,134 screening mammograms in Albuquerque, New Mexico. Radiology 1998;209(2):511–8.

[6] Barlow WE, Lehman CD, Zheng Y, et al. Performance of diagnostic mammography for women with signs or symptoms of breast cancer. J Natl Cancer Inst 2002;94(15):1151–9.

[7] Eltahir A, Jibril JA, Squair J, et al. The accuracy of "one-stop" diagnosis for 1,110 patients presenting to a symptomatic breast clinic. J R Coll Surg Edinb 1999;44(4):226–30.

[8] Dee KE, Sickles EA. Medical audit of diagnostic mammography examinations: comparison with screening outcomes obtained concurrently. AJR Am J Roentgenol 2001;176(3):729–33.

[9] Gennaro G, di Maggio C. Dose comparison between screen/film and full-field digital mammography. Eur Radiol 2006;16(11):2559–66.

[10] Pisano ED, Gatsonis C, Hendrick E, et al. Diagnostic performance of digital versus film mammography for breast-cancer screening. N Engl J Med 2005;353(17):1773–83.

[11] ACR practice guideline for the performance of a breast ultrasound examination. In: ACR practice guidelines and technical standards: ultrasound research (vol. 10). Reston (VA): ACR; 2002. p. 763–5.

[12] Stavros AT, Thickman D, Rapp CL, et al. Solid breast nodules: use of sonography to distinguish between benign and malignant lesions. Radiology 1995;196(1):123–34.

[13] Zonderland HM, Coerkamp EG, Hermans J, et al. Diagnosis of breast cancer: contribution of US as an adjunct to mammography. Radiology 1999;213(2):413–22.

[14] Bassett LW, Kimme-Smith C, Sutherland LK, et al. Automated and hand-held breast US: effect on patient management. Radiology 1987; 165(1):103–8.

[15] Deurloo EE, Tanis PJ, Gilhuijs KG, et al. Reduction in the number of sentinel lymph node procedures by preoperative ultrasonography of the axilla in breast cancer. Eur J Cancer 2003;39(8): 1068–73.

[16] Heywang-Kobrunner SHD, Dershaw D, Schreer I. Diagnostic breast imaging. 2nd edition. New York: Thieme; 2001.

[17] Duffy SW, Tabar L, Chen HH, et al. The impact of organized mammography service screening on breast carcinoma mortality in seven Swedish counties. Cancer 2002;95(3):458–69.

[18] Paci E, Duffy SW, Giorgi D, et al. Quantification of the effect of mammographic screening on fatal breast cancers: the Florence Programme 1990–96. Br J Cancer 2002;87(1):65–9.

[19] Smith RA, Saslow D, Sawyer KA, et al. American Cancer Society guidelines for breast cancer screening: update 2003. CA Cancer J Clin 2003;53(3):141–69.

[20] Dershaw DD. Mammographic screening of the high-risk woman. Am J Surg 2000;180(4):288.

[21] Bazzocchi M, Zuiani C, Panizza P, et al. Contrast-enhanced breast MRI in patients with suspicious microcalcifications on mammography: results of a multicenter trial. AJR Am J Roentgenol 2006;186(6):1723–32.

[22] Kriege M, Brekelmans CT, Boetes C, et al. Differences between first and subsequent rounds of the MRISC breast cancer screening program

for women with a familial or genetic predisposition. Cancer 2006;106(11):2318–26.

[23] Liberman L. Centennial dissertation. Percutaneous imaging-guided core breast biopsy: state of the art at the millennium. AJR Am J Roentgenol 2000;174(5):1191–9.

[24] Liberman L, Goodstine SL, Dershaw DD, et al. One operation after percutaneous diagnosis of nonpalpable breast cancer: frequency and associated factors. AJR Am J Roentgenol 2002; 178(3):673–9.

[25] Liberman L, Feng TL, Dershaw DD, et al. US-guided core breast biopsy: use and cost-effectiveness. Radiology 1998;208(3):717–23.

[26] Liberman L, Sama MP. Cost-effectiveness of stereotactic 11-gauge directional vacuum-assisted breast biopsy. AJR Am J Roentgenol 2000; 175(1):53–8.

[27] Liberman L. Percutaneous image-guided core breast biopsy. Radiol Clin North Am 2002; 40(3):483–500 [vi].

[28] Jackman RJ, Rodriguez-Soto J. Breast microcalcifications: retrieval failure at prone stereotactic core and vacuum breast biopsy—frequency, causes, and outcome. Radiology 2006;239(1): 61–70.

[29] Jackman RJ, Birdwell RL, Ikeda DM. Atypical ductal hyperplasia: can some lesions be defined as probably benign after stereotactic 11-gauge vacuum-assisted biopsy, eliminating the recommendation for surgical excision? Radiology 2002;224(2):548–54.

[30] Lee CH, Carter D, Philpotts LE, et al. Ductal carcinoma in situ diagnosed with stereotactic core needle biopsy: can invasion be predicted? Radiology 2000;217(2):466–70.

[31] Liberman L, Benton CL, Dershaw DD, et al. Learning curve for stereotactic breast biopsy: how many cases are enough? AJR Am J Roentgenol 2001;176(3):721–7.

[32] Pfarl G, Helbich TH, Riedl CC, et al. Stereotactic 11-gauge vacuum-assisted breast biopsy: a validation study. AJR Am J Roentgenol 2002; 179(6):1503–7.

[33] Parker SH, Klaus AJ, McWey PJ, et al. Sonographically guided directional vacuum-assisted breast biopsy using a handheld device. AJR Am J Roentgenol 2001;177(2):405–8.

[34] Philpotts LE, Hooley RJ, Lee CH. Comparison of automated versus vacuum-assisted biopsy methods for sonographically guided core biopsy of the breast. AJR Am J Roentgenol 2003; 180(2):347–51.

[35] Soo MS, Baker JA, Rosen EL. Sonographic detection and sonographically guided biopsy of breast microcalcifications. AJR Am J Roentgenol 2003;180(4):941–8.

[36] Berg WA. Rationale for a trial of screening breast ultrasound: American College of Radiology Imaging Network (ACRIN) 6666. AJR Am J Roentgenol 2003;180(5):1225–8.

[37] LaTrenta LR, Menell JH, Morris EA, et al. Breast lesions detected with MR imaging: utility and histopathologic importance of identification with US. Radiology 2003;227(3):856–61.

[38] Liberman L. Percutaneous magnetic resonance imaging guided biopsy. In: Morris EA, Liberman L, editors. Breast MRI: diagnosis and intervention. New York: Springer, Inc.; 2005. p. 297–315.

[39] Perlet C, Heywang-Kobrunner SH, Heinig A, et al. Magnetic resonance-guided, vacuum-assisted breast biopsy: results from a European multicenter study of 538 lesions. Cancer 2006; 106(5):982–90.

[40] Lehman CD, DePeri ER, Peacock S, et al. Clinical experience with MRI-guided vacuum-assisted breast biopsy. AJR Am J Roentgenol 2005; 184(6):1782–7.

[41] Liberman L, Bracero N, Morris E, et al. MRI-guided 9-gauge vacuum-assisted breast biopsy: initial clinical experience. AJR Am J Roentgenol 2005;185(1):183–93.

[42] Liberman L, Morris EA, Dershaw DD, et al. Fast MRI-guided vacuum-assisted breast biopsy: initial experience. AJR Am J Roentgenol 2003; 181(5):1283–93.

[43] Orel SG, Rosen M, Mies C, et al. MR imaging-guided 9-gauge vacuum-assisted core-needle breast biopsy: initial experience. Radiology 2006;238(1):54–61.

[44] Holland R, Veling SH, Mravunac M, et al. Histologic multifocality of Tis, T1–2 breast carcinomas. Implications for clinical trials of breast-conserving surgery. Cancer 1985;56(5): 979–90.

[45] Orel SG, Schnall MD, Powell CM, et al. Staging of suspected breast cancer: effect of MR imaging and MR-guided biopsy. Radiology 1995;196(1): 115–22.

[46] Fischer U, Kopka L, Grabbe E. Breast carcinoma: effect of preoperative contrast-enhanced MR imaging on the therapeutic approach. Radiology 1999;213(3):881–8.

[47] Bedrosian I, Mick R, Orel SG, et al. Changes in the surgical management of patients with breast carcinoma based on preoperative magnetic resonance imaging. Cancer 2003;98(3):468–73.

[48] Liberman L, Morris EA, Dershaw DD, et al. MR imaging of the ipsilateral breast in women with percutaneously proven breast cancer. AJR Am J Roentgenol 2003;180(4):901–10.

[49] Lee SG, Orel SG, Woo IJ, et al. MR imaging screening of the contralateral breast in patients with newly diagnosed breast cancer: preliminary results. Radiology 2003;226(3):773–8.

[50] Berg WA. Imaging the local extent of disease. Sem Breast Dis 2001;4:153–73.

[51] Quan ML, Sclafani L, Heerdt AS, et al. Magnetic resonance imaging detects unsuspected disease in patients with invasive lobular cancer. Ann Surg Oncol 2003;10(9):1048–53.

[52] Weinstein SP, Orel SG, Heller R, et al. MR imaging of the breast in patients with invasive lobular carcinoma. AJR Am J Roentgenol 2001; 176(2):399–406.

[53] Hwang ES, Kinkel K, Esserman LJ, et al. Magnetic resonance imaging in patients diagnosed with ductal carcinoma-in-situ: value in the diagnosis of residual disease, occult invasion, and multicentricity. Ann Surg Oncol 2003;10(4): 381–8.

[54] Viehweg P, Lampe D, Buchmann J, et al. In situ and minimally invasive breast cancer: morphologic and kinetic features on contrast-enhanced MR imaging. MAGMA 2000;11(3):129–37.

[55] Morris EA, Schwartz LH, Drotman MB, et al. Evaluation of pectoralis major muscle in patients with posterior breast tumors on breast MR images: early experience. Radiology 2000; 214(1):67–72.

[56] Liberman L. Does size matter? Positive predictive value of MRI-detected breast lesions as a function of lesion size. AJR Am J Roentgenol 2006;182(2):426–30.

[57] Morrow M. Role of axillary dissection in breast cancer management. Ann Surg Oncol 1996; 3(3):233–4.

[58] Krag D, Weaver D, Ashikaga T, et al. The sentinel node in breast cancer—a multicenter validation study. N Engl J Med 1998;339(14): 941–6.

[59] Veronesi U, Paganelli G, Viale G, et al. A randomized comparison of sentinel-node biopsy with routine axillary dissection in breast cancer. N Engl J Med 2003;349(6):546–53.

[60] Derossis AM, Fey J, Yeung H, et al. A trend analysis of the relative value of blue dye and isotope localization in 2,000 consecutive cases of sentinel node biopsy for breast cancer. J Am Coll Surg 2001;193(5):473–8.

[61] Lyman GH, Giuliano AE, Somerfield MR, et al. American Society of Clinical Oncology guideline recommendations for sentinel lymph node biopsy in early-stage breast cancer. J Clin Oncol 2005;23(30):7703–20.

[62] Guller U, Nitzsche EU, Schirp U, et al. Selective axillary surgery in breast cancer patients based on positron emission tomography with 18F-fluoro-2-deoxy-D-glucose: not yet!. Breast Cancer Res Treat 2002;71(2):171–3.

[63] van der Hoeven JJ, Hoekstra OS, Comans EF, et al. Determinants of diagnostic performance of [F-18]fluorodeoxyglucose positron emission tomography for axillary staging in breast cancer. Ann Surg 2002;236(5):619–24.

[64] Stadnik TW, Everaert H, Makkat S, et al. Breast imaging. Preoperative breast cancer staging: comparison of USPIO-enhanced MR imaging and 18F-fluorodeoxyglucose (FDC) positron emission tomography (PET) imaging for axillary lymph node staging-initial findings. Eur Radiol 2006;16(10):2153–60.

[65] Kaiser WA, Zeitler E. MR imaging of the breast: fast imaging sequences with and without Gd-DTPA. Preliminary observations. Radiology 1989; 170(3 Pt 1):681–6.

[66] Heywang SH, Wolf A, Pruss E, et al. MR imaging of the breast with Gd-DTPA: use and limitations. Radiology 1989;171(1):95–103.

[67] Mumtaz H, Hall-Craggs MA, Davidson T, et al. Staging of symptomatic primary breast cancer with MR imaging. AJR Am J Roentgenol 1997; 169(2):417–24.

[68] Schelfout K, Van Goethem M, Kersschot E, et al. Contrast-enhanced MR imaging of breast lesions and effect on treatment. Eur J Surg Oncol 2004;30(5):501–7.

[69] Frei KA, Kinkel K, Bonel HM, et al. MR imaging of the breast in patients with positive margins after lumpectomy: influence of the time interval between lumpectomy and MR imaging. AJR Am J Roentgenol 2000;175(6):1577–84.

[70] Orel SG, Reynolds C, Schnall MD, et al. Breast carcinoma: MR imaging before re-excisional biopsy. Radiology 1997;205(2):429–36.

[71] Faverly DR, Hendriks JH, Holland R. Breast carcinomas of limited extent: frequency, radiologic-pathologic characteristics, and surgical margin requirements. Cancer 2001;91(4): 647–59.

[72] Knopp MV. MR mammography with pharmocokinetic mapping for monitoring of breast cancer treatment during neoadjuvant therapy. Magn Reson Imaging Clin N Am 1997;2: 633–58.

[73] Esserman L, Kaplan E, Partridge S, et al. MRI phenotype is associated with response to doxorubicin and cyclophosphamide neoadjuvant chemotherapy in stage III breast cancer. Ann Surg Oncol 2001;8(6):549–59.

[74] Wasser K, Klein SK, Fink C, et al. Evaluation of neoadjuvant chemotherapeutic response of breast cancer using dynamic MRI with high temporal resolution. Eur Radiol 2003;13(1):80–7.

[75] Delille JP, Slanetz PJ, Yeh ED, et al. Invasive ductal breast carcinoma response to neoadjuvant chemotherapy: noninvasive monitoring with functional MR imaging pilot study. Radiology 2003;228(1):63–9.

[76] Gilles R, Guinebretiere JM, Shapeero LG, et al. Assessment of breast cancer recurrence with contrast-enhanced subtraction MR imaging: preliminary results in 26 patients. Radiology 1993;188(2):473–8.

[77] Dao TH, Rahmouni A, Campana F, et al. Tumor recurrence versus fibrosis in the irradiated breast: differentiation with dynamic gadolinium-enhanced MR imaging. Radiology 1993; 187(3):751–5.

[78] Olson JA Jr, Morris EA, Van Zee KJ, et al. Magnetic resonance imaging facilitates breast conservation for occult breast cancer. Ann Surg Oncol 2000;7(6):411–5.

[79] Schorn C, Fischer U, Luftner-Nagel S, et al. MRI of the breast in patients with metastatic disease of unknown primary. Eur Radiol 1999;9(3): 470–3.

[80] Campana F, Fourquet A, Ashby MA, et al. Presentation of axillary lymphadenopathy without detectable breast primary (T0 N1b breast cancer): experience at Institut Curie. Radiother Oncol 1989;15(4):321–5.

[81] Morris EA, Schwartz LH, Dershaw DD, et al. MR imaging of the breast in patients with occult primary breast carcinoma. Radiology 1997;205(2): 437–40.

[82] Orel SG, Weinstein SP, Schnall MD, et al. Breast MR imaging in patients with axillary node metastases and unknown primary malignancy. Radiology 1999;212(2):543–9.

[83] Kuhl CK, Schmutzler RK, Leutner CC, et al. Breast MR imaging screening in 192 women proved or suspected to be carriers of a breast cancer susceptibility gene: preliminary results. Radiology 2000;215(1):267–79.

[84] Warner E, Plewes DB, Shumak RS, et al. Comparison of breast magnetic resonance imaging, mammography, and ultrasound for surveillance of women at high risk for hereditary breast cancer. J Clin Oncol 2001;19(15): 3524–31.

[85] Morris EA, Liberman L, Ballon DJ, et al. MRI of occult breast carcinoma in a high-risk population. AJR Am J Roentgenol 2003;181(3): 619–26.

[86] Warner E, Plewes DB, Hill KA, et al. Surveillance of BRCA1 and BRCA2 mutation carriers with magnetic resonance imaging, ultrasound, mammography, and clinical breast examination. JAMA 2004;292(11):1317–25.

[87] Kriege M, Brekelmans CT, Boetes C, et al. Efficacy of MRI and mammography for breast-cancer screening in women with a familial or genetic predisposition. N Engl J Med 2004; 351(5):427–37.

[88] Morris EA, Harms S. ACR practice guideline for the performance of magnetic resonance imaging (MRI) of the breast. Reston (VA): American College of Radiology; 2004.

[89] ACR breast imaging reporting and data system, breast imaging atlas. Reston (VA): American College of Radiology; 2003.

[90] Abraham D, Jones R, Jones S, et al. Evaluation of neoadjuvant chemotherapeutic response of locally advanced breast cancer by magnetic resonance imaging. Cancer 1998;78(1):91–100.

[91] Partridge SC, Gibbs JE, Lu Y, et al. Accuracy of MR imaging for revealing residual breast cancer in patients who have undergone neoadjuvant chemotherapy. AMJ Am J Roentgenol 2002; 179(5):1193–9.

[92] Partridge SC, Gibbs JE, Lu Y, et al. MRI measurements of breast tumor volume predict response to neoadjuvant chemotherapy and recurrence-free survival. AJR Am J Roentgenol 2005; 184(6):1774–81.

[93] ACRIN. Contrast-enhanced breast MRI for evaluation of patients undergoing neoadjuvant treatment for locally advanced breast cancer: PROTOCOL 6657. Available at: www.acrin. org/6657_protocol.html. Accessed June 19, 2006.

[94] Morris EA. Assessment of residual disease. In: Morris EA, Liberman L, editors. Breast MRI: diagnosis and intervention. New York: Springer; 2005. p. 225.

[95] Negendank W. Studies of human tumors by MRS: a review. NMR Biomed 1992;5:303–24.

[96] Bartella L, Morris EA, Dershaw DD, et al. Proton MR spectroscopy with choline peak as malignancy marker improves positive predictive value for breast cancer diagnosis: preliminary study. Radiology 2006;239(3): 686–92.

[97] Meisamy S, Bolan PJ, Baker EH, et al. Adding in vivo quantitative 1H MR spectroscopy to improve diagnostic accuracy of breast MR imaging: preliminary results of observer performance study at 4.0 T. Radiology 2005;236(2): 465–75.

[98] Bolan PJ, Meisamy S, Baker EH, et al. In vivo quantification of choline compounds in the breast with 1H MR spectroscopy. Magn Reson Med 2003;50(6):1134–43.

[99] Jacobs MA, Barker PB, Bottomley PA, et al. Proton magnetic resonance spectroscopic imaging of human breast cancer: a preliminary study. J Magn Reson Imaging 2004;19(1):68–75.

[100] Roebuck JR, Cecil KM, Schnall MD, et al. Human breast lesions: characterization with proton MR spectroscopy. Radiology 1998;209(1): 269–75.

[101] Yeung DK, Cheung HS, Tse GM. Human breast lesions: characterization with contrast-enhanced in vivo proton MR spectroscopy—initial results. Radiology 2001;220(1):40–6.

[102] Kvistad KA, Bakken IJ, Gribbestad IS, et al. Characterization of neoplastic and normal human breast tissues with in vivo (1)H MR spectroscopy. J Magn Reson Imaging 1999;10(2): 159–64.

[103] Cecil KM, Schnall MD, Siegelman ES, et al. The evaluation of human breast lesions with magnetic resonance imaging and proton magnetic resonance spectroscopy. Breast Cancer Res Treat 2001;68(1):45–54.

[104] Yeung DK, Yang WT, Tse GM. Breast cancer: in vivo proton MR spectroscopy in the characterization of histopathologic subtypes and preliminary observations in axillary node metastases. Radiology 2002;225(1):190–7.

[105] Gribbestad IS, Singstad TE, Nilsen G, et al. In vivo 1H MRS of normal breast and breast tumors using a dedicated double breast coil. J Magn Reson Imaging 1998;8(6):1191–7.

[106] Tse GM, Cheung HS, Pang LM, et al. Characterization of lesions of the breast with proton MR spectroscopy: comparison of carcinomas, benign lesions, and phyllodes tumors. AJR Am J Roentgenol 2003;181(5):1267–72.

[107] Huang W, Fisher PR, Dulaimy K, et al. Detection of breast malignancy: diagnostic MR protocol for improved specificity. Radiology 2004; 232(2):585–91.

[108] Bartella L, Liberman L, Thakur S, et al. Magnetic resonance spectroscopy (MRS) of the breast. Does sensitivity vary with cancer histology? Radiology 2005;237:177.

[109] Bartella L, Thakur S, Morris E, et al. Proton magnetic resonance spectroscopy (MRS) of the breast. Does normal breast parenchyma give a false positive choline peak? Radiology 2005;237:178.

[110] Jagannathan NR, Kumar M, Seenu V, et al. Evaluation of total choline from in-vivo volume localized proton MR spectroscopy and its response to neoadjuvant chemotherapy in locally advanced breast cancer. Br J Cancer 2001;84(8): 1016–22.

[111] Bolan PJ, Snyder CJ, DelaBarre LJ, et al. Preliminary experience with breast 1H MRS at 7Tesla. Proc Int Soc Magn Reson Med 2006;14:580.

[112] Meisamy S, Bolan PJ, Baker EH, et al. Neoadjuvant chemotherapy of locally advanced breast cancer: predicting response with in vivo 1H MR spectroscopy—a pilot study at 4 T. Radiology 2004;233(2):424–31.

[113] Yeung DKW, Yang W-T, Tse GMK. Breast cancer: in vivo proton MR spectroscopy in the characterization of histopathologic subtypes and preliminary observations in axillary node metastases. Radiology 2002;225(1):190–7.

[114] Sharma U, Mehta A, Seenu V, et al. Biochemical characterization of metastatic lymph nodes of breast cancer patients by in vitro 1H magnetic resonance spectroscopy: a pilot study. Magn Reson Imaging 2004;22:697–706.

[115] Seenu V, Pavan Kumar M, Sharma U, et al. Potential of magnetic resonance spectroscopy to detect metastasis in axillary lymph nodes in breast cancer. Magn Reson Imaging 2005; 23:1005–10.

[116] Bathen TF, Sensen LR, Sitter B, et al. MAS MRS: a tool for breast cancer grading? Proc Intl Soc Mag Reson Med 2005;13:130.

[117] Port ER, Yeung H, Gonen M, et al. 18F-2-fluoro-2-deoxy-D-glucose positron emission tomography scanning affects surgical management in selected patients with high-risk, operable breast carcinoma. Ann Surg Oncol 2006;13(5):677–84.

[118] Suarez M, Perez-Castejon MJ, Jimenez A, et al. Early diagnosis of recurrent breast cancer with FDG-PET in patients with progressive elevation of serum tumor markers. Q J Nucl Med 2002; 46(2):113–21.

[119] Jansson T, Westlin JE, Ahlstrom H, et al. Positron emission tomography studies in patients with locally advanced and/or metastatic breast cancer: a method for early therapy evaluation? J Clin Oncol 1995;13(6):1470–7.

[120] Schelling M, Avril N, Nahrig J, et al. Positron emission tomography using [(18)F]Fluorodeoxyglucose for monitoring primary chemotherapy in breast cancer. J Clin Oncol 2000; 18(8):1689–95.

[121] Avril N, Rose CA, Schelling M, et al. Breast imaging with positron emission tomography and fluorine-18 fluorodeoxyglucose: use and limitations. J Clin Oncol 2000;18(20):3495–502.

[122] Murthy K, Aznar M, Thompson CJ, et al. Results of preliminary clinical trials of the positron emission mammography system PEM-I: a dedicated breast imaging system producing glucose metabolic images using FDG. J Nucl Med 2000; 41(11):1851–8.

[123] Rosen EL, Turkington TG, Soo MS, et al. Detection of primary breast carcinoma with a dedicated, large-field-of-view FDG PET mammography device: initial experience. Radiology 2005;234(2):527–34.

[124] Smith-Jones PM, Solit D, Afroze F, et al. Early tumor response to Hsp90 therapy using HER2 PET: comparison with 18F-FDG PET. J Nucl Med 2006;47(5):793–6.

[125] Brem RF, Rapelyea JA, Zisman G, et al. Occult breast cancer: scintimammography with high-resolution breast-specific gamma camera in women at high risk for breast cancer. Radiology 2005;237(1):274–80.

[126] Coover LR, Caravaglia G, Kuhn P. Scintimammography with dedicated breast camera detects and localizes occult carcinoma. J Nucl Med 2004;45(4):553–8.

[127] Jong RA, Yaffe MJ, Skarpathiotakis M, et al. Contrast-enhanced digital mammography: initial clinical experience. Radiology 2003; 228(3):842–50.

[128] Lewin JM, Isaacs PK, Vance V, et al. Dual-energy contrast-enhanced digital subtraction mammography: feasibility. Radiology 2003;229(1): 261–8.

ELSEVIER
SAUNDERS

RADIOLOGIC
CLINICS
OF NORTH AMERICA

Radiol Clin N Am 45 (2007) 69–83

Hodgkin's and Non-Hodgkin's Lymphomas

Jürgen Rademaker, MD

- Clinical and radiologic features
  Hodgkin's disease
  Non-Hodgkin's lymphoma
  Central nervous system lymphoma
  Childhood lymphoma
- Staging
- Assessment of treatment response
- Summary
- References

Lymphomas represent about 4% of the new cases of cancer diagnosed in the United States every year, making them the fifth most common type of cancer and the fifth leading cause of cancer death. Lymphoma can affect any region of the body. Most patients present with lymphadenopathy, focal or diffuse organ involvement, or generalized multi-organ involvement.

Clinical and radiologic features

Hodgkin's disease

The incidence of Hodgkin's disease (HD) is about 4 per 100,000 persons per year, and accounts for less than 1% of all cancers worldwide. New cases of HD in the United States were estimated at 7880 and accounted for 14% of lymphomas [1–3]. HD has a bimodal incidence curve and occurs more frequently in two separate age groups, the first being young adulthood, the second being in those over 50 years old. About one third of people with HD have systemic symptoms, such as low-grade fever, night sweats, weight loss, pruritus, or fatigue [4]. People with a history of infectious mononucleosis have a threefold increased likelihood of developing HD.

During the past 20 years, advances in radiation and chemotherapy increased the cure rate, and now more than 80% of all patients younger than 60 years with newly diagnosed HD are likely to be cured [5]. Selection of the appropriate therapy is based on accurate staging. Patients with early stage disease are treated with abbreviated courses of chemotherapy followed by involved field radiation therapy, whereas those with advanced-stage disease receive a longer course of chemotherapy without radiation therapy. Stage B symptoms and bulky disease (>10 cm) remain the most important prognostic factors in HD.

More than 80% of patients who have HD present with lymphadenopathy above the diaphragm that commonly involves anterior and middle mediastinal nodes with or without disease of the hila (Figs. 1 and 2) [6]. Large mediastinal masses may invade the chest wall and pericardium directly. Hilar adenopathy is uncommon without detectable mediastinal disease. Pleural effusions are often caused by lymphatic or venous obstruction. Secondary involvement of the thyroid or parotid gland is not uncommon, whereas primary involvement is rather rare (Fig. 3).

Pulmonary involvement is found more often in HD than in non-Hodgkin's lymphoma (NHL).

Department of Radiology, Memorial Sloan-Kettering Cancer Center, Cornell University, Weill Medical College, 1275 York Avenue, New York, NY 10021, USA
E-mail address: rademakj@mskcc.org

doi:10.1016/j.rcl.2006.10.006

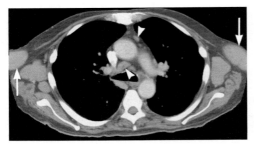

Fig. 1. HD. Imaging findings included axillary *(arrow)* and mediastinal lymphadenopathy *(arrowhead)*.

Nodules (with or without cavitation), reticular nodular infiltrate, ground glass opacities, or irregular consolidations are possible appearances [7,8]. There might be atelectasis secondary to endobronchial or nodal obstruction. Many cases present with hilar lymphadenopathy or mediastinal masses extending into the adjacent lung. Pulmonary involvement at presentation without associated mediastinal or hilar lymphadenopathy is unlikely [9,10]; however, recurrences in the lung may be seen without associated lymphadenopathy.

HD also may affect extranodal tissue by direct invasion or by hematogenous dissemination. The most commonly involved extranodal sides are spleen, lung, liver, and bone marrow. Enlargement of the spleen is not a reliable predictor of disease, although marked enlargement in the setting of other sites of involvement makes splenic lymphoma involvement likely. One third of patients with splenic involvement have normal size spleen, and in one third of those with splenomegaly, the spleen is not involved by tumor. HD with involvement of the kidneys or the gastrointestinal (GI) tract is uncommon. Primary bone lesions are rare,

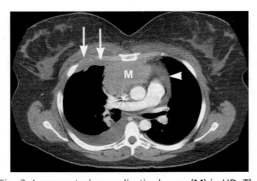

Fig. 2. Large anterior mediastinal mass (M) in HD. The scan demonstrates the growth pattern of the tumor with extension into the right anterior pleural space *(arrows)*. The pericardial effusion is probably from lymphomatous extension into the pericardium *(arrowhead)*. Pleural effusions often result from venous or lymphatic obstruction by enlarged lymph nodes.

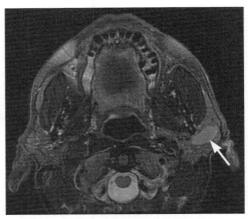

Fig. 3. HD with involvement of the parotid gland. The T2 weighted axial MR imaging scan demonstrates a 2 cm mass *(arrow)* in the superficial aspect of the left parotid gland. The mass enhances after administration of gadolinium (not pictured).

but marrow involvement in cases with advanced disease is not uncommon. Lymph nodes or masses may reveal calcifications after treatment. Calcifications before treatment suggest aggressive disease, such as the nodular sclerosing subtype of HD [11].

Non-Hodgkin's lymphoma

NHL is a heterogenous group of diseases of either B-cell or T-cell origin. NHL represents the second fastest growing cancer in the United States, and the most commonly occurring hematologic cancer. The incidence of NHL in the United States has increased by 50% over the past 15 years, and the cause for this increase is not known. In 2004, new cases of NHL in the United States were estimated at 54,370, resulting in 4% of all cancer deaths.

Overall, NHL has a worse prognosis than HD. Unlike HD, which commonly spreads through contiguous groups of lymph nodes, NHL is infrequently localized at the time of diagnosis and frequently involves extranodal sites of disease.

For decades, NHL was classified by morphology and histology. In 1994, the Revised European-American Lymphoma (REAL) classification introduced additional immunophenotypic, genetic, and clinical characteristics. This system was modified further for the currently accepted classification introduced by the World Health Organization (WHO) [12]. The WHO classification differentiates between B lymphoid neoplasms (including follicular lymphoma and diffuse large B-cell lymphoma) and T- and NK lymphoid neoplasms (including anaplastic large-cell lymphoma) [13]. NHL is actually a complex group of almost 40 distinct entities, and their classification in the WHO classification scheme is summarized in Box 1. The box is included in this radiologic review to illustrate the spectrum of diseases summarized under the name lymphoma. The classification incorporates histologic findings, immunophenotype, cytogenetic, and molecular data. Many diseases are defined better, ultimately helping clinicians better understand and treat disease. Most NHLs develop from B-cells.

Substantial progress has been made in understanding the molecular pathogenesis of several forms of NHL [11,14]. Several forms of NHL are associated closely with an infectious agent, which is not surprising, because most NHLs arise from B-cells. Burkitt's lymphoma is associated with Epstein-Barr virus, MALT lymphoma with *Helicobacter pylori* [15,16], and primary effusion lymphoma with human herpes virus 8, the etiologic agent of Kaposi's sarcoma. Molecular translocations also have been identified for many forms of NHL and not only reflect pathogenesis, but also serve as markers for molecular diagnosis and monitoring. Molecular translocations include translocation t (11;14) for mantle cell lymphoma and translocation t (14;18) for follicular lymphoma [1].

Box 1: World Health Organization classification scheme for lymphoma

B-cell lymphoma/leukemias
Chronic lymphocytic leukemia/small lymphocytic lymphoma
B-cell prolymphocytic leukemia
Lymphoplasmacytic lymphoma/Waldenström's macroglobulinemia
Splenic marginal zone B-cell lymphoma
Hairy cell leukemia
Plasma cell myeloma/plasmocytoma
Extranodal marginal zone B-cell lymphoma of mucosa-associated lymphoid tissue (MALT)
Nodal marginal zone B-cell lymphoma
Follicular lymphoma
Mantle cell lymphoma
Diffuse large B-cell lymphoma
Mediastinal (thymic) large B-cell lymphoma
Primary effusion lymphoma
Burkitt's lymphoma/leukemia
Pre-B-cell lymphoblastic leukemia/lymphoma

T-cell and NK-cell lymphomas/leukemias
T-cell prolymphocytic leukemia
T-cell large granular lymphocytic leukemia
Aggressive NK-cell leukemia
Adult T-cell leukemia/lymphoma (human T lymphotropic virus type 1-positive)
Extranodal NK-cell/T-cell lymphoma, nasal type
Enteropathy type T-cell lymphoma
Hepatosplenic T-cell lymphoma
Subcutaneous panniculitis-like T-cell lymphoma
Blastic NK-cell lymphoma
Mycosis fungoides/Sézary syndrome
Primary cutaneous CD30-positive T-cell lymphoproliferative disorders
Primary cutaneous anaplastic large cell lymphoma
Lymphomatoid papulosis
Angioimmunoblastic T-cell lymphoma
Peripheral T-cell lymphoma, unspecified
Anaplastic large cell lymphoma
Pre-T-cell lymphoblastic leukemia/lymphoma

Hodgkin's lymphoma
Nodular lymphocyte-predominant
Classic Hodgkin's lymphoma
    Nodular sclerosis
    Mixed cellularity
    Lymphocyte depleted
    Lymphocyte rich

Adapted from Harris NL, Jaffe ES, Diebold J, et al. The World Health Organization classification of neoplastic diseases of hematopoietic and lymphoid tissues. Report of the Clinical Advisory Committee meeting, Arlie House, Virginia, November 1997. Ann Oncol 1999;10:1419–32.

Although there are many forms of NHL, the 13 most common types account for 88% of the cases in the United States. The most common forms of NHL in adults in the western world are [4]:

- Diffuse large B-cell lymphoma 31%
- Follicular lymphoma 22%
- Small lymphocytic lymphoma 6%
- Mantle cell lymphoma 6%
- Peripheral T cell lymphoma 6%
- Extranodal marginal zone B-cell lymphoma of MALT type 5%
- Others (including composite lymphomas) 24%

Note that composite lymphoma is defined as simultaneous occurrence of two histologically different types of lymphoma situated in one location.

NHL can be divided into two groups: indolent lymphomas, which grow more slowly and have fewer symptoms (eg, follicular lymphoma, MALT), and aggressive lymphomas, which grow more quickly (eg, diffuse large cell lymphoma, Burkitt's lymphoma, Mantle cell lymphoma). The follicular lymphomas are the most common subtype of indolent NHL. Most of these patients present with advanced disease (stage 3 or 4) and reveal an indolent clinical course with a median survival of 6 to 10 years. Only 10% to 15% of patients have limited disease. It remains controversial whether patients with limited disease can be cured, because relapses occur even after 10 to 20 years. Diffuse large B-cell NHL represents an aggressive type, and at least 40% of patients were cured with standard regimens of chemotherapy and prolonged follow-up [13].

There is a higher incidence of extranodal disease and marrow involvement in patients who have NHL than in patients who have HD. Extranodal lymphatic tissue like Waldeyer's ring or spleen and nonlymphatic organs like liver, GI tract [17–19], lung, bone, and CNS often are involved with NHL. Parotid and thyroid gland (Fig. 4), breast, bones, testes, or leptomeninges (Fig. 5) may be involved [20–26]. Certain forms of lymphoma like primary effusion lymphoma/body cavity lymphoma, enteropathy-type T-cell lymphoma, or MALT lymphoma might present with localized and rather typical imaging findings [17–19,27].

Pulmonary involvement and pleural disease may be seen without mediastinal involvement. Solid pleural masses are infrequent but may be encountered with NHL. Isolated chest wall soft tissue masses are not common and are usually a manifestation of NHL.

Involvement of liver (Fig. 6) or spleen [28] (Fig. 7A) may present with focal lesions, and the imaging features are similar to metastatic disease. Diffuse involvement of liver and spleen is more

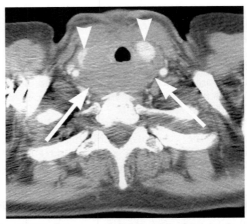

Fig. 4. Diffuse large cell lymphoma with involvement of the thyroid and spleen (not pictured). Small amount of regular thyroid tissue *(arrowhead)* is depicted within the large neck mass *(arrow)*.

difficult to detect despite advances in imaging [29]. Enlargement of the liver is suggestive of infiltration. Enlargement of the spleen is not a reliable predictor of disease, although marked enlargement in the setting of other sites of involvement makes splenic lymphoma involvement likely.

Small bowel, stomach, or colon often are involved with NHL [30], and disease may be multicentric. The stomach is the most commonly involved organ in primary and secondary lymphoma (Fig. 8). Secondary involvement of the pancreas also is seen often in patients who have NHL [31] (Fig. 9). Renal involvement with

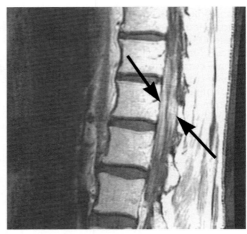

Fig. 5. Leptomeningeal lymphoma. Sagittal T1 weighted MR scan after administration of gadolinium reveals plaque-like and confluent leptomeningeal disease *(arrow)* along the lower thoracic spinal cord and conus medullaris.

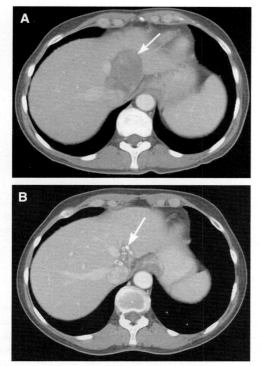

Fig. 6. Residual mass in large cell lymphoma. The initial scan from 2003 *(A)* revealed a large heterogeneous low-attenuation mass involving the caudate lobe extending to the confluence of the hepatic veins *(arrow)*. Three years after treatment, there is a much smaller partially calcified residual mass in the apex of the liver *(B, arrow)*.

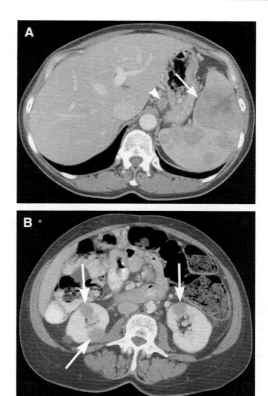

Fig. 7. Diffuse large-cell lymphoma with splenic involvement *(A, arrow)*, paragastric lymphadenopathy *(A, arrowhead)*, retroperitoneal lymphadenopathy (not pictured), and enhancing bilateral renal masses *(B, small arrow)*.

NHL may occur as solid masses (see Fig. 7B), diffuse infiltrations with nephromegaly, or by invasion of retroperitoneal disease [32]. The genitourinary tract is very rarely involved at presentation. Retroperitoneal and mesenteric disease [33] may present with subtle findings mimicking peritoneal carcinomatosis, with enlarged lymph nodes, or with conglomerate masses (Figs. 10–12).

There is an increased incidence of NHL in immunocompromised patients, such as patients with AIDS or patients receiving immunosuppressive medications for an organ transplant [34–36]. Extranodal sites (GI tract, central nervous system [CNS],

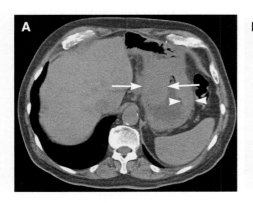
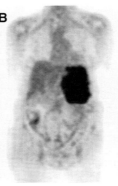

Fig. 8. Gastric NHL (MALT lymphoma). *(A)* Stomach with a large lesser curvature mass *(arrows)* and circumferential thickening of the gastric wall *(arrowheads)*. *(B)* Positron emission tomography (PET) with F18-FDG usually does not visualize extranodal B-cell lymphoma of the mucosa-associated lymphoid tissue (MALT)-type. This is a rare case of a FDG-avid MALT lymphoma (SUV 17.5) (different patient than patient in *A*).

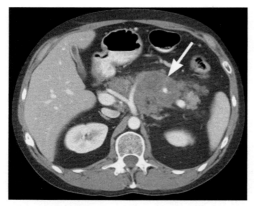

Fig. 9. Retroperitoneal NHL with secondary involvement of the pancreas *(arrow)*.

liver, bone marrow, lung) are most involved commonly.

Central nervous system lymphoma

Most primary CNS lymphomas are NHL. With an increasing incidence in both the immunocompetent and immunocompromised populations, primary CNS lymphoma represents 1% of all lymphomas and as many as 16% of all primary brain tumors. HIV infection and AIDS, congenital causes of immunodeficiency (such as IgA deficiency), and immunosuppressive therapy after organ transplantation are associated with greater risk for developing CNS lymphoma.

In the immunocompetent patient, lymphoma is usually a solitary, supratentorial lesion with homogeneous enhancement. Lesions may cross the corpus callosum in a butterfly pattern. Highly packed abnormal cells are thought to be responsible for the high density of these lesions in unenhanced

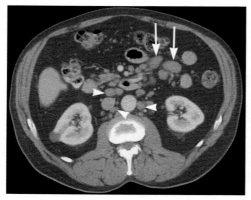

Fig. 10. Extensive mesenteric *(arrow)* and retroperitoneal *(arrowhead)* lymphadenopathy in a patient with NHL. Lymphoma is the most common malignancy resulting in mesenteric lymphadenopathy. Right kidney with small cyst.

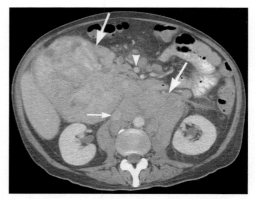

Fig. 11. Large bulky retroperitoneal lymphoma *(arrow)*. Note how the masses displace vessels such as the inferior vena cava *(short arrow)* and the superior mesenteric vein *(arrowhead)*.

CT and for the often slightly hypointense signal intensity on T2 weighted MR images.

In the immunocompromised patient, the presence of multiple lesions is more common, and the lesions more often display irregular margins, heterogeneity, and ring enhancement. In the immunocompromised population, it is difficult to distinguish a primary CNS lymphoma from the more common cerebral toxoplasmosis.

Primary leptomeningeal lymphoma often reveals unremarkable neuroimaging examinations, nonspecific findings, or discrete masses or faint enhancement. Leptomeningeal lymphoma occurs most often in combination with solitary intracerebral lesions; primary leptomeningeal lymphoma (without other, intracerebral or extracerebral lymphomatous deposits) is rare [37,38] (see Figs. 5 and 13).

Childhood lymphoma

Approximately 1700 children in the United States are diagnosed annually with lymphoma. In general, NHL is slightly more common than HD. In children younger than 15 years of age, NHL is slightly more common. In children older than 15 years and adolescents, HD becomes more common.

Table 1 compares the most important features of HD and NHL in pediatric patients. Childhood NHL has a high incidence of lymphoma in the GI tract, solid abdominal viscera including the pancreas and kidneys [39], and extranodal sites in the head and neck. The number of relevant forms of NHL is much smaller than in adult patients; Burkitt's lymphoma, large cell lymphoma and T-cell lymphoma are the most common.

Presentation of children with Burkitt's lymphoma includes an abdominal mass (70%),

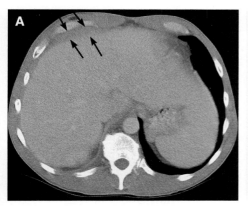

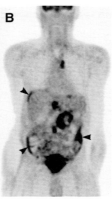

Fig. 12. Follicular and diffuse large cell lymphoma with mediastinal, retroperitoneal, and peritoneal manifestations (composite histology: two different histologies in the same biopsy site). (A) CT reveals peritoneal tumor growth between liver and diaphragm *(arrowhead)*. (B) PET reveals mediastinal and retroperitoneal manifestations. Note the sheet-like implants in the peritoneal cavity *(arrowhead)*.

enlarged nodes in neck or pharynx (25%), pleural effusion (22%), bone involvement (10%), and mediastinal or hilar nodes (7%). Intussusception in teenagers or children with Burkitt's lymphoma is not an uncommon presentation.

T-cell lymphoma commonly involves the thymus (Fig. 14). T-cell lymphoma and T-cell leukemia are differentiated by the degree of bone marrow involvement but have similar radiographic features.

Staging

Accurate staging allows minimization of toxic therapies (such as extended field radiation or overly aggressive chemotherapy), thereby decreasing the risk of secondary malignancies, which exceeds 10% in historical series of patients with early-stage HD [40]. Ann Arbor staging is the staging system for lymphoma, both in HD and NHL.

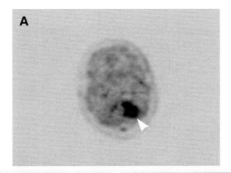

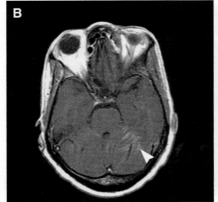

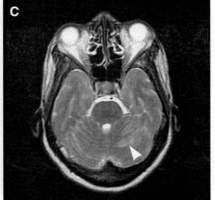

Fig. 13. Leptomeningeal lymphoma in a patient with skin lymphoma and lymphadenopathy. (A) PET revealed increased uptake in the left tentorium cerebellae (arrowhead). The corresponding axial T1 weighted MR imaging scan after administration of gadolinium reveals leptomeningeal enhancement *(B, arrowhead)* with corresponding T2 hyperintensity in the T2 weighted MR imaging scan *(C, arrowhead)*.

Table 1: **Comparison of Hodgkin's disease and non-Hodgkin's lymphoma in pediatric patients**

Feature	Hodgkin's disease	Non-Hodgkin's lymphoma
Age	Mostly >10 years	Any age in children
Stage at diagnosis	Mostly localized	Commonly widespread
Constitutional symptoms	Alter prognosis	Do not affect prognosis
Central nervous system involvement	Rare	Occurrence increases with AIDS
Mediastinal involvement	Most common with nodular sclerosing Hodgkin's disease	Most common with lymphoblastic lymphoma
Gastrointestinal involvement	Rare	Occurs
Abdominal nodal involvement	Can be small or large, mesenteric rare	Usually enlarged, mesenteric common
Bone involvement	Rare	Occurs
Marrow involvement	Rare	Common

It initially was developed for HD, but it has some use in NHL [4].

The staging classification was modified after a 1988 meeting in Cotswold (UK) (Table 2) [41]. The staging system is based on numerous factors, including the involved sites, whether the involved lymph nodes are on one or both sides of the diaphragm, or whether there is extranodal involvement. In NHL, prognosis also depends on factors like the histological type, and this classification is of less value. Imaging remains crucial for staging, and standard imaging examinations include chest radiography, CT, MR imaging and fluorine-18-deoxyglucose (FDG)-positron emission tomography (PET). Lymphography does not significantly contribute to staging [22,42,43].

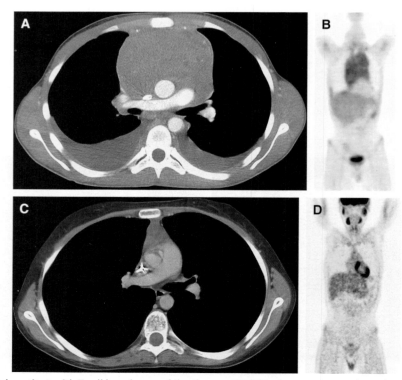

Fig. 14. Pediatric patient with T-cell lymphoma of the thymus. CT *(A)* before treatment shows large heterogenous anterior mediastinal mass and bilateral pleural effusions. There is increased FDG uptake in the mediastinum *(B)*. CT *(C)* and PET *(D)* after treatment show marked improvement. (*From* Sara Abramson, MD, New York, NY.)

Table 2: **Cotswold staging classification**

Stage	Description
Stage I	Involvement of a single lymph node region or lymphoid structure (eg, spleen, thymus, Waldeyer's ring) or involvement of a single extralymphatic site (IE)
Stage II	Involvement of two or more lymph node regions on the same site of the diaphragm (II) or localized contiguous involvement of only one extranodal organ or side and its regional lymph nodes with or without other lymph node regions on the same side of the diaphragm (IIE) Note: The number of anatomic regions involved may be indicated by a subscript (eg, II3).
Stage III	Involvement of lymph node regions on both sides of the diaphragm (III), which also may be accompanied by involvement of the spleen (IIIS) or by localized contiguous involvement of only one extranodal organ side (IIIE) or both (IIISE)
Stage IV	Disseminated (multifocal) involvement of one or more extranodal organs or tissues, with or without associated lymph node involvement or isolated extralymphatic organ involvement with distant (nonregional) nodal involvement
Designations applicable to any disease stage	
A	No symptoms
B	Fever (temperature >38°C), night sweats, unexplained loss of more than 10% of body weight during the previous 6 months.
X	Bulky disease
E	Involvement of a single extranodal site that is contiguous or proximal to the known nodal site

Involvement of hilar nodes on both sides constitutes stage II disease.
Bulky mediastinal disease has been defined as a thoracic ratio of maximum transverse mass diameter greater than or equal to one third of the internal transverse thoracic diameter measured at the T5/6 intervertebral disk level on chest radiography. Other authors have designated a lymph node mass measuring 10 cm or more in greatest dimension as bulky disease.
Evidence of invasion of adjacent structures such as bone, chest wall, or lung is an important consideration, as this may influence management. For example, a mediastinal or hilar mass that invades the adjacent lung is classified as IIE, whereas pulmonary involvement separate from adenopathy represents stage IV.

Clinical staging of NHL in children is less important, because all cases are considered to have disseminated disease, even if the radiologic findings suggest localized disease. Staging of NHL uses the St. Jude Children's Research Hospital model (**Box 2**) [44,45], which is slightly simpler than the St. Jude Children's Research Hospital model [45]. The clinical staging of HD uses the Ann Arbor/Cotswold classification (see **Table 2**). Clinical issues and radiologic features of HD in pediatric patients are very similar to those of HD in adult patients.

Most studies evaluating FDG-PET in lymphoma include patients who have diffuse large B-cell NHL or HD. FDG-PET accurately detected disease in patients who had diffuse large cell B cell NHL, mantle cell lymphoma, follicular lymphoma, and HD [46]. PET was less reliable at detecting small lymphocytic NHL [47]. Recent studies [48] suggest that FDG-PET is useful for detecting and staging marginal zone lymphoma, contradicting prior studies [47]. Combined PET/CT is a more accurate test than either of its individual components and is probably better than side-by-side viewing of images

from both modalities [49]. For the evaluation of lymph node involvement, PET/CT and contrast-enhanced CT had sensitivities of 98% and 88% and specificities of 100% and 86%, respectively [50].

Review of the literature reveals a limited number of studies that have addressed primary staging of lymphoma with FDG-PET. FDG-PET adds substantially to the staging information obtained using other radiologic methods (**Fig. 15**) [51–55]. The use of a PET staging work-up appears to lead to a change in stage in approximately 15% to 40% of patients [2,50,55]. About half of such changes in disease stage led to modifications of therapy [2].

Assessment of treatment response

Tumor measurements on an axial cross-sectional imaging modality should be made as biperpendicular measurements in the axial plane (ie, the longest axial diameter by the largest perpendicular diameter). Diffuse, ill-defined lesions such as perirenal infiltration in NHL or pulmonary lymphatic spread are not measurable, but should be described [56].

Box 2:   St. Jude staging system for childhood non-Hodgkin's lymphoma

Stage I
A single tumor (extranodal) or single anatomic area (nodal), with the exclusion of the mediastinum or abdomen

Stage II
A single tumor (extranodal) with regional node involvement
Two or more nodal areas on the same side of the diaphragm
Two single (extranodal) tumors with or without regional node involvement on the same side of the diaphragm
A primary gastrointestinal tract tumor, usually in the ileocecal area, with or without involvement of associated mesenteric nodes only

Stage III
Two single tumors (extranodal) on opposite sides of the diaphragm
Two or more nodal areas above and below the diaphragm
All primary intrathoracic tumors (mediastinal, pleural, and thymic)
All extensive primary intra-abdominal disease
All paraspinal or epidural tumors, regardless of other tumor side(s)

Stage IV
Any of the previous with initial central nervous system and/or bone marrow involvement

(*From* Murphy S. Childhood non-Hodgkin's lymphoma. N Engl J Med 1978;299:1446–8; with permission.)

Standardized guidelines for response assessment are important to facilitate interpretation of data and for comparison of the results among various clinical trials.

The International workshop criteria (IWC) from 1999 are used widely and accepted for response assessment of NHL. They are summarized in Box 3 [57]. These criteria are based primarily on CT, although bone marrow biopsy and clinical and biochemical information also are considered.

Response criteria for HD [41] are slightly different from the NHL response criteria. These response criteria were not included in this article, because application of the NHL response criteria is also appropriate; the NHL response criteria are used by many centers, including the author's institution.

Some of the response criteria in Box 3 appear subtle but have implications for the interpretation of data and comparison of results. A complete response in NHL requires that all involved lymph nodes return to normal size, and this might not be achieved in all lymph nodes because of fibrosis or necrosis. These patients with mildly enlarged lymph nodes after treatment might show a high

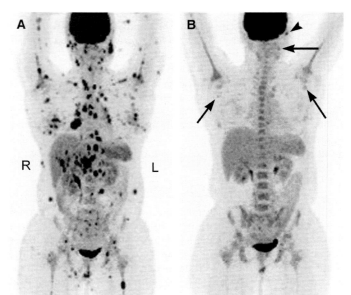

Fig. 15. T cell lymphoma. *(A)* PET reveals multiple hypermetabolic lesions above and below the diaphragm and within several bones. The highest standardized uptake values (SUVs) measured 24.3 (left proximal femur). Many of these nodes had normal size on cross-sectional imaging. *(B)* After treatment, there is a significant decrease in intensity and extent of previously noted lesions. Note activity in bilateral axillary and cervical nodes *(arrows)* and in the parotid gland *(arrowhead)*. Diffuse bone marrow uptake is likely a post-treatment effect.

> **Box 3:** **Criteria of response for non-Hodgkin's lymphoma (often also used for Hodgkin's disease)**
>
> *Complete remission (CR)*
> Complete disappearance of all detectable clinical and radiological evidence of disease
> All nodal masses to have decreased to normal (<1.5 cm in diameter for nodes that were >1.5 cm before therapy). If the nodes were initially between 1 and 1.5 cm, they must have decreased to 1 cm or by more than 75% of the sum of the products of the diameter of the nodes (SPD).
> The spleen, if previously enlarged on CT, must be normal, and any focal lesions should have resolved. Similarly, the liver and kidney, if previously involved, must have returned to normal.
> If the marrow was involved, it must be clear. Marrow biopsy and not imaging is used for this criterion.
>
> *Complete remission—unconfirmed/uncertain (CRu)*
> As in first and third point, but with a residual mass greater than 1.5 cm, which must have regressed by more than 75% from the original size. Individual nodes that were confluent must have decreased by more than 75% of pretherapy SPD.
>
> *Partial response (PR)*
> More than a 50% decrease in SPD of the six largest nodes or masses. These nodes should be from different areas of the body if possible, including the mediastinum and retroperitoneum.
> No increase in the size of other nodes, liver or spleen
> Any splenic or hepatic lesions should have decreased by 50%.
> Involvement of other organs is assessable but not measurable disease.
> No new side of ascites
>
> *Stable disease (SD)*
> Less than partial response but not progressive disease
>
> *Progressive disease (PD)*
> Appearance of new lesions, or an increase of more than 50% in established lesions
> Increase of more than 50% in the greatest diameter of any previously identified node that was greater than 1 cm
>
> (*Adapted from* Cheson BD, Horning SJ, Coiffier B, et al. Report of an international workshop to standardize response criteria for non-Hodgkin lymphomas. NCI Sponsored International Working Group. J Clin Oncol 1999:17:1244–53.)

response rate, and they might be cured. Still, they would not be classified as patients with a complete response. As a result, a publication about a successful treatment regimen might show a relatively low rate of complete response.

FDG-PET is superior to CT in differentiation of viable tumor, necrosis, and fibrosis. Combined IWC and PET-based assessment appears to better discriminate between complete response and partial response [58].

> **Box 4:** **Proposed response criteria for assessment of non-Hodgkin's lymphoma and Hodgkin's disease**
>
> This classification refers to patients who have PET-avid disease at initial staging, and it is based on recent advances including in PET and immunohistochemistry. CR unconfirmed (CRu) is no longer included. PET does not replace biopsy before initiating new therapy.
>
> *Complete remission*
> No signs or symptoms of disease
> PET-negative in a PET avid lymphoma, or negative CT in a not predictably PET avid lymphoma
> Normal bone marrow by morphology, or if indeterminate, negative by immunohistochemistry, flow cytometry or molecular genetic studies
>
> *Partial remission*
> At least 50% decrease in tumor size, but PET positive at prior PET-avid sites
> Bone marrow is irrelevant if positive pretreatment.
>
> *Stable disease*
> Neither partial remission nor progressive disease, PET positive only at prior sites of disease
>
> *Progressive/relapsed disease*
> At least 50% increase in disease or new lesions that are PET-positive if PET-avid lymphoma
>
> (*Adapted from* Cheson BD, Pfistner B, Juweid ME, et al. Recommendations for revised response criteria for malignant lymphoma. J Clin Oncol 2006;18S:7507.)

Seven years after the publication of the IWC criteria, there is need of revision of the currently used response criteria in lymphoma [59]. Meetings of the International Harmonization Project (IHP) in 2005 and 2006 stressed the importance of the introduction of PET and PET/CT for response assessment. The proposed new criteria are summarized in Box 4 [60]. For predictably PET-avid histologies (eg, diffuse large B-cell NHL, Hodgkin's lymphoma, and follicular and mantle cell lymphoma), PET pretreatment is encouraged strongly to define sites of disease, but it is not required. Any response on CT with normalization on PET would be considered as complete remission.

A major indication for FDG-PET is the evaluation of treatment response after completion of therapy, especially in patients who have residual masses, where it is unclear whether these masses represent tumor persistence (Fig. 16). Residual masses seen after treatment represent a mixture of fibrosis and necrotic tumor but may sometimes represent viable tumor. Serial CT, initially performed at 2- to 3-month intervals, is the most widely used method for following residual masses.

FDG-PET is proving to provide important, clinically relevant information about response to treatment and prognosis.

A positive PET scan at completion of treatment is a poor prognostic factor (despite imaging findings on CT) and warrants close follow-up or additional procedures. Persistently positive PET scans during and after chemotherapy appear to have a high sensitivity for predicting subsequent relapse [61].

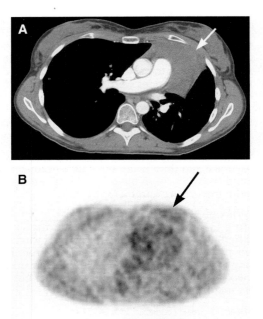

Fig. 16. Large residual mass in a patient with HD treated with chemotherapy and radiation to the mediastinum. *(A)* Axial CT scan reveals a large left upper anterior mediastinal mass that involves the adjacent pericardium *(arrow)*. *(B)* The corresponding PET scan shows minimal FDG activity (SUV 1.6), probably because of post-therapy changes *(arrow)*.

A negative PET scan at completion of treatment predicts a high likelihood for relapse-free survival [62].

Patients who have a negative PET scan after two cycles of treatment for early-stage favorable disease

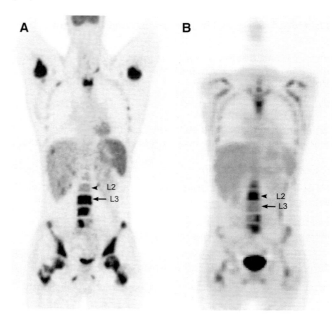

Fig. 17. Burkitt's lymphoma with multiple bone lesions before *(A)* and after *(B)* treatment. The L3 vertebral body *(arrow)* is affected by lymphoma and shows high metabolic activity before treatment and no activity after treatment. The L2 vertebral body *(arrowhead)* was not affected by lymphoma. After treatment and administration of growth factor, there is mild metabolic activity caused by bone marrow hyperproliferation. The L4 and L5 vertebral bodies reveal a mosaic pattern; the right side of these vertebral bodies was affected by lymphoma, but the left side was not affected and shows marrow response after administration of hematopoietic growth factor.

are considered for an abbreviated course of chemo-therapy alone, whereas those with a positive PET scan require standard treatment with a combination of chemotherapy and radiation therapy. This approach needs to be validated by larger studies [62,63].

It should be noted that discordant findings between PET and other imaging modalities often remain unresolved, because biopsy usually is not done. The performance of PET varies in different regions; the highest sensitivity was found in the thorax (91%) and the lowest in the abdomen/pelvis (75%) [63].

There is a considerable overlap in the standardized uptake values (SUV) of indolent and aggressive NHL, with a relatively wide range of SUVs observed even within the same histologic subtype. Despite this overlap, the following two statements seem to be reasonable: An SUV of at least 13 indicates a high likelihood of aggressive histology, and an SUV of no more than 6 is very likely associated with indolent histology.

False-positive findings at FDG-PET other than in residual masses may be caused by rebound thymic hyperplasia or infectious or inflammatory processes. The diffusely increased bone marrow uptake often observed after treatment or administration of hematopoietic growth factor is usually caused by bone marrow stimulation and should not be misinterpreted as lymphomatous involvement (Fig. 17).

Summary

This article reviewed the clinical features of HD and NHL, common imaging features, the staging of lymphoma, and the role of FDG-PET in the assessment of patients with lymphoma. The significant changes that have occurred in the diagnosis and management of lymphoma over the past 20 years were emphasized.

References

[1] Fisher RI. Overview of non-Hodgkin's lymphoma: biology, staging, and treatment. Semin Oncol 2003;30:3–9.

[2] Schiepers C, Filmont JE, Czernin J. PET for staging of Hodgkin's disease and non-Hodgkin's lymphoma. Eur J Nucl Med Mol Imaging 2003; 30(Suppl 1):S82–8.

[3] Lu P. Staging and classification of lymphoma. Semin Nucl Med 2005;35:160–4.

[4] DeVos S. Historical overview and current state of art in diagnosis and treatment of lymphoma and Hodgkin's disease. PET Clinics 2006;1:203–17.

[5] Connors JM. State-of-the-art therapeutics: Hodgkin's lymphoma. J Clin Oncol 2005;23:6400–8.

[6] Sharma A, Fidias P, Hayman LA, et al. Patterns of lymphadenopathy in thoracic malignancies. Radiographics 2004;24:419–34.

[7] Guermazi A, Brice P, de Kerviler E, et al. Extranodal Hodgkin's disease: spectrum of disease. Radiographics 2001;21:161–79.

[8] Sider L, Weiss AJ, Smith MD, et al. Varied appearance of AIDS-related lymphoma in the chest. Radiology 1989;171:629–32.

[9] Graham BB, Mathisen DJ, Mark EJ, et al. Primary pulmonary lymphoma. Ann Thorac Surg 2005; 80:1248–53.

[10] Ferraro P, Trastek VF, Adlakha H, et al. Primary non-Hodgkin's lymphoma of the lung. Ann Thorac Surg 2000;69:993–7.

[11] Apter S, Avigdor A, Gayer G, et al. Calcification in Lymphoma occurring before therapy: CT features and clinical correlation. AJR Am J Roentgenol 2002;178:935–8.

[12] Harris NL, Jaffe ES, Diebold J, et al. The World Health Organization classification of neoplastic diseases of the hematopoietic and lymphoid tissues. Report of the Clinical Advisory Committee meeting, Airlie House, Virginia, November, 1997. Ann Oncol 1999;10:1419–32.

[13] Cheson BD. What is new in lymphoma? CA Cancer J Clin 2004;54:260–72.

[14] Hennessy BT, Hanrahan EO, Daly PA. Non-Hodgkin's lymphoma: an update. Lancet Oncol 2004;5:341–53.

[15] Ahmad A, Govil Y, Frank BB. Gastric mucosa-associated lymphoid tissue lymphoma. Am J Gastroenterol 2003;98:975–86.

[16] An SK, Han JK, Kim YH, et al. Gastric mucosa-associated lymphoid tissue lymphoma: spectrum of findings at double-contrast gastrointestinal examination with pathologic correlation. Radiographics 2001;21:1491–504.

[17] Byun JH, Ha HK, Kim AY, et al. CT findings in peripheral T cell lymphoma involving the gastrointestinal tract. Radiology 2003;227:59–67.

[18] Kim YH, Lim HK, Han JK, et al. Low-grade gastric mucosa-associated lymphoid tissue lymphoma: correlation of radiographic and pathologic findings. Radiology 1999;212: 241–8.

[19] Lee HJ, Im JG, Goo JM, et al. Peripheral T-cell lymphoma: spectrum of imaging findings with clinical and pathological features. Radiographics 2003;23:7–28.

[20] Mengiardi B, Honegger H, Hodler J, et al. Primary lymphoma of bone: MRI and CT characteristics during and after successful treatment. AJR Am J Roentgenol 2005;184:185–92.

[21] Mussurakis S, Carleton PJ, Turnbull LW. MR imaging of primary non-Hodgkin's breast lymphoma: a case report. Acta Radiol 1997;38: 104–7.

[22] Rademaker J. Diagnostic imaging modalities for assessment of lymphoma with special emphasis on CT, MRI, and ultrasound. PET Clinics 2006; 1:219–30.

[23] Ochsner HC, Moser RH. Ivory vertebra. AJR Am J Roentgenol 1933;29:635–7.

[24] Liberman L, Giess CS, Dershaw DD, et al. Non-Hodgkin's lymphoma of the breast: imaging characteristics and correlation with histopathology. Radiology 1994;192:157–60.

[25] Zicherman JM, Weissman D, Gribbin C, et al. Primary diffuse large B cell lymphoma of the epididymis and testis. Radiographics 2005;25:243–8.

[26] Krishnan A, Shirkhoda A, Tehranzadeh J, et al. Primary bone lymphoma: radiographic MR imaging correlation. Radiographics 2003;23:1371–87.

[27] Miketic LM, Chambers TP, Lembersky BC. Cutaneous -cell lymphoma: value of CT in staging and determining prognosis. AJR Am J Roentgenol 1993;160:1129–32.

[28] Lieberman S, Libson E, Maly B, et al. Imaging-guided percutaneous splenic biopsy using a 20- or 22-gauge cutting-edge core biopsy needle for the diagnosis of malignant lymphoma. AJR Am J Roentgenol 2003;181:1025–7.

[29] Catalano O, Matarazzo I, Hawru J. Contrast-enhanced sonography of the spleen. AJR Am J Roentgenol 2005;184:1150–6.

[30] Macari M, Balthazar EJ. CT of bowel wall thickening: Significance and pitfalls of interpretation. AJR Am J Roentgenol 2001;176:1105–16.

[31] Merkle EM, Bender GN, Brambs HJ. Imaging findings in pancreatic lymphoma: differential aspects. AJR Am J Roentgenol 2000;174:671–5.

[32] Urban BA, Fishman EK. Renal lymphoma: CT patterns with emphasis on helical CT. Radiographics 2000;20:197–212.

[33] Lucey BC, Stuhlfaut JW, Soto JA. Mesenteric lymph nodes seen at imaging: causes and significance. Radiographics 2005;25:351–65.

[34] Blaes AH, Peterson BA, Bartlett N, et al. Rituximab therapy is effective for post-transplant lymphoproliferative disorders after solid organ transplantation: results of a phase II trial. Cancer 2005;104:1661–7.

[35] Claudon M, Kessler M, Champigneulle J, et al. Lymphoproliferative disorders after renal transplantation: role of medical imaging. Eur Radiol 1998;8:1686–93.

[36] Scarsbrook AF, Warakaulle DR, Dattani M, et al. Post-transplantation lymphoproliferative disorder: the spectrum of imaging findings. Clin Radiol 2005;60:47–55.

[37] Slone HW, Blake JJ, Shah R, et al. CT and MRI findings of intracranial lymphoma. AJR Am J Roentgenol 2005;184:1679–85.

[38] Erdag N, Bhorade RM, Alberico RA, et al. Primary lymphoma of the central nervous system: typical and atypical CT and MR imaging appearances. AJR Am J Roentgenol 2001;176:1319–26.

[39] Chepuri NB, Strouse PJ, Yanik GA. CT of renal lymphoma in children. AJR Am J Roentgenol 2003;180:429–31.

[40] Ng AK, Bernardo MV, Weller E, et al. Second malignancy after Hodgkin's disease treated with radiation therapy with or without chemotherapy: long-term risks and risk factors. Blood 2002;100:1989–96.

[41] Lister TA, Crowther DM, Sutcliffe SB, et al. Report of a committee convened to discuss the evaluation and staging of patients with Hodgkin's disease: Cotswolds meeting. J Clin Oncol 1989;7:1630–6.

[42] North LB, Wallace S, Lindell MM, et al. Lymphography for staging lymphomas: is it still a useful procedure? AJR Am J Roentgenol 1993;161:867–9.

[43] Guermazi A, Brice P, Hennequin C, et al. Lymphography: an old technique retains its usefulness. Radiographics 2003;23:1541–60.

[44] Murphy S. Childhood non-Hodgkin's lymphoma. N Engl J Med 1978;299:1446–8.

[45] Kaste SC, Shulkin BL. 18F-fluorodeoxyglucose PET/CT in childhood lymphoma. PET Clinics 2006;1:265–73.

[46] Elstrom R, Guan L, Baker G, et al. Utility of FDG-PET scanning in lymphoma by WHO classification. Blood 2003;101:3875–6.

[47] Jerusalem G, Beguin Y, Najjar F, et al. Positron emission tomography (PET) with 18F-fluoro-deoxyglucose (18F-FDG) for the staging of low-grade non-Hodgkin's lymphoma (NHL). Ann Oncol 2001;12:825–30.

[48] Beal KP, Yeung HW, Yahalom J. FDG-PET scanning for detection and staging of extranodal marginal zone lymphomas of the MALT type: a report of 42 cases. Ann Oncol 2005;16:473–80.

[49] von Schulthess GK, Steinert HC, Hany TF. Integrated PET/CT: current applications and future directions. Radiology 2006;238:405–22.

[50] Schaefer NG, Hany TF, Taverna C, et al. Non-Hodgkin's lymphoma and Hodgkin's disease: coregistered FDG PET and CT at staging and restaging—do we need contrast-enhanced CT? Radiology 2004;232:823–9.

[51] Metser U, Goor O, Lerman H, et al. PET-CT of extranodal lymphoma. AJR Am J Roentgenol 2004;182:1579–86.

[52] Bar-Shalom R. Normal and abnormal patterns of 18F-Fluorodeoxyglucose PET/CT in lymphoma. PET Clinics 2006;1:231–42.

[53] Podoloff DA, Macapinlac HA. PET and PET/CT in the management of lymphomas. PET Clinics 2006;1:243–50.

[54] Even-Sapir E, Lievshitz G, Perry C, et al. Fluorine-18 Fluorodeoxyglucose PET/CT patterns of extranodal involvement in patients with non-Hodgkin's lymphoma and Hodgkin's disease. PET Clinics 2006;1:251–63.

[55] Bangerter M, Moog F, Buchmann I, et al. Whole-body 2-[18F]-fluoro-2-deoxy-D-glucose positron emission tomography(FDG-PET) for accurate staging of Hodgkin's disease. Ann Oncol 1998;9:1117–22.

[56] Padhani AR, Husband JE. Are current tumour response criteria relevant for the 21st century. Br J Radiol 2000;73:1031–3.

[57] Cheson BD, Horning SJ, Coiffier B, et al. Report of an international workshop to standardize response criteria for Non-Hodgkin Lymphomas. NCI Sponsored International Working Group. J Clin Oncol 1999;17:1244–53.

[58] Juweid ME, Wiseman GA, Vose JM, et al. Response assessment of aggressive non-Hodgkin's lymphoma by integrated International Workshop Criteria and fluorine-18-fluorodeoxyglucose positron emission tomography. J Clin Oncol 2005;23:4652–61.

[59] Guermazi A, Juweid ME. Commentary: PET poised to alter the current paradigm for response assessment of non-Hodgkin's lymphoma. Br J Radiol 2006;79:365–7.

[60] Cheson BD, Pfistner B, Juweid ME, et al. Recommendations for revised response criteria for malignant lymphoma. J Clin Oncol 2006;18S: 7507.

[61] Hutchings M, Loft A, Hansen M, et al. FDG-PET after two cycles of chemotherapy predicts treatment failure and progression-free survival in Hodgkin's lymphoma. Blood 2006;107:52–9.

[62] Hutchings M, Mikhaeel NG, Fields PA, et al. Prognostic value of interim FDG-PET after two or three cycles of chemotherapy in Hodgkin's lymphoma. Ann Oncol 2005;16:1160–8.

[63] Jerusalem G, Beguin Y, Fassotte MF, et al. Whole-body positron emission tomography using 18F-fluorodeoxyglucose compared to standard procedures for staging patients with Hodgkin's disease. Haematologica 2001;86: 266–73.

RADIOLOGIC
CLINICS
OF NORTH AMERICA

Radiol Clin N Am 45 (2007) 85–118

ELSEVIER
SAUNDERS

Update on Colorectal Cancer Imaging

Marc J. Gollub, MD*, Lawrence H. Schwartz, MD,
Tim Akhurst, MD

- ■ Screening
  - *Fecal occult blood test*
  - *Sigmoidoscopy*
  - *Fecal DNA analysis*
  - *Barium enema: time to put it to rest?*
  - *Colonoscopy*
  - *CT colonography (virtual colonoscopy)*
- ■ Diagnosis and staging
  - *Barium enema*
- *CT*
  - *Virtual colonoscopy*
  - *Newer imaging methods*
- ■ Primary and recurrent rectal cancer
  - *Positron emission tomography in rectal cancer*
- ■ Radiologic follow-up and treatment monitoring
- ■ Summary
- ■ References

Worldwide, colorectal cancer (CRC) is the third most frequently occurring cancer in both sexes, but it ranks second in developed countries [1]. In the United States, cancer is the second most common cause of death after heart disease and causes one in four deaths. The American Cancer Society (ACS) estimates 1,399,790 new cases of cancer in 2006. About 148,610 of these will be of colon or rectum. An estimated 55,170 deaths caused by CRC are expected in 2006. Because of screening and premalignant polyp removal, CRC incidence rates have been decreasing since 1985. Because of improvements in survival, mortality rates have also been decreasing an average of 1.8% per year. If CRC is diagnosed at an early stage, the prognosis is favorable with 5-year survival rates exceeding 90% [2].

The risk of CRC increases with age, with most cases diagnosed after age 50, and a median age in the mid-70s. The lifetime risk for CRC is approximately 5% to 6%. Several risks factors for the development of CRC have been identified that could be altered, including obesity, physical inactivity, smoking, heavy alcohol consumption, a diet high in red meat, and inadequate intake of fruits and vegetables. Protective effects may be gained from regular use of nonsteroidal anti-inflammatory drugs, including aspirin, estrogen and progestin hormone therapy, and 3-hydroxy-3-methylglutary coenzyme A reductase inhibitors (cholesterol-lowering drugs). These drugs, however, are not currently recommended for prevention [3].

More than 80% of CRC cases arise from adenomatous polyps; however, less than 1% of adenomatous polyps smaller than 1 cm become cancer. Polyps 10 to 20 mm in size have an approximately 4% risk of carcinoma and a 21% risk of high-grade dysplasia. Subcentimeter polyps have a much lower risk ($\leq 1\%$) for carcinoma and high-grade dysplasia (3%–5%) [4].

About 80% of CRC occurs in patients at average risk (no known risk factors and age 50 or greater) and 20% occur in those with a family history of

Department of Radiology, Weill Medical College of Cornell University, Memorial Sloan-Kettering Cancer Center, Room C276F, 1275 York Avenue, New York, NY 10021, USA
* Corresponding author.
E-mail address: gollubm@mskcc.org (M.J. Gollub).

0033-8389/07/$ – see front matter © 2006 Elsevier Inc. All rights reserved.
radiologic.theclinics.com

doi:10.1016/j.rcl.2006.10.003

CRC in a first-degree relative. Of this latter group, a small proportion (6%) is associated with genetic syndromes, such as familial adenomatous polyposis and hereditary nonpolyposis CRC. Others at higher risk include those with long-standing ulcerative colitis and those with a personal history of large adenomatous polyps or CRC or a family history of adenomatous polyps diagnosed before age 60.

There have been exciting new developments in CRC research since the last monograph on CRC in the *Radiologic Clinics of North America* [5]. Most are beyond the scope of this article:

1. Further understanding and delineation of molecular and genetic details in the adenoma-carcinoma sequence of mutations, including microsatellite instability markers and DNA mismatch repair genes
2. Development of fecal DNA assays for screening
3. Development of more effective chemotherapy [6]
4. Rapid development and maturation of CT colonography (CTC, also known as virtual colonoscopy)
5. Rapid technologic evolution of multislice helical CT imaging and higher field strength MR imaging magnets (3 T) with phased array coils
6. New and improved methods of liver metastasis diagnosis and treatment, such as microbubble contrast agents in ultrasound and radiofrequency ablation techniques in interventional radiology, respectively
7. Exponential increase in understanding, use, and reimbursement for positron emission tomography (PET), now combined with CT (fusion technology)
8. Greater publicity and public awareness of this preventable cancer killer through more widespread screening efforts and media coverage.

Screening

Screening persons at risk for CRC to detect precancerous polyps differs from screening for tumors like breast or cervical cancer. Whereas the mammogram and the Papanicolau smear are single examinations that are widely accepted and used and for which little overall controversy remains, for CRC there continues to be several available screening examinations and various different strategies recommended by several health care advisory committees (Table 1).

Existing clinical trials for CRC screening have not directly compared different screening approaches for clinical effectiveness or cost-effectiveness and have not tested starting and stopping ages. In an analysis of seven publications using simulation analyses, Pignone and coworkers [7] found that any of the commonly recommended screening strategies for adults age 50 years or greater reduce mortality from CRC. The cost per life-year saved for CRC screening ranges from $10,000 to $25,000 and compares favorably with other commonly endorsed preventative health care interventions, such as screening mammography. There have been no conclusions on the most cost-effective strategy.

Various options exist because no single test shows unequivocal superiority. Although this allows patients a choice, perhaps promoting greater compliance, these choices might result in confusion. This might in part explain why less than 40% [8] of screen-eligible patients in the United States have ever undergone CRC screening. More probable explanations for underscreening include embarrassment, fear, and aversion to the colonic cleansing required for some examinations [9].

Recent increases in public awareness, in part through the publicity surrounding sports personalities like Darryl Strawberry and media personalities like Katie Couric, have finally brought screening for CRC to the forefront. Nonetheless, efforts must still increase exponentially to help recruit the millions of people at risk who still go unscreened.

Indirect studies have demonstrated that as many as 95% of cancers arise from colorectal adenomas along the adenoma-carcinoma sequence [10]. Because this process has been estimated to take an average of 10 years to occur (polyp dwell time), there is ample time during which screening can be performed, and ample opportunity to prevent deaths caused by this leading cancer killer [11].

For the estimated 12,000,000 American adults each year [12] who become eligible for screening, by virtue of turning age 50, without other known risk factors (so-called "average risk"), numerous options are available, including the fecal occult blood test, sigmoidoscopy, colonoscopy, barium enema, fecal DNA assay, and CTC.

Fecal occult blood test

Four randomized controlled trials of serial fecal occult blood test conducted in Minnesota, the United Kingdom, Sweden, and Denmark involving more than 300,000 subjects followed for up to 18 years has consistently demonstrated that serial fecal occult blood test reduces colorectal mortality from 15% to 33% [10,13]. The test suffers from many false-positive and false-negative results, however, with a reported sensitivity for detection of CRC in the range of 27% to 57%, and as low as 8% for adenoma [14]. Rare red meat and some vegetables and fruits containing peroxidase can cause false-positive results. Nonbleeding CRC and polyps

Table 1: Screening recommendations for colorectal cancer and polyps

Risk category	Screening method	Age to begin screening
Average risk	Choose one of the following Fecal occult blood testing annually Flexible sigmoidoscopy every 5 years Fecal occult blood testing annually and flexible sigmoidoscopy every 5 years[a] Double-contrast barium enema every 5 to 10 years[b] Colonoscopy every 10 years	50 years
Family history	Choose one of the following Colonoscopy every 10 years Double-contrast barium enema every 5 to 10 years	40 years or 10 years before cancer was diagnosed in the youngest affected family member, whichever is earlier 5 years
Hereditary nonpolyposis colorectal cancer	Colonoscopy every 1 to 3 years Genetic counseling Consider genetic testing	21 years
Familial adenomatous polyposis	Flexible sigmoidoscopy or colonoscopy every 1 to 2 years Genetic counseling Consider genetic testing	Puberty
Ulcerative colitis	Colonoscopy with biopsies for dysplasia every 1 to 2 years	Seven to eight years after the diagnosis of pancolitis 12 to 15 years after the diagnosis of left-sided colitis

[a] Some experts recommend combining annual fecal occult blood testing with flexible sigmoidoscopy every 5 years.
[b] Rigid proctoscopy is recommended as an adjunctive examination to allow adequate visualization of the distal rectum. Flexible sigmoidoscopy may be necessary to evaluate tortuous or spostic signoid color.
From Read TE, Kodner IJ. Colorectal cancer: risk factors and recommendations for early detection. Am Fam Physician 1999;59:3803–92; with permission. Copyright ©1999 American Academy of Family Physicians. All rights reserved.

(the majority) and tumors in persons ingesting vitamin C can cause false-negative fecal occult blood test results. Most people with a positive test do not have CRC, but are subjected to the risk, cost, and discomfort associated with colonoscopy. Furthermore, compliance rates in the largest trials were below 60% [11,14]. Recent evidence, comparing the immunohistochemical tests for a single monoclonal antibody agglutinating with hemoglobin A showed a higher specificity and sensitivity for human hemoglobin than the guaiac-based fecal occult blood test [14]. Finally, stool obtained during a digital rectal examination is inadequate to screen for fecal occult blood, and despite its widespread use, this type of testing is not recommended.

Sigmoidoscopy

Flexible sigmoidoscopy provides direct visualization of a portion of the colon and suspicious lesions can be removed. It is a very safe procedure with only two perforations reported in a retrospective review of 49,501 examinations [10]. Only 65% to 75% of adenomatous polyps and 40% to 65% of CRC, however, are within the reach of the 60-cm flexible sigmoidoscope. In fact, recent observational studies from colonoscopy suggest that one half of all advanced adenomas (>1 cm) and cancers in the proximal colon are missed on sigmoidoscopy [10]. This explains why this type of examination has been referred to in the radiology community as tantamount to performing a unilateral mammogram to screen for breast cancer [15]. The sensitivity of sigmoidoscopy for CRC and large polyps is 96% and for small polyps 73%. The specificity for CRC and large polyps is 94% and for small polyps 92%. Nonetheless, no completed, large, randomized controlled trials have demonstrated the effectiveness of sigmoidoscopy in the prevention of CRC death. Only indirect evidence from case-control studies supports its effectiveness. Mortality reductions of between 59% and 80% have been reported [13]. Two ongoing studies, the National Cancer Institute Prostate, Lung, Colorectal and Ovarian screening trial and the UK Flexiscope Trial, will assess 60-cm flexible sigmoidoscopy in more than 250,000 subjects. The US Agency for Health Care Policy and Research recommends flexible sigmoidoscopy every 5 years. Colonoscopy should follow sigmoidoscopy when factors associated with an increased risk for proximal neoplasia are present, including age >65 years, a polyp with villous histology, adenoma ≥ 1 cm, multiple distal adenomas, and a family history of CRC. Current evidence suggests that the risk of advanced neoplasia in persons with only a distal hyperplastic polyp is not greater than those without distal polyps.

The reduction in CRC mortality using a combined approach of fecal occult blood test and sigmoidoscopy has never been studied in a randomized trial, but two randomized controlled trials have reported that the addition of a one-time fecal occult blood test to sigmoidoscopy increased the detection of CRC from 70% to 76%. The ACS and other agencies recommend a yearly fecal occult blood test in combination with sigmoidoscopy every 5 years as one method of screening. This option continues to be viewed as inferior if colonoscopy resources are available, because direct visualization of the entire colon is only possible with colonoscopy [11].

Fecal DNA analysis

The molecular genetics of CRC were initially popularized by molecular biologists in the late 1980s [16]. Eighty-five percent of CRC result from chromosomal instability, with mutations involving the adenomatous polyposis coli gene, the p53 tumor-suppressor gene, and the K-ras oncogene. The other 15% arise from loss of genes involved in DNA mismatch repair, manifested by microsatellite instability. A recent study comparing a fecal-based, multitarget DNA panel with Hemoccult II in asymptomatic adults 50 years of age or older who were at average risk for CRC revealed a sensitivity four times that of the Hemoccult test (51.6% versus 12.9%, $P = .003$) for invasive cancer and more than twice as sensitive as the Hemoccult for advanced adenoma (40.8% versus 14.1%, $P < .001$) without a loss of specificity (94.4% for fecal DNA versus 95.2% for Hemoccult II) [8]. The increased detection of non-advanced adenoma from 11% to 15% was not significant. In previous studies, not exclusively confined to asymptomatic patients, the sensitivity for detection of cancer has ranged from 37% to 71%. In this and other studies, most lesions detected by colonoscopy were not detected by either test. Although colonoscopy is superior to other tests, the Preventive Services Task Force has determined that

no single test or strategy for CRC screening can be endorsed on the basis of currently available data. Although the fecal DNA test has a low sensitivity, potentially limiting its use as a one-time test for cancer, like the Hemoccult test, its use at more frequent intervals might be as effective as a more sensitive test used infrequently, such as colonoscopy. More studies are needed at this time. The ACS, at the time of this writing, does not yet include this test in its screening recommendations. Reasons may include (1) a wide confidence interval of sensitivity of 35% to 68% at a 95% probability; (2) higher cost; and (3) acceptability (patients must collect and refrigerate an entire bowel movement).

Barium enema: time to put it to rest?

Double-contrast barium enema (DCBE) is included in the screening recommendations of the ACS at 5-year intervals. The rationale for its inclusion includes its cost-effectiveness [17] and wide availability. It is less sensitive at detecting colonic neoplasms than colonoscopy, and cannot remove polyps. Although to date randomized controlled trials are not available to determine if screening by DCBE reduces mortality from CRC, DCBE detects most advanced adenomas and cancers [10]. In the National Polyp Study, however, the sensitivity for polyps even as large as 1 cm or greater was approximately 50%. Many false-negative results are found for smaller polyps, but their clinical importance is questionable [18]. A case-control study did reveal a 33% reduction in CRC death, but confidence intervals were wide [19]. In a nonrandomized study of 2193 consecutive CRC cases in a community practice the sensitivity of DCBE for cancer was 85% compared with colonoscopy of 95% [20]. Finally, an investigation that received a lot publicity and caused a lot of uproar in the radiology community [21,22], and which may have done more to harm the reputation of the DCBE than warranted, was a prospective study in a surveillance population compared with colonoscopy as a gold standard. Here, DCBE detected only 39% of polyps identified at colonoscopy, including 21% of polyps 5 mm or smaller, 53% of adenomatous polyps 6 to 10 mm in size, and only 48% of those >1 cm in size. Some of the limitations of this study included the presence of only 23 lesions greater than 1 cm in 973 patients, the risk of extrapolating data from a surveillance population to a screening population, and the lack of generalizability of results derived from expert academic centers to community practice. Additionally, the high completion rate of colonoscopy in this study and the 3:1 ratio of male to female patients may not reflect a true screening situation in the average community practice. Use of sensitivity statistics from a one-time screening examination also ignores the potential for subsequent detection of early lesions on repeat screening studies [17]. Finally, as the authors of this same study admit, "screening and diagnostic tests are judged not only on the basis of their accuracy in detecting and ruling out lesions but also on the basis of their safety, convenience, acceptance by patients, cost and cost-effectiveness, as well as on the number of physicians needed to conduct the examination properly" [23].

A survey performed in collaboration with the National Cancer Institute, the Centers for Disease Control and Prevention, and the Centers for Medicare and Medicaid Services published in 2002 found evidence to support the claims of a continuing trend of colonoscopy replacing DCBE as an initial colorectal examination since 1980. Although the benefits of colonoscopy are well known and publicized, in this survey of 1718 primary care physicians and 381 nationally representative radiologists, 75% of radiologists but only 33% of primary care physicians rated DCBE as a "very effective" modality. Furthermore, despite high ratings by both groups, fewer than 10% of radiologists and fewer than 10% of primary care physicians reported that colonoscopy should be or was the screening approach most often recommended to their patients. Single-contrast barium enema is less sensitive than DCBE, and alone is not recommended as a screening strategy [18].

Colonoscopy

There are no randomized control studies evaluating whether colonoscopy screening alone reduces the incidence or mortality from CRC in people at average risk. But two large cohort studies, the Italian Multicenter Study [24] and the National Polyp Study [25], revealed a reduction in CRC incidence compared with nonconcurrent control groups. The National Cancer Institute is now sponsoring a study of colonoscopy screening (Prostate, Lung, Colorectal and Ovarian). The trial began in 1993 and closed to accrual in 2001, with screening continuing until 2006 and follow-up anticipated for 10 years thereafter. The study includes nearly 155,000 men and women aged 55 to 74 [26]. The ACS and others recommend screening colonoscopy every 10 years based on data extrapolated from sigmoidoscopy studies showing a protective effect of endoscopy up to 10 years [11]. In addition, Medicare instituted reimbursement of screening colonoscopy as of July 2001.

The test is performed with a 160-cm flexible endoscope. A recent large study of screening colonoscopy resulted in a completion rate of 98% of patients with a mean procedure time of 30 minutes [27], but completion rates of 75% to 96% have been reported elsewhere [17,18]. The safety of the test has been well-established, but the rate of perforation and death is not trivial. Perforation or hemorrhage is reported to occur in 1 of 500 examinations with fatality in 1 of 5000 [28]. By comparison, for barium enema, important complications of any type arise in 1 of 10,000 cases and the perforation rate is reported to be 1 of 25,000 cases with death in 1 of 55,000 [29]. Although colonoscopy is considered the criterion standard for detecting CRC and adenomas, it is an imperfect examination. Up to 6% of advanced adenomas were missed in an oft-quoted series of back-to-back examinations performed by two expert examiners. Miss rates were 13% for adenomas 6 to 9 mm and 27% for those below 5 mm [30]. More recent data using the newly developed CTC have challenged previously undisputed claims of excellent accuracy in colonoscopy. Using a method known as "segmental unblinding," a second colonoscopic inspection is made in a segment with a positive finding at CTC. With this new standard, Pickhardt and coworkers revealed a colonoscopic miss rate of 10% for polyps ≥ 10 mm [31,32].

Reported sensitivities for colonoscopy are 96.7% for cancer, 85% for large polyps, and 78.5% for small polyps, with a specificity of 98% for all lesions [33]. Although it is the only technique that offers screening, diagnosis, and therapeutic management of the entire colon in one procedure, it involves greater cost, risk, and inconvenience to the patient than other screening tests, all important features to be taken into consideration for any screening test.

Finally, two recent trends and two new developments warrant mentioning. First, misuse of this expensive resource, specifically, unwarranted repeat colonoscopy or short interval surveillance for insignificant hyperplastic polyps or even mucosal tags, has been documented by the US National Cancer Institute survey regarding postpolypectomy surveillance [34]. In an era in which waiting lists for colonoscopy exist in parts of the country this practice may result in even further decreased rates of screening [35]. Second, the recent introduction of intravenous propofol, a deep sedative hypnotic medication, administered by an anesthesiologist (and adding significantly to the cost of the procedure) has resulted in fewer incomplete colonoscopies in the authors' institution and likely on a national basis. Two new exciting colonoscopic developments beyond the scope of this article include the use of endoscopic mucosal resection, whereby at colonoscopy solution is injected submucosally before polypectomy, and chromoendoscopy, in which characterization of mucosal topography is used to predict histology. The reader is referred to Saitoh and coworkers [36].

CT colonography (virtual colonoscopy)

This new technology (described further later) is not as yet approved for use as a screening test. No randomized controlled studies are available investigating the ability of CTC to reduce CRC morbidity. Until recently, no screening studies were available to evaluate the efficacy of CTC, and the accuracy of the test had to be extrapolated from multiple studies using primarily surveillance-type populations.

The appeal of CTC in the screening setting derives from the fact that the examination is a noninvasive CT scan that uses no sedatives or contrast media, and could provide an attractive alternative for many patients who refuse to or cannot undergo colonoscopy. Because it is an imaging test only, and cannot remove polyps, its role is limited compared with colonoscopy.

The first and largest screening study performed by Pickhardt and coworkers [37] at three United States military hospitals revealed that CTC performed as well as or better than optical colonoscopy in a same-day back-to-back correlative comparison of 1233 asymptomatic subjects at average risk for CRC. Five experienced radiologists and 17 experienced colonoscopists were involved. Sensitivity for adenomatous polyps was 94% for CTC versus 92% for optical colonoscopy at the 8-mm diameter threshold and 96% for CTC versus 88% for optical colonoscopy at the 10-mm threshold size. The accuracy of CTC for adenomatous polyps on a per-patient basis was 92% for 8 mm and 96% for 10 mm. CTC depicted 54 (91.5%) of 59 advanced neoplasms, whereas optical colonoscopy depicted 52 (88.1%). The negative predictive value of CTC was 99% for adenomas 8 mm or larger. The authors were the first to use a primary three-dimensional interpretation method after fecal tagging with barium and meglumine diatrizoate, followed by electronic subtraction of labeled stool and fluid using a commercially available, US Food and Drug Administration–approved computer. The technique of segmental unblinding (see later) allowed separate validation of both CTC and colonoscopy. These results closely mimicked or improved on a large number of preceding studies performed in surveillance or mixed-type populations, using combined two-dimensional and three-dimensional interpretations, without fecal tagging and electronic subtraction (Table 2) [2,38,39]. A coincident study, not performed in a screening population and using older technology with less reader experience [40], led to much argument and deliberation in the literature, and served well to point out the necessity of attention to detail (ie, slice thickness, polyp nomenclature, and reader experience) required to achieve robust and reliable results, and to point out the existence of a steep radiologist's learning curve for CTC [41]. Nonetheless, as of this writing, no other large study in screening subjects has been performed to validate the Pickhardt study.

Other screening trials now in progress include a large multicenter trial launched by the American College of Radiology Imaging Network to test two-dimensional versus three-dimensional accuracy in 2600 subjects. The Special Interest Group in Gastrointestinal and Abdominal Radiology (United Kingdom) will compare CTC with barium enema and colonoscopy in 4500 patients. The Italian Multicenter Study on Accuracy of CT Colonography will enroll 3550 patients.

Because of the novelty of this technique, cost-effectiveness has only been able to be investigated using various statistical models [42–44]. Taking into account compliance, the cost of care from missed polyps, the avoidance of perforations and other factors, and assuming optimal sensitivity and specificity for CTC, some investigators have determined that the cost of CTC has to be significantly lower than colonoscopy (up to 54% less) to be cost effective [42].

Numerous studies have looked at patient comfort and preference for CTC versus colonoscopy [45] and found varying results. In a recent study testing preference immediately after each test and 5 weeks later, CTC with bowel relaxants was preferred over colonoscopy [46].

Although CTC is noninvasive, potentially serious adverse events have been reported in 0.08% of symptomatic patients and perforations have occurred in 0.05% to 0.059% [47,48]. By comparison, the colonoscopy perforation rate reported in the same and similar hospitals was 0.13%, suggesting a much lower risk with CTC [47].

Finally, use of a screening test that uses radiation must address concerns regarding potential radiation-induced cancers. According to one investigator, the best estimate for the absolute lifetime cancer risk using the typical scanner (prone and supine scans, for one CTC only) is about 0.14% in a 50 year old and half of that in a 70 year old. Multiple interval examinations increase these values [49].

Diagnosis and staging

The diagnosis of CRC is definitively made at histopathologic examination using biopsy or surgical specimens, although radiographic appearances can be pathognomonic. Most often, colonic malignancy is discovered through asymptomatic screening examinations; during endoscopic examinations done for symptoms; as incidental discovery on imaging tests; by clinical examination revealing signs of intestinal blood loss (hematochezia, or tarry stools); or as a result of abnormal blood tests indicating anemia or elevated carcinoembryonic antigen (CEA). Once discovered or suspected, confirmation and simultaneous staging are the roles most often conferred on CT, MR imaging, ultrasound, CTC, and DCBE. The radiologist must describe tumor size; location; depth of local wall penetration, if feasible; involvement of nodes; spread to other organs; and associated complications, such as obstruction, hemorrhage, abscess formation, inflammation, perforation and the like (within the limitations of the modality). In the following subsections, each modality is reviewed with respect to expected appearances and pitfalls in detecting and staging CRC and its relative accuracy in staging.

Staging of CRC has evolved to the use of tumor, node, metastasis system (Table 3), rather than the Duke's classification or the modified Duke's (Astler-Collin's) system. These latter systems are not discussed. The tumor, node, metastasis system results in stage groupings for which prognostic and survival statistics are published (Table 4). The stages and associated survival statistics are based on pathologic staging not radiologic assessments (eg, pT1; pathologic T1 not uT1; ultrasound stage T1).

Barium enema

The role of the single-contrast barium enema or the DCBE in diagnosing and staging known or suspected CRC is threefold: (1) it can be used to diagnose colon cancer in those patients undergoing screening or work-up of symptoms; (2) it can be used to complete the total colon examination in cases of incomplete colonoscopy, a role traditionally reserved for barium enema, but now largely replaced by CTC; and (3) it can simply confirm a suspected diagnosis of CRC from other imaging or clinical tests when colonoscopy is not available, not affordable, or not preferred by the patient. Although it is inferior to colonoscopy in the detection of small polyps, large polyps, and cancers, it has many advantages including lower cost, lack of necessity for sedation, greater safety, and wider availability. Furthermore, because colonoscopy can occasionally miss lesions, these two examinations may be viewed as complementary, the development of CTC notwithstanding. It is unfortunate that the explosive technologic imaging revolution has resulted in a diminishing cadre of highly skilled radiologists who perform and teach these worthwhile examinations. Nonetheless, with scrupulous attention to good colonic cleansing and with rigorous fluoroscopic-radiographic technique, described in detail elsewhere [50], most polyps and cancers can be detected with DCBE.

The detection of adenomatous polyps, which may undergo malignant transformation through the adenoma-carcinoma sequence, and the detection of neoplasms is the primary goal. Most polyps never become CRC [51], and the risk is related to polyp size. Only about 1% of polyps less than 10 mm harbor CRC, whereas 10% to 20% of adenomas 10 to 20 mm in diameter and 40% to 50% of those greater than 20 mm in diameter harbor adenocarcinoma.

Small, classic, hyperplastic polyps, often effaced by distention, are not important to detect, because they are not believed to undergo this transformation (a recently described hyperplastic polyposis syndrome of "serrated" adenomas is one exception, but these are larger lesions) [52].

Adenomas are classified as tubular, tubulovillous, or villous at histologic examination. The greater the amount of the villous component, the greater is the risk of malignant degeneration. Polyps may be flat, sessile, or pedunculated (Fig. 1). A pedunculated polyp with a stalk longer than 2 cm is rarely associated with invasive carcinoma. On DCBE, sessile polyps on the dependent surface appear as filling defects in a pool of barium. Those on the nondependent surface are etched in white and appear as ring shadows (Fig. 2). These can at times be confused with diverticula, but the "bowler-hat" appearance with the dome of the hat pointed inward toward the colon lumen distinguishes these from diverticula [53]. The most common entity confused with polyps is stool. Even in a well-prepared colon, one or two fragments of fecal residue may persist, requiring rotation and repositioning or gentle palpation of the patient (Fig. 3). Villous adenomas have a higher risk of malignant degeneration. They are recognized by their granular or reticular appearance because of the filling of the interstices on the polyp surface (Fig. 4). Carpet-lesions, a particularly worrisome diffuse type of villous tumor, may be hard to recognize and may be confused for stool. These may protrude very little into the colon lumen [53]. Flat-lesions are a diagnosis de rigueur of late, because of the recognition that these may easily be missed at colonoscopy and CTC. These are important and controversial lesions. It is estimated that 36% of adenomas in European populations and 22.7% of adenomas in the United States population may be flat [54,55]. Controversy surrounds reports that these are more likely to have advanced dysplasia compared with protuberant polyps. One problem, learned from the CTC literature, is the inconsistent distinction of these from, for example, sessile lesions. A small study of flat adenomas found that their detection was limited at DCBE compared with colonoscopy [56].

Table 2:   Literature survey of CT colonoscopy

		Per polyp sensitivity %			
	N patients	Overall	Detection of polyps <6 mm	Detection of polyps 6–9 mm	Detection of polyps >9 mm
Rockey et al, 2005	614	—	—	60	64
Chung et al, 2005	51	90	84	94	100
Cotton et al, 2004	600	12.7	7.6	22.7	51.9
Macari et al, 2004	186	27.7	14.7	46.2	90.9
Van Gelder et al, 2004	249	51.8	40.6	76.7	77.8
Macari et al, 2004	68	21.4	11.5	52.9	100
Hoppe et al, 2004	92	42.6	25.4	57.9	70.6
Pickhardt et al, 2003	1233	—	—	83.6	92.2
Iannaccone et al, 2003	158	70.3	51.4	83.3	100
Johnson et al, 2003	703	—	—	47.1	46.3
Pineau et al, 2003	205	46.8	29.4	75	77.8
Taylor et al, 2003	54	48.4	37.5	75	100
Ginnerup Pedersen et al, 2003	144	—	—	73.7	92.3
Yee et al, 2003	182	69.9	60.3	79.8	92.7
Munikrishnan et al, 2003	61	75.8	53.3	83.3	100
Laghi et al, 2002	165	78.4	50	82.4	91.7
Gluecker et al, 2005	50	22.4	2.4	33.3	81.8
Lefere et al, 2002	100	77.5	56.5	90.3	100
Macari et al, 2002	105	32.6	12.1	70.4	92.9
McFarland et al, 2002	70	—	—	36.1	68.1
Yee et al, 2001	300	77.5	66.9	81.8	94.1
Hara et al, 2001	237	—	—	—	—
Spinzi et al, 2001	96	57.8	—	—	61.5
Fletcher et al, 2000	180	60.1	—	47.2	75.2
Morrin et al, 2000	81	—	32.9	64.5	90.9
Mendelson et al, 2000	53	27.5	17.5	22.2	72.7
Macari et al, 2000	42	37.5	20	60	100
Morrin et al, 2000	34	—	—	—	—
Fenlon et al, 1999	100	71.3	66.7	89.7	90.9
Rex et al, 1999	46	22	11.1	42.9	50
Dachman et al, 1998	44	46.7	7.7	33.3	83.3
Royster et al, 1997	20	91.4	66.7	90	100
Hara et al, 1997	70	37.4	25.9	57.1	70

From Mulhall BP, Veerpan GR, Jackson JL. Meta-analysis: computed tomographic colonography. Ann Intern Med 2005;142:635–650; with permission.

Most CRC are detected on DCBE, and are either semiannular or annular (Fig. 5). Fewer than 10% appear as polypoid or carpet lesions [53]. False-negative examinations do occur when lesions are overlooked because of perceptive error from overlapping bowel loops (Fig. 6). Overlooked carcinomas in the rectum may occur if the rectal tube or balloon obscures the mucosa. Attention to technique avoids these errors (Fig. 7).

Rarely, other abnormalities may mimic annular CRC, such as amoeboma or histoplasmoma [57]. In the authors' oncologic population, slow-growing secondary malignancies, such as ovarian cancer, have occasionally been seen to mimic the annular appearance of primary CRC (Fig. 8). Because 5% of patients with CRC have a synchronous lesion, every attempt should be made to examine the entire colon at DCBE when one nonobstructive lesion is found. Single-contrast barium enema has been shown to be inferior to DCBE. Although a large annular lesion may be very well appreciated, smaller malignancies can be missed in the barium pool even with systematic compression [58]. The use of single-contrast barium enema (or water soluble–based contrast enema) is best reserved for the elderly and infirm and those cases in which there is a question of obstruction, perforation, or anastomotic leak. Barium enema plays a minimal role in the diagnosis of recurrent CRC. Most cases arise extraluminally next to or distant from the regions of resection of the primary tumor, rather than at the anastomosis. For

Table 2: (continued)

	Per patient sensitivity %		Detection of polyps 6–9 mm		Detection of polyps of >9 mm	
Overall	Patients with cancer	Overall specificity %	Sensitivity %	Specificity %	Sensitivity %	Specificity %
—	78	—	51	—	59	96
—	—	—	—	—	—	—
20.5	75	90.5	30.3	93.1	54.8	95.9
—	—	83.1	—	—	—	—
62.1	—	30.6	—	—	83.9	92
—	—	89.7	—	—	—	98.5
73.3	87.5	—	—	—	95	98.5
—	—	—	—	—	93.8	96
96	100	96.5	—	—	—	—
—	—	—	52.2	91.2	47.9	97.5
61.8	—	70.7	—	—	90	94.6
64.5	83.3	—	50	—	90	100
—	—	—	82.4	—	95.7	—
90.4	—	82.4	—	—	—	—
74.3	96.6	96.2	—	—	—	—
93	100	—	—	—	—	—
—	—	90.5	—	—	—	—
86	—	—	91.3	92.2	100	100
57.6	100	87	—	—	—	—
—	—	—	71.3	—	87.5	—
93.9	100	56.5	95.2	—	100	—
—	—	—	—	—	67.9	95.5
—	87.5	—	—	—	—	—
—	—	—	—	—	85.4	92.9
—	—	—	72.7	96.6	87.5	100
—	—	—	—	—	—	—
—	100	—	—	—	—	—
82.4	100	83.7	94	92	96	96
45.5	—	—	42.9	—	80	88.9
43.8	—	89.3	—	—	—	—
—	95	—	—	—	—	—
—	—	—	—	—	75	90.5

this reason, CT or PET is of greater use than luminal investigations, such as barium enema or colonoscopy.

CT

Extrahepatic disease

CT technology has evolved rapidly from incremental to single-slice helical to 4-, 8-, 16-, 64-, and 256-slice multidetector scanners now commercially available. Images obtained from 16-slice (or greater) scanners can be near-isotropic (ie, nearly perfectly cubical voxels without distortion of anatomy). This allows for so-called "volumetric imaging" during a single breathhold in many instances covering the entire chest, abdomen, and pelvis. The acquisition of ultrathin slices (typically 0.5, 0.625, or 0.75 mm depending on the vendor) allows reformation of images in any plane without loss of resolution (isotropic) [59]. This technologic advance, allowing multiplanar postprocessing, puts CT on par with or ahead of (because of better spatial resolution) MR imaging. Nonetheless, a remaining advantage of MR imaging is the lack of ionizing radiation.

Faster CT scanning requires faster injection rates, smaller volumes, the use of saline bolus chasers, more concentrated iodine contrast agents, and longer delays between injection time and scan time. For a complete discussion on this topic the reader is referred to the review by Brink [60]. Various CT angiographic techniques can be used for preoperative liver assessment (discussed later).

Although CT scan is widely used for preoperative staging of CRC, there is no consensus on its use in

Table 3:   TNM staging system for colorectal cancer

Stage	Definition
Primary tumor (T)	
TX	Primary tumor cannot be assessed
T0	No evidence of primary tumor
Tis	Carcinoma *in situ:* intraepithelial or invasion of lamina propria
T1	Tumor invades submucosa
T2	Tumor invades muscularis propria
T3	Tumor invades through muscularis propria into the subserosa or into nonperitonealized pericolic or perirectal tissues
T4	Tumor perforates visceral peritoneum or directly invades other organs or structures
Regional lymph nodes (N)[a]	
NX	Regional lymph nodes could not be assessed
N0	No regional lymph node metastases
N1	Metastases in one to three regional lymph nodes
N2	Metastases in four or more regional lymph nodes
Distant metastases (M)	
MX	Distant metastases could not be assessed
M0	No distant metastases
M1	Distant metastases
Extent of resection (R)[b]	
RX	Presence of residual tumor cannot be assessed
R0	No residual tumor
R1	Microscopic residual tumor
R2	Macroscopic residual tumor

[a] A tumor nodule greater than 3 mm in diameter in perirectal or pericolic adipose tissue without histologic evidence of a residual lymph note in the nodule is classified as residual lymph node metastases; however, a tumor nodule up to 3 mm in diameter is classified in the T category as discontinuous extension (ie, T3)
[b] Cases not considered R0 (complete resection) if the following are evident: non-en-bloc resection; radial or bowel margin positive for disease; residual lymph node disease; or NX (incomplete resection)
From Nelson H, Petrelli N, Carlin A, et al. Guidelines 2000 for colon and rectal surgery. J Natl Cancer Inst 2001;93:8; with permission.

preoperative scanning of patients with intraperitoneal colon cancer. Although detection of primary colon lesions is usually made by colonoscopy or barium enema, the increased use of CT for a variety of gastrointestinal symptoms is such that the radiologist may be the first to detect CRC based on CT findings. CT is most useful for detecting metastatic disease and regional tumor extension. Complications, such as obstruction, perforation, and fistula, can be readily visualized. CT is also useful in identifying recurrences, evaluating anatomic relationships, documenting normal postoperative anatomy, and confirming the absence of new lesions during and after therapy. A recent study of CT in 130 Veterans Administration patients to determine clinical use and cost-effectiveness found disease previously unknown to the surgeon as follows: demonstration of local extension (9%); demonstration of metastases (15%); unsuspected vascular abnormalities (10%); second malignancies (4%); and other pathology (13%). The investigators determined that the preoperative scan directly aided operative planning in 43 (33%) cases; actually altered management (surgery canceled) in six cases (5%); and led to qualitatively different care in 16%. The sensitivity and specificity for all metastases were 75% and 99%, respectively. For liver metastases these were 90% and 99%, respectively [61]. Furthermore, a cost savings of $24,000 was realized over 5 years.

Patients undergo scanning using multidetector scans after the ingestion of oral contrast and the intravenous injection of an equivalent dose of 45 g of

Table 4:   Colon cancer 5-year survival rates

Stage	%
Stage I	93
Stage IIA	85
Stage IIB	72
Stage IIIA	83
Stage IIIB	64
Stage IIIC	44
Stage IV	8

I, T1,2,N0M0; IIA, T3 N0M0; IIB, T4N0M0; IIIA, T1,2N1M0; IIIB, T3,4N1M0; IIIC, any T, N2M0; IV, any T, any N, M1.
Reprinted with the permission of the American Cancer Society, Inc. All rights reserved.

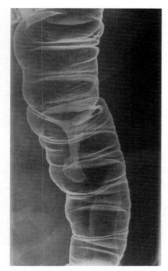

Fig. 1. Double-contrast barium enema reveals a pedunculated left colon polyp with a long stalk.

iodine in the form of low or iso-osmolar contrast medium. Routine scans are currently acquired at 0.625-mm or 1.25-mm slice thickness, during a single breathhold, in the portal venous phase of liver enhancement and reconstructed axially for viewing at 5-mm or thinner slices. Oral contrast can be given the night before to opacify the colon, or can be given rectally, but this is not routinely indicated, because primary disease has usually already been confirmed. Reformatted images may also be used if determined helpful.

The primary lesion, unless sizable, may not be seen unless the colon has been previously cleansed, an unusual scenario. Even in the uncleansed colon

on routine CT, polypoid or annular lesions can be well-appreciated because of their enhancement and more solid appearance compared with stool (Fig. 9). Associated findings, such as lymphadenopathy, peritoneal implants (Fig. 10), tumor penetration through the bowel wall, and colonic obstruction, can be well-appreciated. Tumor appearances may vary from a discrete mass narrowing the lumen, to bowel wall thickening (see Fig. 10), to a necrotic mass appearing much like an abscess. In cases of associated inflammation and microperforation, the primary differential diagnosis is perforated diverticulitis. The presence of lymph nodes may help distinguish tumors from diverticulitis, whereas many other findings are shared by both [62]. Tumors may intussuscept and be easily recognized in longitudinal (Fig. 11) or axial plane. Mucinous tumors may be quite bulky. If mucinous colonic or appendiceal tumors perforate, patients may present with pseudomyxoma peritonei at CT (Fig. 12). Pericolic tumor extension can be suggested (T3 disease) on CT when the fat planes are blurred, but this appearance is not specific, nor is it sensitive. Inflammation or deep ulceration may cause blurred fat planes. Normal fat planes may be seen with microscopic penetration of the muscularis propria.

Peritoneal surfaces may be involved with tumor in up to 10% to 15% of patients at the time of diagnosis of CRC, and 40% to 70% of patients with recurrent CRC [63]. Although CT may currently be the best modality to detect early disease, it remains limited, even with helical technology and thin slices. CRC peritoneal tumor nodules less than 1 cm were detected in 9% to 24% of 25 patients in a recent study in which non–picture archiving and communications system observation methods

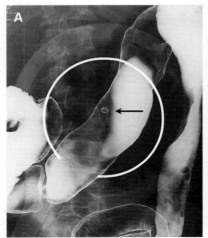
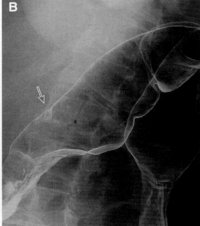

Fig. 2. (*A*) Double-contrast barium enema reveals a ring-like density etched-in-white in the transverse colon representing a polyp viewed en face (*arrow*). (*B*) More oblique view reveals a small pedunculated polyp (*arrow*).

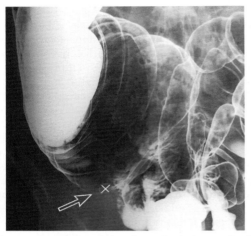

Fig. 3. A fecal filling defect (*arrow*) mimics a polyp in the cecum (confirmed at colonoscopy).

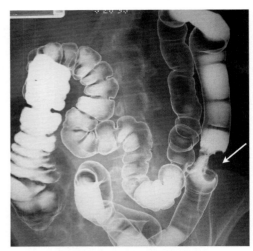

Fig. 5. Double-contrast barium enema reveals an annular or apple-core–type appearance indicating primary colon cancer (*arrow*).

were used. Overall, for all sizes, two radiologists detected only 60% to 76% of peritoneal implants with a poor interobserver agreement level. Surprisingly, these poor results are little improved from the pre-helical CT era where up to one third of peritoneal metastases were missed in patients undergoing staging laparoscopy for gastric adenocarcinoma [64]. It is expected that with the use of multidetector scanners and picture archiving and communications system for reviewing images, greater accuracy can be achieved.

CT provides the best resolution of any known imaging modality and is the first choice for lung nodule detection. Despite its high sensitivity, specificity is quite poor. In a recent series of high-risk oncologic patients with nodules 3 cm or less (75%

were equal or less than 1 cm), in only 60% of patients with a solitary nodule and in only 64% of patients with multiple nodules were the nodules malignant [65].

CRC may recur in between 37% and 44% of patients after curative resection, usually within 2 years. Local recurrence accounts for 19% to 48%, whereas distant metastases account for 25% to 44%. Multiple sites of recurrence are most common and local and distant recurrences are more common in rectal tumors. Local recurrences most often occur in the perianastomotic tissues or lymph nodes and may not be appreciated with luminal examinations like colonoscopy or barium enema. A recent study of recurrent CRC by CTC found that 46 of 51 local recurrences were in the extraluminal soft tissues [66]. It is critical to optimize the ability of CT to detect recurrence at anastomoses and perianastomotic tissues by ensuring a well-distended colon. CT is invaluable in assessing the response to chemotherapy through measurement of index lesions in the lung, liver, lymph nodes, or peritoneum.

Hepatic metastatic disease
CT scanning performed with the newer multidetector scanners may be timed to obtain images of the liver during both the hepatic arterial phase and the portal venous phase of hepatic parenchymal enhancement. This may improve both lesion visualization and characterization. The use of multidetector CT scanning with isotropic voxels allows for images to be reconstructed in any plane in both phases of contrast administration. For imaging of hepatic metastases, this generally permits better segmental visualization of the metastases relative to

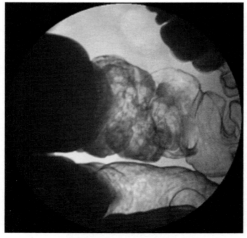

Fig. 4. Large filling defect in sigmoid colon with a typical lacy, reticulated surface pattern, representing a villous adenoma.

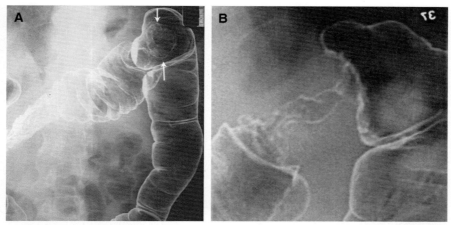

Fig. 6. (A) In the splenic flexure there is an abnormality that is not clearly characterized because of overlapping segments (*arrows*). (B) Rotating the patient reveals the pathognomonic appearance for a primary neoplasm.

hepatic arterial and portal venous structures. This may aid the surgeon for preoperative planning of resection of liver metastases [67,68]. The appearance of colorectal metastases to the liver depends in large part on both the phase of contrast administration in which the scanning is performed and the overall vascularity of the tumor. In general, colorectal metastases appear on CT scan as well-defined areas of low attenuation compared with normal hepatic parenchyma in the portal venous phase of enhancement (Fig. 13A). In the arterial phase, colorectal metastases may show rim enhancement with a relatively hyperdense rim. Some larger colorectal metastases may demonstrate central areas of low attenuation likely representing necrosis or cystic change. Hepatic metastases may be associated with calcification or the development of

calcification [69]. Overall, in a meta-analysis, the CT sensitivity for hepatic metastases was reported as 72% based on analysis in 1747 patients in 25 publications [70]. Overall CT has been shown to have a detection rate of 85.1% with a positive predictive value of 96.1% and a false-positive rate of 3.9%. Some entities that may be confused with colorectal metastases include hemangioendothelioma, hemangioma, hepatic peliosis, biliary adenoma, biliary hamartoma, and periportal fibrosis [71,72].

CT may also be performed during arterial portography. Before the advances in multidetector CT and MR imaging this technique was considered the most sensitive for lesion detection. CT arterial portography, however, is used less routinely with advances in other imaging modalities and because it

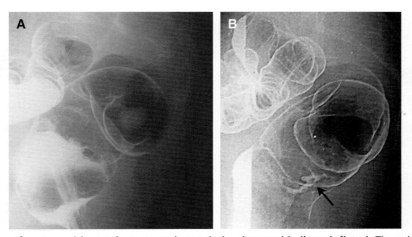

Fig. 7. (A) View of rectum with rectal enema catheter tip in place and balloon inflated. There is no apparent abnormality. (B) After removal of the catheter an irregular lesion is revealed on the lateral wall (*arrow*). This represented rectal carcinoma.

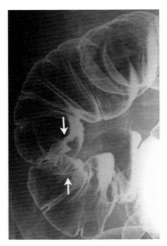

Fig. 8. In the ascending colon, near the ileocecal valve location, an annular mass is noted (*arrows*). This represented gradual circumferential invasion from an extrinsic ovarian peritoneal implant in the colic gutter.

is an invasive and costly procedure. It remains an option in the imaging armamentarium, especially for problem-solving cases or in difficult patients.

Virtual colonoscopy

This CT examination (also known as CT colonography) of the air-filled colon was first described by Vining and coworkers [73] in 1994 as a result of newly available software, which allowed perspective volume rendering (fly-through) of CT data for the first time. Since that time, there has been rapid development and improvement in the software, CT scanner hardware, computer processing speed and storage capabilities; the understanding of colonic cleansing preparations; reader-strategies and reader experience; and greater public awareness of the extent and importance of detecting colon polyps and colon cancer. This radiologic test has

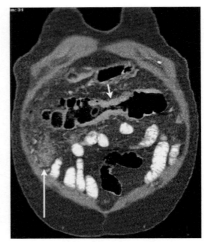

Fig. 10. Coronal-reformatted image in a different patient with a mid-transverse colon primary colon cancer manifested by wall thickening and luminal narrowing (*short arrow*). Note also the peritoneal infiltration (*long arrow*), representing extracolonic metastasis.

contributed greatly the public's awareness of radiologists and their role in cancer care.

Although created with the ultimate goal of becoming a more acceptable screening test for CRC, current indications, based on extensive evidence-based research, include a superior alternative to barium enema for total colon examination [74], especially in the setting of incomplete colonoscopy [75]; evaluation of the colon proximal to an obstructing neoplasm [76]; and as an alternative total colon examination in patients with comorbid factors precluding conventional colonoscopy (eg, on warfarin, pulmonary fibrosis, or allergic to sedatives) or in those who refuse this or other screening tests. It has also been suggested that it is useful in staging primary [77] and recurrent [78] colon cancer.

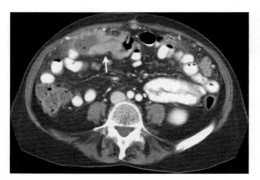

Fig. 9. Axial contrast-enhanced CT reveals a transverse colon mass (*arrow*) with wall thickening and narrowing of the lumen, consistent with tumor.

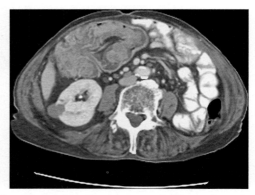

Fig. 11. Axial contrast-enhanced CT reveals a mass within the colon accompanied by mesenteric fat and vessels indicating an intussuscepting carcinoma.

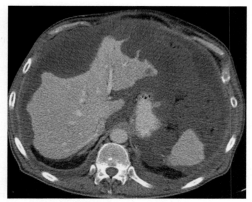

Fig. 12. Axial CT scan demonstrating scalloping of the liver surface, peritoneal fluid, and omental low-density mass indicative of pseudomyxoma peritonei in a patient with a perforated appendiceal carcinoma.

Advantages of CTC over colonoscopy include its noninvasiveness, lack of need for sedation, lower cost, and ability to detect significant extracolonic abnormalities and more accurate lesion location. Its main disadvantage is an inability to obtain biopsy material, because it is a noninvasive imaging test.

Using single breathhold helical thin-slice acquisitions (typically 1.25–2.5 cm, pitch 0.9–1.375) after undergoing an accepted colonic cleansing preparation (preferably a dry preparation rather than a wet preparation [79]) patients are scanned in prone and supine positions to redistribute retained fluid or mobile stool particles. Room air or carbon dioxide is insufflated by a physician, nurse, the patient themselves, or an automated pump until good colonic distention is achieved as ascertained with baseline and repeated low-dose scout topograms (Fig. 14). Carbon dioxide is theorized to be reabsorbed more rapidly and to be more comfortable for the patient after the examination is completed (based on older barium enema literature). Automated insufflation seems to allow better colonic insufflation over manual insufflation of CO_2, but to date comfort studies comparing similar administration methods have not determined if air or CO_2 is more acceptable to patients [80]. The use of bowel relaxants (glucagon in the United States and hyoscine-N-Butylbromide in Europe) has been suggested to improve distention and patient comfort, with some investigations showing no improvement [81] and others suggesting improved distention and greater patient comfort [82].

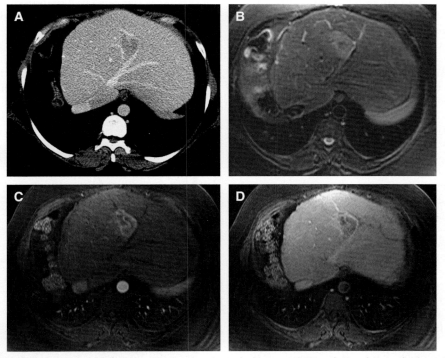

Fig. 13. (*A*) CT demonstrating a left lobe colorectal metastasis. Note on CT its relationship to the hepatic vein. (*B*) MR image demonstrating a left lobe colorectal metastasis. Note hyperintensity of fat-suppressed T2. (*C*) MR image demonstrating a left lobe colorectal metastasis. Note heterogeneous early enhancement postgadolinium. (*D*) MR image demonstrating a left lobe colorectal metastasis Note heterogeneous delayed enhancement postgadolinium.

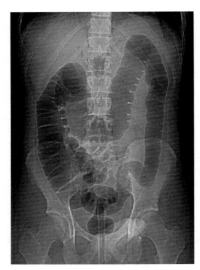

Fig. 14. Supine CT scout tomograph after rectal CO_2 automated insufflation reveals a gas-density well-outlined colon.

Raw data are reconstructed with 50% to 60% overlap for two-dimensional reformatted images in sagittal and coronal planes and for high-quality virtual endoscopic views. Using either a primary two-dimensional, confirmed with three-dimensional, or primary three-dimensional (vice versa) type reading strategy [37], including two-dimensional axial images viewed at lung window level, the entire colon is perused in both supine and prone positions for the presence of polyps or masses. Recently, fecal tagging has been developed to overcome the pitfall of stool particles appearing as polyps, because these do not always contain air or remain mobile [83]. Novel visualization techniques, such as virtual dissection views (Fig. 15), are undergoing continued investigation to determine the most accurate and time-efficient mode of interpreting results [84]. Computer-assisted detection is also being applied to data sets to improve accuracy and reader efficiency with some success [85].

Numerous issues are evolving as the technology and approach undergo changes. Radiation-exposure can be quite low in a screening setting because of the intrinsic contrast between air and soft tissue. Typical doses for CTC are between 3.6 and 12.2 mSv for both acquisitions [86] with microamperage as low as 10 mA being reported to produce diagnostic images [87]. Patient comfort studies compared with colonoscopy have varied, with generally good results in favor of high acceptance for CTC [88,89]. Reimbursement by the Center for Medicare and Medicaid Services continues to evolve based on evidence in the literature. Coverage varies with local

carriers, but has been good in the setting of incomplete colonoscopy. Screening is not covered, and probably awaits addition of CTC to the ACS screening recommendations list. Several HMOs have, however, begun to cover for screening CTC based on aggressive local lobbying and evidence-based publications [90].

Finally, an international symposium meets each year in Boston to review and present developments in CTC and in addition has formed a consortium of experts with recommendations for reader training; standards of examination performance (see also ACR standards [91]); and a new CT Colonography Reporting and Data System coding assignment with recommended follow-up intervals [92]. Although this system has yet to be validated with long-term studies, it is a good start to standardizing communication between radiologists, clinical colleagues, and patients.

Filling defects in the colon may represent polyps (Fig. 16); masses (Fig. 17); stool; inverted diverticula; mucosal; mural or extramural masses; or normal structures, such as the ileocecal valve or complex folds [93]. The two-dimensional images, when adequately thin, demonstrate air in stool and particle mobility between prone and supine images. Furthermore, a smooth round or lobulated morphology can be seen in both stool and polyps, but geometric or irregularly angled borders almost always represents stool.

Many pitfalls exist, such as desiccated and adherent stool particles. The three-dimensional images are useful to distinguish true polyps from folds (Fig. 18), but do not show surface details to allow distinction of stool from polyps (Fig. 19), other than morphologic observations, such as acute

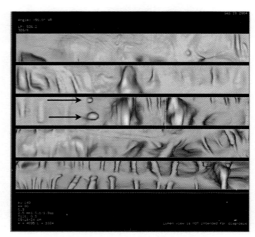

Fig. 15. Virtual dissection view of entire colon visualizing 45 degrees of the wall. Note two larger polyps (*arrows*) in this patient with familial adenomatous polyposis.

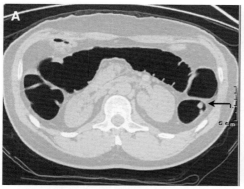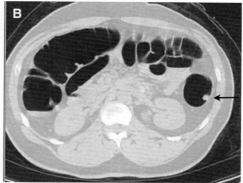

Fig. 16. (*A*) Prone axial CT colonography images (viewed at lung-window settings) demonstrating a left colon polyp (*arrow*). (*B*) Supine axial CT colonography images (viewed at lung-window settings) demonstrating a left colon polyp (*arrow*).

angles, not characteristic of polyps. Flat polyps may be harder to detect with CTC if the wall of the bowel is not observed at soft tissue windows, because using lung-type windows the reader is relying on gross protrusions into the air-filled lumen (Fig. 20).

The main limitation to detection of polyps and masses in the colon is retained stool or fluid, as is the case for other investigations of the colon, albeit some of this material can be suctioned at colonoscopy. The development of fecal-tagging followed by electronic subtraction has begun to overcome this limitation. Here, oral barium and water-soluble contrast agents are added to the colonic-cleansing regimen in varying amounts to label stool and retained liquid. Based on higher attenuation at CT, these can be electronically subtracted using specialized software, and underlying polyps and masses can be discovered (Fig. 21). Another strategy to overcome a poor colon preparation is the addition of intravenous contrast to enhance polyps and masses and make their presence more conspicuous

in the presence of nonenhancing stool or copious fluid [94]. Efforts are underway to develop more acceptable, noncathartic colon preparations (or no cleansing preparation at all [95]) with fecal tagging combined with electronic stool subtraction to enhance patient compliance with screening for CRC [95,96]. As reader experience improves, colon-cleansing preparations become more tolerable, and a greater number of informed patients seek colorectal screening, CTC will likely play an expanding role in the diagnosis of colon cancer, and more importantly in the detection of precancerous polyps.

MR imaging can also be used for virtual colonoscopy with either a bright-lumen technique using rectally administered water spiked with a paramagnetic contrast agent and imaging with T1-weighted sequences [97], or with a dark-lumen technique using rectal water or air alone and intravenous paramagnetic contrast, using ultrafast three-dimensional gradient-echo acquisitions [98]. A recent small study showed this technique could diagnose all lesions 10 mm and greater and 16 of 18 lesions 6 to 9 mm in size compared with colonoscopy. No lesions 5 mm or less were able to be seen [99]. Clearly, in younger patients who would receive frequent surveillance for ulcerative colitis or familial polyposis, the lack of ionizing radiation with this technique offers an intriguing advantage, but larger studies with cost-effectiveness analyses are awaited.

Ultrasound

Transabdominal ultrasound is the mainstay of evaluation of the liver in many countries throughout the world. Ultrasound evaluation affords a low cost tool for evaluation and screening of patients with suspected liver metastases. At ultrasound, most hepatic metastases are hypoechoic. Some may have areas of other sonographic patterns including

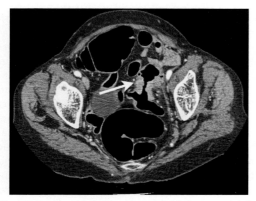

Fig. 17. Supine axial CT colonographic image with intravenous contrast, viewed at soft tissue window setting, reveals an annular sigmoid carcinoma (*arrow*).

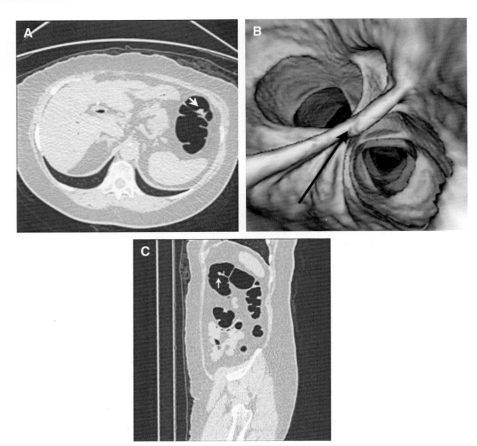

Fig. 18. (*A*) Prone axial image from CT colonography examination viewed at lung window setting reveals an apparent filling defect at the splenic flexure (*arrowhead*), caused by doubling up of the wall at the inner point of the fold to create a pseudomass. (*B*) Virtual colonoscopic (three dimensional) view pointed at abnormality reveals that it is a fold right at the point of turn (*arrow*). (*C*) Sagittal reformatted image, viewed at lung-window setting, clearly depicts location at splenic flexure of colon (*arrow*).

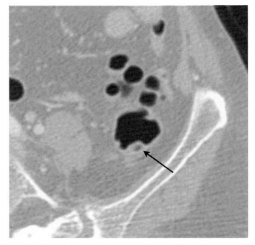

Fig. 19. Axial supine image from CT colonography, viewed at lung-window settings, shows that an apparent mass at virtual colonoscopy contains air (*arrow*), revealing its fecal nature.

cystic, calcific, or mixed echogenic patterns. The most common pattern of metastases to the liver is that of multiple lesions with hypoechoic halos. Some other metastases to the liver may be echogenic, depending on the tumor's vasculature and origin. Transabdominal ultrasound generally has a relatively low sensitivity for the detection of liver metastases [100]. It is for this reason that it is currently not an accepted tool for preoperative planning for liver surgery but may be used as an adjunct to CT and MR imaging to evaluate the liver and especially to look at the vasculature and biliary tree. Several new technical developments in ultrasound including power Doppler and microbubble contrast agents have improved both detection and characterization of solid liver lesions [101]. Contrast-enhanced ultrasound may be useful for differentiating hepatic tumors, especially malignant from benign ones by their differing enhancement patterns.

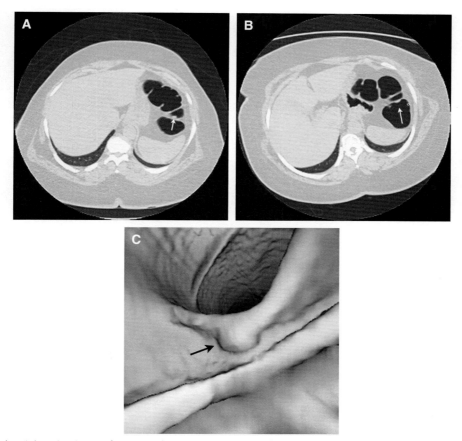

Fig. 20. (A) Axial supine image from CT colonography shows a small filling defect in splenic flexure (*arrow*), representing a flat adenoma. (B) Axial prone image of same area reveals lack of movement of same filling defect (*arrow*). (C) Virtual colonoscopic view of flat adenoma adjacent to a fold (*arrow*).

MR imaging

MR imaging is an imaging technique that uses strong magnetic fields and radiofrequency pulses to create an image with outstanding spatial resolution and tissue contrast. Certain nuclei have a magnetic moment because they are composed of an odd number of protons and neutrons. When placed in a strong magnetic field, these nuclei align with the field and rotate, or spin (precess) about the axis of the magnetic field. The frequency of precession (the Larmor frequency) depends on the specific nuclei and the field strength of the magnet.

Most commonly, the hydrogen nucleus is imaged because of its abundance in the body and its high gyromagnetic ratio compared with other nuclei. When hydrogen nuclei in a strong magnetic field are excited by the addition of a radiofrequency pulse, these nuclei gain energy. When the radiofrequency pulse is turned off, the nuclei return to their resting state and emit the previously absorbed energy at the same frequency. The magnitude of the emitted signal and the time it takes for the nuclei

to return to the resting state depend on certain intrinsic properties of the nuclei, which include the nuclear spin density (or proton density); longitudinal relaxation; transverse relaxation; and flow. The longitudinal (or T1) relaxation time is a measure of the time of the precessing nuclei to return to their baseline state (ie, oriented parallel to the magnetic field) after the radiofrequency pulse has been turned off. The transverse (or T2) relaxation time is a measure of the loss of signal in the plane orthogonal to the long axis of the magnetic field because of the loss of phase coherence between the protons.

Recent advancements in MR imaging hardware, software, and contrast agents have made a major impact on imaging of the liver. Conventional spin echo pulse sequences have been replaced by faster sequences. The use of the phased-array surface coil technology allows for images to be acquired with higher signal-to-noise, larger matrices, smaller fields of view, and thinner slices. Because of these technologies, almost all liver imaging is now done in a breathhold fashion.

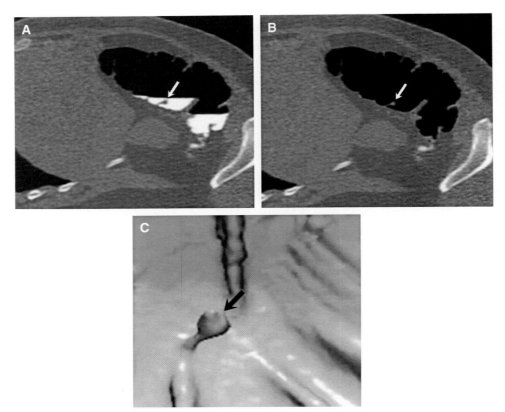

Fig. 21. (*A*) Sagittal reformatted image of right colon from CT colonography performed after fecal tagging. High-attenuation fluid labeled by administration of meglumine diatrizoate obscures underlying colon lumen and wall (*arrow*). (*B*) After electronic computer subtraction, air density is restored to this region revealing an unsubtracted, unlabeled (true) abnormality characterized by a small stalk and polyp head (*arrow*). (*C*) Virtual colonoscopic view of small colonoscopically proved pedunculated polyp (*arrow*). (*From* Pickhardt PJ, Choi JH. Electronic cleansing and stool tagging in CT colonography: advantages and pitfalls with primary three-dimensional evaluation. AJR Am J Roentgenol 2003;181:799–805; with permission.)

Contrast enhancement is also routinely used to evaluate for colorectal metastases to the liver. Gadolinium-diethylenetriamine pentaacetic acid is used routinely to improve hepatic lesion detection and characterization. Other liver-specific contrast agents have been recently introduced further to improve hepatic lesion detection and characterization. For instance, mangafodipir trisodium is a hepatocyte-selective contrast agent that is taken up by normal hepatocytes. Normal liver parenchyma shows increased signal on T1-weighted post–mangafodipir trisodium images. Superparamagnetic iron oxide is another liver contrast agent, but it is specific for the reticuloendothelial system. Iron oxide causes signal loss within the liver on T2-weighted images. Liver metastases do not take up the iron oxide; there is an increase in the contrast of the metastases relative to the liver. The literature is replete with studies comparing all modalities for evaluation of liver metastases. For instance, in one prospective staging study comparing CT, CT arterial portography, and MR imaging, the sensitivity and specificity for MR imaging was 82% and 93%, respectively, which was not statistically better than CT and CT arterial portography [102].

Hepatic metastases may have many different appearances on MR images. On T2-weighted images, most metastases are hyperintense relative to normal hepatic parenchyma (see Fig. 13B). They may be homogeneous or heterogeneous. On T1-weighted images, most hepatic metastases are hypointense. Metastases tend to have irregular borders and may demonstrate a halo or ring with central hyperintensity and lower signal around the periphery. This halo pattern has been attributed to peritumoral edema or peritumoral tumor infiltration. Following gadolinium enhancement, metastases show heterogeneous uptake of contrast (Fig. 13C, D). Classically, rim-enhancement with peripheral washout is seen with dynamic gadolinium-enhanced MR imaging [103,104].

In terms of the value of MR imaging of the liver in staging patients for hepatic resection, a recent study has concluded that MR imaging detected not only all resectable cases as determined by other imaging modalities, but three additional cases that were not deemed resectable with other modalities. The real question that remains is, what is the true medical and economic value of the additional identification of a subset of patients who can potentially go on to surgical resection [105]. The relative value versus cost must be carefully considered. Overall, MR imaging of the liver plays a major role in lesion characterization and problem solving. It is also important in hepatobiliary imaging for staging and potentially assessing response to therapy.

Positron emission tomography

PET refers to the acquisition of anatomic and metabolic data by a PET camera. The most commonly used radiotracer used for PET imaging is 18-F fluorodeoxyglucose (FDG). FDG is an analogue of glucose that is transported by glucose transporters and phosphorylated by hexokinase to FDG-6-phosphate. The polar nature of FDG-6-phosphate reduces the capacity of the molecule to diffuse out of a cell and the stereochemistry of FDG is such that it is not a substrate for any further metabolism. The net effect is a quantifiable, objective measure of the rate of metabolism from the time of injection to the time of imaging. In general, cancer cells have an accelerated glucose metabolism [106]. Many of the pathophysiologic and cellular processes that lead to or result from inflammation are mimicked by oncogenesis. FDG imaging for cancer is rendered less specific because both inflammation and oncogenesis are associated with accelerated glucose metabolism. Newer agents are being investigated but need Food and Drug Administration approval.

One distinct advantage of PET imaging over anatomic imaging is that quantitative results are generated; this allows assessment and reassessment of locoregional metabolism before and after treatment (the hypothesis being that measurable alterations in FDG metabolism reflect the biologic processes induced by a treatment, before a structural change occurs). Reliable imaging with FDG requires consistency and use of strict practice guidelines to ensure dependability and reproducibility. A large amount of data is acquired and quantitative results are generated. Examples of good practice guidelines include injection of adequate amounts of radioactivity and imaging for a sufficient period of time to ensure images are of sufficient quality for interpretation and analysis. If semiquantitative measures of FDG uptake are to be used for patient follow-up, such as the standardized uptake value, the same measure (eg, maximum uptake within a region of interest versus average uptake) should be used. Consistency in postinjection image acquisition times for subsequent FDG PET scans is necessary to generate biologically relevant semiquantitative information; the same can be said for the use of the same camera with the same reconstruction algorithm. Strict adherence to institutional standards for patient elevated blood glucose (eg, >150 mg/mL) is recommended so that rescheduling of patients is done if proper levels do not exist.

FDG PET imaging has a role in the preoperative evaluation of patients with a biologically aggressive primary and in patients with suspected recurrence to exclude unexpected distant metastases. There is also a role of FDG PET in the work-up of patients with occult disease manifesting solely as an elevated CEA level. The early FDG PET literature was remarkably consistent across many tumor types whereby the addition of FDG imaging to conventional imaging led to management change in about one third of all cases. There have been significant changes in the technology of cross-sectional imaging devices in the last 10 years with the widespread implementation of multislice CT scanners and higher field strength MR imaging machines. The increment in PET acquisition technology has been comparatively small over the interim with modest changes in sensitivity and resolution of PET devices. It is likely that the clinical impact of the addition of PET data alone has lessened as the performance of other modalities has improved. The greatest innovation in PET imaging devices has not been the PET device itself but rather the successful deployment of PET-CT scanners that are fully integrated allowing generation of anatomically coregistered or fused images. Although difficult to quantify, it is generally accepted that anatomically coregistered imaging improves the interpretation of both the PET and CT data. A representative case in which a peritoneal lesion was missed on CT (Fig. 22A) reveals that it was detected on FDG fusion images (Fig. 22B). Finally, an important and emerging role exists for PET imaging in treatment monitoring.

A further extension of this is to use FDG PET imaging at an early time point in the course of treatment to determine if otherwise toxic therapy is resulting in an expected fall in glucose metabolism. This technique has been used in other tumor types and parameters associated with good outcomes have been described [107–109].

A classic indication for CRC imaging with FDG PET is CEA elevation with a negative CT examination. It has been shown that there is a correlation between metabolically active tumor bulk as measured by PET and CEA level [110]. As more and more CT scans are performed using multislice helical technology, the false-negative rate on CT

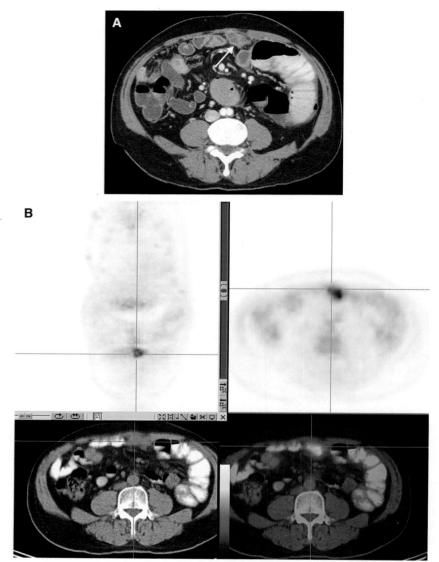

Fig. 22. (*A*) Axial contrast-enhanced CT scan showing a peritoneal implant (*arrow*) mimicking unfilled intestine. (*B*) PET-CT fusion image four-quadrant screen revealing coronal (*upper left*) and axial (*upper right*) PET, and unfused CT (*lower left*) and fused PET-CT (*lower right*) with grid lines indicating FDG avid peritoneal implant missed on CT (see *A*).

imaging is falling, in part because images are acquired faster reducing motion artifacts, and thinner slices are used, increasing sensitivity for small tumor deposits. Isolated CEA elevation with a negative conventional (CT) imaging study is now a rare scenario. A report of 272 cases of CRC that underwent FDG PET imaging found only 15 such cases, of which 14 had true-positive FDG scans, and one was false-positive. There were four patients who had symptoms, a negative work-up, and a normal CEA level, and four of whom had cases of positive FDG PET scans, of which three were false-positive

[111]. Resection of CRC metastases with or without adjuvant hepatic arterial pump therapy has led to extraordinary success with long-term follow-up demonstrating up to 60% 10-years survival [112]. Correct selection of patients for local therapy is dependent on adequate preoperative imaging, of which FDG PET plays an important role. Early studies suggested approximately 30% to 40% of patients would have their management altered on the basis of a preoperative FDG PET scan [113]. These numbers seem similar today [114]. The major role FDG plays in the staging of these patients is in the

identification of extrahepatic disease, rather than staging the liver itself. In those patients receiving chemotherapy within 6 months of surgery, the authors found that FDG uptake was the strongest predictor of postoperative survival in patients who had liver resections for CRC [115].

Research continues at a rapid pace into further refining measures of metabolic activity and into the use of more tissue or disease-specific radionuclides. Investigations such as these have opened up a whole new exciting field of molecular imaging, of which PET leads the way into the future with the goal of more accurate and earlier disease detection and treatment monitoring.

Newer imaging methods

Exciting advances are occurring in colonic imaging, mainly in the setting of endoscopic visualization. These have been developed with the knowledge that up to 27% of small adenomas remain undiagnosed at colonoscopy [30,116]. Chromoendoscopy in combination with high-magnification colonoscopy for in vivo prediction of histology using a pit-pattern technique has been successful. Near-infrared spectroscopy (Raman effect) during endoscopy can allow distinction of hyperplastic from adenomatous polyps. Optical coherence tomography uses light waves to obtain two-dimensional cross-sectional images of the layers of the gastrointestinal tract. Based on light scattering this can distinguish adenomas from hyperplastic polyps. Finally, confocal laser microscopy can now be combined with videoendoscopy using fiber bundle technology, and after the injection of fluorescein sodium has been shown to predict the presence of colonic neoplasia with high accuracy [117]. Clearly these techniques are in their infancy, but they may provide more histospecific imaging of CRC, albeit on a submacroscopic or microscopic level beyond the confines of the specialty of radiology.

Primary and recurrent rectal cancer

Because of its extraperitoneal location, close proximity to other organs, higher rate of recurrence, higher morbidity, amenability to different treatment strategies, and requirement for subspecialized surgery, rectal cancer is addressed separately from colon cancer in this section.

Approximately 45,000 cases of rectal cancer are diagnosed each year, representing about one third of new cases of CRC. Recurrent disease is more common in the rectum than in the colon and can result in pain, immobility, and prolonged hospitalization. Furthermore, a unique surgical challenge presents because of the confined anatomic space, often demanding subspecialization by colorectal surgeons, for whom expertise in sphincter-preserving operations is a must.

Important structures must be considered in the radiologic and clinical staging of primary and recurrent disease including the mesorectal fascia; pelvic sidewall muscles (pyriformis, obturator internus); the levator ani muscles (puborectalis, pubococcygeus, iliococcygeus); the internal and external anal sphincter muscles; nerves (sciatic, autonomic and sacral roots); sacrum; genitourinary organs; and iliac vessels.

The staging of rectal cancer is identical to colon cancer, but surgical treatment differs. For tumors-in-situ and T1 lesions, patients can undergo transanal excision. For T2-T3 tumors that do not involve the anal sphincters or levator ani, patients can undergo anterior resection or an abdominoperineal resection if these structures are involved. Pelvic exenteration is often needed if T4 disease is present. In patients with a wide pelvis, laparoscopic surgery can sometimes be performed. The total mesorectal excision has become the standard operation for curative intent and removes the rectum with its surrounding fascia and lymph nodes in an intact package. Staging using the tumor, node, metastasis system has been shown to be somewhat limited for prognosis. T3 lesions, which are close to the circumferential resection margin (CRM, bulky lesions), have a higher risk of recurrence and a three-fold higher death rate than smaller T3 lesions [118].

Treatment of rectal surgery differs between northern Europe and other parts of the world, including the United States. The use of preoperative chemoradiation is currently considered the standard of care for T3-T4 or node-positive disease because it downstages disease, decreases local recurrence, and allows sphincter-preserving surgery. In northern Europe, however, a short course of preoperative radiation therapy alone is given, because it is believed that the total mesorectal excision is adequate to prevent recurrence in most patients. If a close margin (1 mm by MR imaging) exists between tumor and the CRM, these higher-risk patients may get neoadjuvant chemotherapy in addition. As such, determination of the CRM is more important for treatment decisions in northern Europe. In the United States and elsewhere, it is recognized that this can predict prognosis, but this information does not affect treatment because all patients get chemotherapy and radiation if they are T3-T4 or node-positive.

Most rectal tumors are diagnosed by the digital rectal examination. It has an accuracy of 67% to 83% [119] and gives a surgeon an idea of the location, bulkiness, and fixation of the tumor, but can lead to understaging in 47% of cases. It provides only indirect evidence about sphincter infiltration.

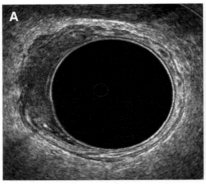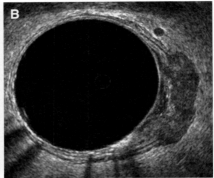

Fig. 23. Endorectal ultrasound image obtained with a radial probe revealing hypoechoic masses seemingly disrupting all layers in two different patients, and representing pathologically proved T2 (*A*) and T3 disease (*B*). (Courtesy of W. Douglas Wong, MD, New York, NY.)

Recently, MR imaging has been found to be more accurate at predicting an involved CRM compared with digital rectal examination with a specificity of 84% versus 29% [120].

Endorectal ultrasound (ERUS) is the most established and preferred modality for T-staging of rectal cancer. It is usually part of the initial digital rectal examination performed by surgeons, although in some centers it is performed by radiologists. Its accuracy is 80% to 90%. It is limited in distinguishing between T2 and early T3 disease (Fig. 23), and recently, based on data from the authors' institution, a modification of the staging system has been proposed whereby uT2–early uT3 lesions are classified as uTy wherein pathologic features and nodal status determine need for neoadjuvant therapy [121]. Another limitation of ERUS is its limited ability to visualize the mesorectal fascia. Tumor overstaging occurs in 11% to 18% of cases and understaging in 5% to 13% of cases [121]. For nodal staging, the ERUS accuracy is 64% to 83%. The main limitation is the use of size criteria (as for other structural imaging modalities). One study found that two thirds of metastatic nodes in CRC were <5 mm. Overstaging occurs in 5% to 22% (inflammatory enlargement) and understaging in 2% to 25% (nodes beyond the range of the probe). At the authors' institution, nodes that are 3 mm or more, round, hypoechoic, and in the appropriate location are regarded as potentially positive (Fig. 24).

In comparison, even when optimized with rectal contrast, glucagon, and prone thin-slice imaging, CT is limited for local staging because of its inherent low soft tissue contrast (Fig. 25), which does not allow for accurate approximation of T stage unless there is gross invasion of adjacent organs (T4), and even here many false-positive cases are seen (Fig. 26). Errors are usually caused by incorrect diagnosis of pyriform muscle, pelvic floor, or sacral invasion. A meta-analysis of 83 published studies

of rectal cancer between 1980 and 1998 compared the performance characteristics of ERUS, MR imaging, endorectal MR imaging, and CT for T and N staging and found that CT performed poorly compared with other modalities with a T-stage sensitivity of 78%, specificity of 63%, and accuracy of 73% compared with ERUS, the most accurate (sensitivity of 93%, specificity of 78%, and accuracy of 87%). CT performed poorly for nodes with a sensitivity of 52%, specificity of 78%, and accuracy of 66% compared with ERUS (sensitivity of 71%, specificity of 76%, and accuracy of 74%). This is likely caused by the reliance on size criteria at CT, whereas at ultrasound one can use some additional morphologic criteria, such as shape and echogenicity. T-stage sensitivity on CT is even more limited in those studies in which preoperative radiation was used (probably because of blurring of fat planes) [122]. Another meta-analysis of 90 studies between 1985 and 2002 found no statistically significant difference in the receiver operating characteristic curves between CT, ERUS, and MR imaging for nodal staging, but found superiority of ERUS for perirectal soft

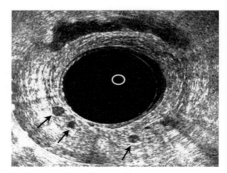

Fig. 24. Endorectal ultrasound image revealing several rounded hypoechoic lymph nodes in the mesorectal fascia (*arrows*). (Courtesy of W. Douglas Wong, MD, New York, NY.)

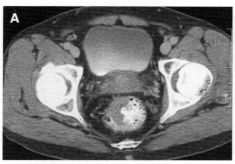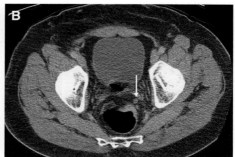

Fig. 25. (A) Supine pelvic CT scan after administration of rectal barium revealing semiannular rectal carcinoma along right wall. (B) Prone pelvic CT scan in a different patient after administration of rectal air and intravenous glucagon revealing sessile carcinoma at 12- to 2-o'clock position with adjacent mesorectal lymph node enlargement (*arrow*).

tissue invasion. CT sensitivity for N staging on average was 55% [123]. Little data exist on performance characteristics for multidetector helical CT. A recent prospective two-reader study of 55 patients using four-row multislice CT found higher average accuracy's for T, N, and overall stage compared with nonhelical studies. Coronal and sagittal two-dimensional reformatted images improved performance even more. For example, T-stage accuracy increased from 81%/77% to 98%/90% (P = .02) for two readers; N-stage accuracy increased from 73%/71% to 96%/80% (P = .01); and overall clinical stage accuracy also increased significantly [124]. N staging is particularly difficult after chemoradiotherapy because of blurring of fat planes. In the authors' study of 78 patients with ERUS T3-T4 or N-positive disease who received 5040 Gy and 5-fluorouracil–based therapy and underwent pretherapy and 6-week posttherapy optimized multidetector helical CT scans, followed by total mesorectal excision resection and whole-mount

pathologic specimens, two radiologists in consensus achieved an overall accuracy of only 65% in determining involved mesorectal lymph nodes, with a good interobserver agreement (k = 0.64, unpublished data).

MR imaging displays superior soft tissue contrast to CT. It has excellent resolution and can depict the entire mesorectum. This is possible using phased-array coils, small fields of view, fast T2-weighted sequences, stronger magnetic gradients, and thinner sections. Nonetheless, limitations do exist for distinction between T2 and early T3 lesions, because stranding into the mesorectal fat may represent inflammation and be overstaged as T3 or microscopic tumor extending into this fat may not be seen and be understaged as T2. Furthermore, nodal staging is limited because of the use of size criteria as for other morphologic imaging modalities. In the Kwok meta-analysis, overall T-stage accuracy was

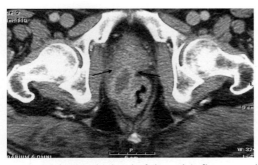

Fig. 26. Axial CT at the level of the pelvic floor reveals an ovoid ring-enhanced mass lesion arising from the rectum in a patient with known rectal primary carcinoma and seemingly inseparable from the prostate gland (*arrow*). After abdominoperineal resection and partial prostatectomy, no tumor was seen invading the prostate at histopathology.

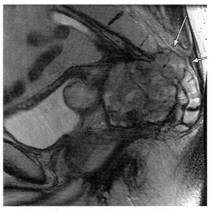

Fig. 27. Sagittal fast spin echo (FSE) T2-weighted pelvic MR image using pelvic 8-channel phased-array coil (TR/TE of 470/107, NEX = 1, 4-mm thickness, matrix 256 × 192) revealing a large mass of the rectum invading the sacrum (*arrows*).

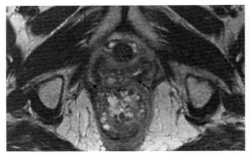

Fig. 28. Axial FSE T2-weighted MR image (TR/TE of 500/104, NEX 1, 4-mm thickness, 256 × 256) revealing a bulky low rectal tumor invading anteriorly obliterating (*arrows*) the posterior vaginal muscular wall (low T2 signal).

82% with a sensitivity of 86% and a specificity of 77%. For N staging the sensitivity was 76%, specificity 80%, and accuracy 74%. In publications that used endorectal coil MR imaging, accuracy's were higher, but limitations still exist in coil design such that stenotic or proximal tumors cannot always be easily imaged. Cases of overstaging and understaging were seen in from 6% to 13% for both phased-array and endorectal coil MR imaging.

Recent data support MR imaging as an overall superior modality to stage rectal cancer. Use of newly defined criteria for nodes by one investigator was found to allow N-stage sensitivity of 85% and specificity of 97%. Compared with ERUS and digital rectal examination, MR imaging was superior in terms of clinical benefit, cost-effectiveness, assessment of depth of invasion, lymph node involvement, and CRM status [125].

Because of the importance of the CRM in determination of treatment in certain European centers, the Magnetic Resonance Imaging and Rectal Cancer European Equivalence Study from 11 European centers investigated the use of MR imaging as a preoperative tool compared with histopathology for its ability to predict the CRM. Abstracted early data, not as yet comprehensively published, indicated 95% accuracy in predicting a clear CRM (tumor greater than 1 mm from the CRM) compared with histopathology. MR imaging was equivalently accurate in determining tumor depth compared with histopathology to within an error of 0.5 mm [126].

At the authors' institution, an eight-channel phased array coil is used with a 1.5-T magnet. The authors perform fast spin echo T2-weighted axial, oblique axial (angled perpendicular to the rectal lumen and sacrum), sagittal, and coronal images and T1-weighted axial fat-saturation images and sagittal T1-weighted gradient echo type gadolinium-enhanced perfusion images. Local staging of primary tumor can be well depicted with small field of view, 512 × 512 matrix images, using several signal averages, not requiring breathholding (Figs. 27–31).

Recurrent rectal cancer occurs in 4% to 30% of patients and is isolated in 25% to 50%. It can be difficult to detect with CT and even on clinical examination. It often involves major structures. Survival is usually 3 to 6 months without treatment. Surgery is advised to avert morbidity and prolong survival but only if an R0 resection (no gross or microscopic residual disease) can be achieved [127]. MR imaging is superior to CT to predict invasion (sensitivity 97% versus 70%), but both can falsely predict muscle invasion. The distinction between tumor and scar tissue related to recent surgery or radiation may be quite difficult and can often be aided by PET imaging (see later). Although MR imaging can distinguish between muscle and tumor using gadolinium enhancement differences, errors can be caused by briskly enhancing scar (immature fibrosis) within 1 year of surgery. Furthermore, low

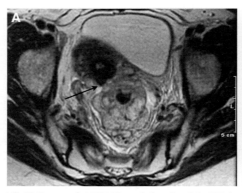
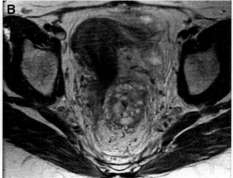

Fig. 29. (*A*) Oblique axial FSE T2-weighted pelvic MR image through mid-pelvis demonstrating rectal tumor extending into perirectal soft tissues and invading cervical stroma (*dark T2 ring, arrow*). (*B*) Standard axial FSE T2-weighted MR image at same level reveals uncertain relationship with cervix, seen now in obliquity.

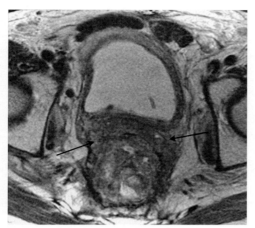

Fig. 30. Axial FSE T2-weighted pelvic MR image showing bulky rectal tumor invading and obliterating normal high T2 signal fluid appearance of seminal vesicles (*arrows*).

T2-weighted signal masses do not always represent pure fibrosis. At histologic examination, biopsies of low T2 areas have also contained malignant cells. Tumor may also be desmoplastic, and atypically low in signal on T2-weighted sequences [128]. In a study of 139 rectal MR imaging examinations at the authors' institution, 46 patients had localized disease and 33 had pathologic correlation. A total of 133 of 156 areas of recurrence were agreed on by two radiologists (85% concordance). In 77 pathologically proved involved organs at curative resection in 33 patients, using MR imaging the authors identified 72 (93.5%) and missed 5 (6.5%). The

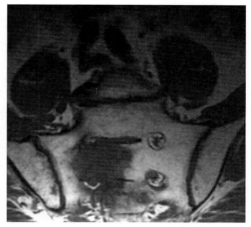

Fig. 32. Coronal FSE T2-weighted pelvic MR image (TR/TE of 4466/105, NEX 1, 4-mm thickness, 256 × 192) reveals intermediate signal tumor metastasis invading sacrum and sacral nerve roots.

false-positive rate was 15.58% and the false-negative rate was 4.58% (Figs. 32–34) (Lawrence Schwartz, unpublished data). Prediction of invasion of the bladder, prostate, and sacral periosteum when not grossly obvious can be limited. Seminal vesicle invasion may be the easiest to predict because of replacement of high-signal T2 fluid by tumor (Fig. 35).

Positron emission tomography in rectal cancer

Low rectal cancers represent a particular patient population that may behave differently from the remainder of patients with CRC. The low rectum has lymphatic drainage to inguinal nodes and the more common pelvic side wall and intra-abdominal nodes. The venous drainage of the low rectum may bypass the liver, and lead to increase in pulmonary metastases in this group. For these very reasons a recent investigation found that FDG PET-CT altered treatment plans in patients with untreated rectal cancers 38% of the time primarily by detecting disease in inguinal nodes [129] with most occult disease found in tumors within 6 cm of the anal verge. A case of rectal cancer with inguinal nodes is presented in Fig. 36.

Induction chemotherapy or induction chemoradiation therapy is often given to patients with advanced rectal cancer to downstage disease, allow sphincter-preservation, and decrease local recurrence rates. A number of groups have investigated the use of posttreatment, preoperative FDG PET in the prediction of local control and overall survival. It is hypothesized that a positive FDG scan posttreatment may portend a biologically more

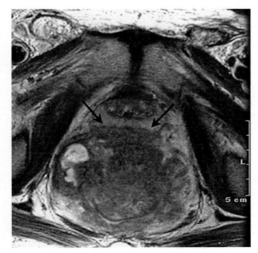

Fig. 31. Axial FSE T2-weighted pelvic MR image reveals a large intermediate signal rectal mass with extension to the peripheral zone of the prostate (*arrows*).

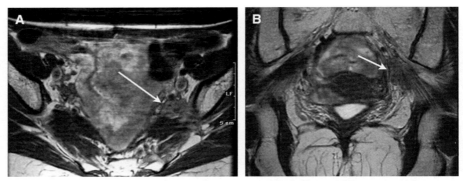

Fig. 33. (A) Axial FSE T2-weighted pelvic MR image revealing a mass invading the left sciatic nerve at the greater sciatic foramen (*arrow*). (B) Coronal FSE T2-weighted pelvic MR image revealing a mass invading the left sciatic nerve (*arrow*) at the greater sciatic foramen in a different patient.

aggressive or less chemosensitive–type tumor. In contradistinction, if complete pathologic responses to therapy can be predicted by PET, surgery might in theory be avoided. It seems that FDG PET is the current gold standard in determining the response to induction treatment [130] and prognosis [131].

Radiologic follow-up and treatment monitoring

Surgery is the mainstay of therapy for CRC. Seventy percent to 80% of patients have tumors that can be resected with curative intent. Adjuvant radiation therapy, chemotherapy, or both are useful in

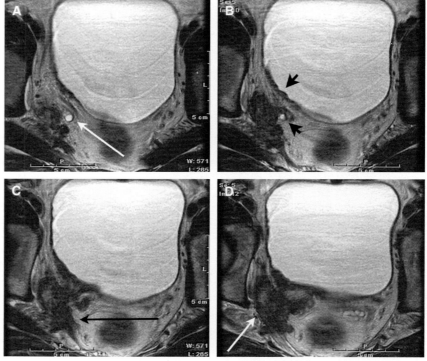

Fig. 34. (A) Axial FSE T2-weighted pelvic MR image revealing a low-signal infiltrative mass invading the right ureter (*arrow*). (B) Axial FSE T2-weighted pelvic MR image revealing a low-signal infiltrative mass invading the right ureter and right bladder wall (*arrowheads*). (C) Axial FSE T2-weighted pelvic MR image revealing a low-signal infiltrative mass invading the right pelvic sidewall (*arrow*). (D) Axial FSE T2-weighted pelvic MR image revealing a low-signal infiltrative mass invading the right pelvic sidewall (*arrow*).

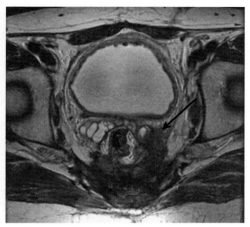

Fig. 35. Axial FSE T2-weighted pelvic MR image revealing recurrent low-signal tumor in the presacral space growing anteriorly to invade the left seminal vesicle (*arrow*).

selected patients. Among patients who have undergone resection for localized disease, the 5-year survival rate is 90%. The rate is only 65% if lymph node metastases are present. Thirty percent to 40% of patients recur within the first 2 to 3 years

[132,133]. The most common sites of relapse are the liver, the local site, the abdomen, and the lung.

Current recommendations for follow-up after resection include (1) physician visits every 3 to 6 months for 3 years with decreasing frequency thereafter; (2) colonoscopy every 3 to 5 years depending on findings, with continued surveillance after 5 years; and (3) serum CEA levels every 3 to 6 months for 5 years [133].

CEA elevation is associated with disease recurrence in 60% to 70% of cases. Most often these recurrences are found to be unresectable anyway. As such, it has been estimated that if all patients were subjected to CEA surveillance, only 0.7% would be cured by CEA-directed second-look surgery [132].

Because in part of the lack of evidence-based data regarding the efficacy of imaging for surveillance, the American Society of Clinical Oncology and the National Comprehensive Cancer Network do not recommend CT imaging for surveillance, whereas the European Society of Medical Oncology recommends liver ultrasound annually for 3 years.

In the first prospective randomized multicenter controlled clinical trial performed of its type, it has been shown that more intensive follow-up of

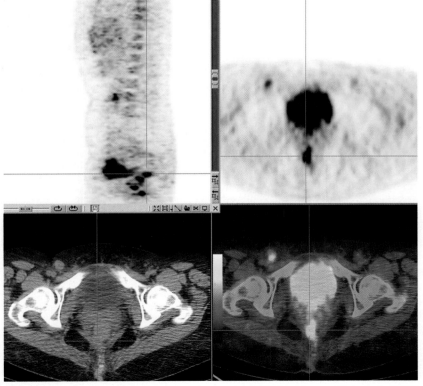

Fig. 36. Fusion PET-CT in low rectal cancer demonstrating sagittal PET showing multiple foci of FDG avidity in the rectum (*upper left*), rectal and right inguinal activity (axial, *upper right*), nonfused CT (*lower left*), and fused PET-CT (*lower right*) with enlarged inguinal nodes and mildly prominent lower rectum corresponding to area of tumor.

patients with stage II CRC and of rectal tumors specifically can lead to higher overall survival compared with simple surveillance. "Intensive follow-up" was defined as the addition of CT, ultrasound, and colonoscopy to routine clinical examination, CEA, and other blood tests. More intensive surveillance also led to a higher proportion of resectable tumor recurrence [134], but the difference in median survival (50 months versus 35 months) did not reach statistical significance, possibly because of a small sample size. Other studies may have been similarly underpowered to detect a true difference between intensive and standard monitoring. Large randomized studies are required to address this question.

At several institutions, including our own , oncologists typically obtain annual CT scans of the abdomen and pelvis for the first 3 years, but this is not based on any formal assessment of utility. Further larger studies are needed to confirm that this is a cost-effective and clinically effective strategy in terms of overall survival and quality of life.

For patients at higher risk, such as those with familial adenomatous polyposis, hereditary nonpolyposis CRC, or ulcerative colitis, guidelines for more frequent endoscopy exist, but there are no formal imaging recommendations.

Summary

The role of imaging in the screening, diagnosis, staging, and restaging of CRC is vast, ranging from detection of precancerous minute adenomas using colonoscopy or virtual colonoscopy to accurate confirmation and restaging of recurrent disease using the exquisite resolution of MR imaging and the highly sensitive metabolic imaging technique of PET scanning. Equally encouraging is the continual evolution and recreation of new roles for radiology, such as refinements in lymph node MR imaging with iron oxide agents and the potential to fuse imaging modalities (eg, PET and CTC [135]), which introduces and expands the role that molecular imaging may play in diagnosis and perhaps ultimately in therapy.

Although the understanding of the development and progression of CRC has come a long way, huge hurdles lay ahead in the ability to access and screen large numbers of average-risk individuals. Until such time as that is achieved, this all too preventable neoplasm will continue to be a leading cancer killer.

References

[1] Spann S, Levin B, Rozen P, et al. Colorectal cancer: How big is the problem, why prevent it and how might it present? In: Rozen P, Young G, Levin B, editors. Colorectal cancer in clinical practice: prevention, early detection and management. London: Martin Dunitz; 2002. p. 1–13.

[2] Mulhall BP, Veerappan GR, Jackson JL. Meta-analysis: computed tomographic colonography. Ann Intern Med 2005;142:635–50.

[3] American Cancer Society. Cancer facts and figures 2006. Atlanta: American Cancer Society; 2006.

[4] Nusko G, Mansmann U, Partzsch U, et al. Invasive carcinoma in colorectal adenomas: multi-variate analysis of patient and adenoma characteristics. Endoscopy 1997;29:626–31.

[5] Gore RM, Gelfand DW, Smith C, et al. Colorectal cancer: clinical and pathologic features, screening strategies, radiologic diagnosis and radiologic staging. Radiol Clin north Am 1997; 35:403–87.

[6] Goldberg RM, Sargent DJ, Morton RF, et al. A randomized controlled trial of fluorouracil plus leucovorin, irinotecan and oxaliplatin combinations in patients with previously untreated metastatic colorectal cancer. J Clin Oncol 2004;1:23–30.

[7] Pignone M, Saha S, Hoerger T, et al. Cost-effectiveness analysis of colorectal cancer screening: a systematic review for the US Preventive Services Task Force. Ann Intern Med 2002;137:96–104.

[8] Imperiale TF, Ransohoff DF, Itzkowitz SH, et al. Fecal DNA versus fecal occult blood for colorectal-cancer screening in an average-risk population. N Engl J Med 2004;351:2704–14.

[9] Ristvedt SL, McFarland EG, Weinstock LB, et al. Patient preferences for CT colonography, conventional colonoscopy, and bowel preparation. Am J Gastroenterol 2003;98:578–85.

[10] Muto T, Bussey HJ, Morson BC. The evolution of cancer of the colon and rectum. Cancer 1975;36:2251–70.

[11] Winawer SJ, Fletcher RF, Rex D, et al. Colorectal cancer screening and surveillance: clinical guidelines and rationale. Update based on new evidence. Gastroenterology 2003;124:544–60.

[12] Ferrucci JT. Virtual colonoscopy for colon cancer screening: further reflections on polyps and politics. AJR Am J Roentgenol 2003;181:795–7.

[13] Hawk ET, Levin B. Colorectal cancer prevention. J Clin Oncol 2005;23:378–91.

[14] Mak T, Lalloo F, Evans DGR, et al. Molecular stool screening for colorectal cancer. Br J Surg 2004;91:790–800.

[15] Podolsky DK. Going the distance: the case for true colorectal cancer screening. N Engl J Med 2000;343:207–8.

[16] Fearon ER, Vogelstein B. A genetic model for colorectal tumorigenesis. Cell 1990;61:759–67.

[17] Levine MS, Glick SN, Rubesin SE, et al. Double-contrast barium enema examination and colorectal cancer: a plea for radiologic screening. Radiology 2002;222:313–5.

[18] Winawer SJ, Stewart ET, Zauber AG, et al. A comparison of colonoscopy and double-

contrast barium enema for surveillance after polypectomy. N Engl J Med 2000;342:1766–72.

[19] Scheitel SM, Ahlquist DA, Wollan PC, et al. Colorectal cancer screening: a community case-control study of proctosigmoidoscopy, barium enema radiography, and fecal occult blood test efficacy. Mayo Clin Proc 1999;74:1207–13.

[20] Rex DK, Rahmani EY, Haseman JH, et al. Relative sensitivity of colonoscopy and barium enema for detection of colorectal cancer in clinical practice. Gastroenterology 1997;112:17–23.

[21] Fletcher RH. The end of barium enemas? [editorial]. N Engl J Med 2000;342:1823–4.

[22] Glick SN. Comparison of colonoscopy and double-contrast barium enema, correspondence. N Engl J Med 2000;343:1728–30.

[23] Winawer SJ, Fletcher RH, Miller L, et al. Colorectal cancer screening: clinical guidelines and rationale. Gastroenterology 1997;112:594–642.

[24] Citarda F, Tomaselli G, Capocaccia R, et al. Efficacy in standard clinical practice of colonoscopic polypectomy in reducing colorectal cancer incidence. Gut 2001;48:812–5.

[25] Winawer SJ, Zauber AG, Ho MN, et al. Prevention of colorectal cancer by colonoscopic polypectomy: The National Polyp Study Workgroup. N Engl J Med 1993;329:1977–81.

[26] National Cancer Institute Web site. Available at: http://www.nci.nih.gov/cancertopics/factsheet/ColorectalPLCO.

[27] Lieberman DA, Weiss DG, Bond JH, et al. Use of colonoscopy to screen asymptomatic adults for colorectal cancer. N Engl J Med 2000;343:162–8.

[28] Habr-Gama A, Waye JD. Complications and hazards of gastrointestinal endoscopy. World J Surg 1989;13:193–201.

[29] Blakeborough A, Sheridan MB, Chapman AH. Complications of barium enema examinations: a survey of UK consultant radiologists 1992 to 1994. Clin Radiol 1997;52:142–8.

[30] Rex DK, Cutler CS, Lemmel GT, et al. Colonoscopic miss rates of adenomas determined by back-to-back colonoscopies. Gastroenterology 1997;112:24–8.

[31] Lieberman D. Quality and colonoscopy: a new imperative. Gastrointest Endosc 2005;61:392–4.

[32] Pickhardt PJ, Nugent PA, Mysliwiec PA, et al. The adenoma miss rate at optical colonoscopy: a novel assessment using virtual colonoscopy as a separate reference standard. Ann Intern Med 2004;141:352–9.

[33] Smith RA, Cokkinides V, von Eschenbach AC, et al. American Cancer Society Guidelines for early detection of cancer. CA Cancer J Clin 2002;52:8–22.

[34] Mysliwiec PA, Brown ML, Klabunde CN, et al. Are physicians doing too much colonoscopy? A national survey of colorectal surveillance after polypectomy. Ann Intern Med 2004;141:264–71.

[35] Seeff LC, Manninen DL, Dong FB, et al. Is there endoscopic capacity to provide colorectal cancer screening to the unscreened population in the United States? Gastroenterology 2004; 127:1841–4.

[36] Saitoh Y, Obara T, Watari J, et al. Invasion depth diagnosis of depressed type early colorectal cancers by combined use of videoendoscopy and chromoendoscopy. Gastrointest Endosc 1998; 48:362–70.

[37] Pickhardt PJ, Choi JRC, Hwang I, et al. Computed tomographic virtual colonoscopy to screen for colorectal neoplasia in asymptomatic adults. N Engl J Med 2003;349:2191–200.

[38] Halligan S, Altman DG, Taylor SA, et al. CT colonography in the detection of colorectal polyps and cancer: systematic review, meta-analysis, and proposed minimum data set for study level reporting. Radiology 2005;237: 893–904.

[39] Banerjee S, Van Dam J. CT colonography for colon cancer screening. Gastrointest Endosc 2006; 63:121–33.

[40] Cotton PB, Durkalski VL, Pineau BC, et al. Computed tomographic colonography (virtual colonoscopy): a multicenter comparison with standard colonoscopy for detection of colorectal neoplasia. JAMA 2004;291:1713–9.

[41] Ferrucci JT. Colonoscopy: virtual and optical-another look, another view. Radiology 2005; 235:13–6.

[42] Sonnenberg A, Delco F, Bauerfeind P. Is virtual colonoscopy a cost-effective option to screen for colorectal cancer? Am J Gastroenterol 1999;94:2268–74.

[43] Ladabaum U, Song K, Fendrick AM. Colorectal neoplasia screening with virtual colonoscopy: when, at what cost, and with what national impact? Clin Gastroenterol Hepatol 2004;2: 554–63.

[44] Heitman S, Fong A, Dean S, et al. Cost-effectiveness study of CT colonography versus colonoscopy using decision analysis. [abstract]. Gastroenterology 2004;126:A202.

[45] van Gelder RE, Florie J, Stoker J. Colorectal cancer screening and surveillance with CT colonography: current controversies and obstacles. Abdom Imaging 2005;30:5–12.

[46] van Gelder RE, Birnie E, Florie J, et al. Patient experience and preference with CT colonography and conventional colonoscopy: a five-week follow-up study. Radiology 2004;233: 328–37.

[47] Burling D, Halligan S, Slater A, et al. Potentially serious adverse events at CT colonography in symptomatic patients: national survey of the United Kingdom. Radiology 2006;239: 464–71.

[48] Sosna J, Blachar A, Amitai M, et al. Colonic perforation at CT colonography: assessment of risk in a multicenter large cohort. Radiology 2006; 239:457–63.

[49] van Gelder RE, Nio CY, Florie J, et al. Computed tomographic colonography compared with

colonoscopy in patients at increased risk for colorectal cancer. Gastroenterology 2004;127: 41–8.

[50] Rubesin SE, Levine MS, Laufer I, et al. Double-contrast barium enema examination technique. Radiology 2000;215:642–50.

[51] Eide TJ. Colorectal polyps: a symposium. World J Surg 1991;15:1–56.

[52] Torlakovic E, Snover DC. Serrated adenomatous polyposis in humans. Gastroenterology 1996; 100:748–55.

[53] Levine MS, Rubesin SE, Laufer I, et al. Diagnosis of colorectal neoplasms at double-contrast barium enema examination. Radiology 2000;216:11–8.

[54] Rembacken BJ, Fujii T, Cairns A, et al. Flat and depressed colonic neoplasms: a prospective study of 1000 colonoscopies in the UK. Lancet 2000;355:1211–4.

[55] Saitoh Y, Waxman I, West AB, et al. Prevalence and distinctive biologic features of flat colorectal adenomas in a North American population. Gastroenterology 2001;120:1657–65.

[56] Fujiya M, Maruyama M. Small depressed neoplasms of the large bowel: radiographic visualization and clinical significance. Abdom Imaging 1997;22:325–31.

[57] Lee JT, Dixon MR, Murrell Z, et al. Colonic histoplasmosis presenting as colon cancer in the non immunocompromised patient: report of a case and review of the literature. Am Surg 2004;70:959–63.

[58] Ott DJ, Chen YM, Gelfand DW, et al. Single-contrast vs double-contrast barium enema in the detection of colonic polyps. AJR Am J Roentgenol 1986;146:993–6.

[59] Prokop M. Image processing and display techniques. In: Prokop M, Galnski M, editors. Spiral and multislice computed tomography of the body. Sttugart: Thieme; 2003. p. 45–82.

[60] Brink JA. Contrast optimization and scan timing for single and multidetector-row computed tomography. J Comput Assist Tomogr 2003; 27(Suppl 1):S3–8.

[61] Mauchley DC, Lynge DC, Langdale LA, et al. Clinical utility and cost-effectiveness of routine preoperative computed tomography scanning in patients with colon cancer. Am J Surg 2005; 189:512–7.

[62] Chintapalli KN, Esola CC, Chopra S, et al. Pericolic mesenteric lymph nodes: an aid in distinguishing diverticulitis from cancer of the colon. AJR Am J Roentgenol 1997;169:1253–5.

[63] De Bree E, Koops W, Kroger R, et al. Peritoneal carcinomatosis from colorectal or appendiceal origin: correlation of preoperative CT with intraoperative findings and evaluation of interobserver agreement. J Surg Oncol 2004;86:64–73.

[64] Burke EC, Karpeh MS, Conlon KC, et al. Laparoscopy in the management of gastric adenocarcinoma. Ann Surg 1997;225:262–7.

[65] Ginsberg MS, Griff SK, Go BD, et al. Pulmonary nodules resected at video-assisted thoracoscopic surgery: etiology in 426 patients. Radiology 1999;213:277–82.

[66] You YT, Chien CRC, Wang JY, et al. Evaluation of contrast-enhanced computed tomographic colonography in detection of local recurrent colorectal cancer. World J Gastroenterol 2006;12:123–6.

[67] Fetita C, Lucidarme O, Preteux F, et al. CT hepatic venography: 3D vascular segmentation for preoperative evaluation. Med Image Comput Assist Interv Int Conf 2005;8(Pt 2):830–7.

[68] Sahani D, Mehta A, Blake M, et al. Preoperative hepatic vascular evaluation with CT and MR angiography: implications for surgery. Radiographics 2004;24:1367–80.

[69] Easson AM, Barron PT, Cripps C, et al. Calcification in colorectal hepatic metastases correlates with longer survival. J Surg Oncol 1996;63:221–5.

[70] Kinkel K, Lu Y, Both M, et al. Detection of hepatic metastases from cancers of the gastrointestinal tract by using noninvasive imaging methods (US, CT, MR imaging, PET): a meta-analysis. Radiology 2002;224:748–56.

[71] Abdelmoumene A, Chevallier P, Chalaron M, et al. Detection of liver metastases under 2 cm: comparison of different acquisition protocols in four row multidetector-CT (MDCT). Eur Radiol 2005;15:1881–7.

[72] Valls C, Andia E, Sanchez A, et al. Hepatic metastases from colorectal cancer: preoperative detection and assessment of resectability with helical CT. Radiology 2001;218:55–60.

[73] Vining DJ, Gelfand DW, Bechtold RE, et al. Technical feasibility of colon imaging with helical CT and virtual reality [abstract]. AJR Am J Roentgenol 1995;162:194.

[74] Johnson CD, MacCarty RL, Welch TJ, et al. Comparison of the relative sensitivity of CT colonography and double-contrast barium enema for screen detection of colorectal polyps. Clin Gastroenterol Hepatol 2004;2:314–21.

[75] Macari M, Berman P, Dicker M, et al. Usefulness of CT colonography in patients with incomplete colonoscopy. AJR Am J Roentgenol 1999; 173:561–4.

[76] Fenlon HM, McAneny DB, Nunes DP, et al. Occlusive colon carcinoma: virtual colonoscopy in the preoperative evaluation of the proximal colon. Radiology 1999;210:423–8.

[77] Neri E, Giusti P, Battolla L, et al. Colorectal cancer: role of CT colonography in preoperative evaluation after incomplete colonoscopy. Radiology 2002;223:615–9.

[78] Fletcher JG, Johnson CD, Krueger WR, et al. Contrast-enhanced CT colonography in recurrent colorectal carcinoma: feasibility of simultaneous evaluation for metastatic disease, local recurrence, and metachronous neoplasia in colorectal carcinoma. AJR Am J Roentgenol 2002; 178:283–90.

[79] Macari M, Lavelle M, Pedrosa I, et al. Effect of different bowel preparations on residual fluid at CT colonography. Radiology 2001;218:274–7.

[80] Burling D, Taylor SA, Halligan S, et al. Automated insufflation of carbon dioxide for MDCT colonography: distension and patient experience compared with manual insufflation. AJR Am J Roentgenol 2006;186:96–103.

[81] Yee J, Hung RK, Akerkar GA, et al. The usefulness of glucagon hydrochloride for colonic distinction in CT colonography. AJR Am J Roentgenol 1999;173:169–72.

[82] Taylor SA, Halligan S, Goh V, et al. Optimizing colonic distention for multi-detector row CT colonography: effect of hyoscine butylbromide and rectal balloon catheter. Radiology 2003; 229:99–108.

[83] Lefere PA, Gryspeerdt SS, Dewyspelaere J, et al. Dietary fecal tagging as a cleansing method before CT colonography: initial results polyp detection and patient acceptance. Radiology 2002;224:393–403.

[84] Hoppe H, Quattropani C, Spreng A, et al. Virtual colon dissection with CT colonography compared with axial interpretation and conventional colonoscopy: preliminary results. AJR Am J Roentgenol 2004;182:1151–8.

[85] Summers RM, Jerebko AK, Franaszek M, et al. Colonic polyps: complementary role of computer-aided detection in CT colonography. Radiology 2002;225:391–9.

[86] van Gelder RE, Venema HW, Serlie IW, et al. CT colonography at different radiation dose levels: feasibility of dose reduction. Radiology 2002; 224:25–33.

[87] Cohnen M, Vogt C, Beck A, et al. Feasibility of MDCT Colonography in ultra-low-dose technique in the detection of colorectal lesions: comparison with high-resolution video colonoscopy. AJR Am J Roentgenol 2004;183:1355–9.

[88] Edwards JT, Mendelson RM, Fritschi L, et al. Colorectal neoplasia screening with CT colonography in average-risk asymptomatic subjects: community-based study. Radiology 2004;230: 459–64.

[89] Gluecker TM, Johnson CD, Harmsen WS, et al. Colorectal cancer screening with CT colonography, colonoscopy, and double-contrast barium enema examination: prospective assessment of patient perceptions and preferences. Radiology 2003;227:378–84.

[90] Pickhardt PJ, Taylor AJ, Johnson GL, et al. Building a CT colonography program: necessary ingredients for reimbursement and clinical success. Radiology 2005;235:17–20.

[91] Practice Guidelines ACR, Colonography CT. 10/01/05, p. 295–9. Available at: http://www.acr.org/s_acr/bin.asp?TrackID=&SID=1&DID=14802&CID=1848&VID=2&DOC=File.PDF.

[92] Zalis ME, Barish MA, Choi JR, et al. Working Group on Virtual Colonoscopy. CT colonography reporting and data system: a consensus proposal. Radiology 2005;236:3–9.

[93] Macari M, Bini EJ, Jacobs SL, et al. Filling defects at CT colonography: pseudo- and

diminutive lesions (the good), polyps (the bad), flat lesions, masses, and carcinomas (the ugly). Radiographics 2003;23:1073–91.

[94] Morrin MM, Farrell RJ, Kruskal JB, et al. Utility of intravenously administered contrast material at CT colonography. Radiology 2000;217:765–71.

[95] Lefere P, Gryspeerdt S, Baekelandt M, et al. Laxative-free CT colonography. AJR Am J Roentgenol 2004;183:945–8.

[96] Iannaccone R, Laghi A, Catalano C, et al. Computed tomographic colonography without cathartic preparation for the detection of colorectal polyps. Gastroenterology 2004;127: 1300–11.

[97] Luboldt W, Bauerfeind P, Wildermuth S, et al. Colonic masses: detection with MR colonography. Radiology 2000;216:383–8.

[98] Luboldt W, Bauerfeind P, Wildermuth S, et al. Contrast optimization for assessment of colonic wall and lumen in MR colonography. J Magn Reson Imaging 1999;9:745–50.

[99] Ajaj W, Pelster G, Vogt F, et al. Dark lumen MR colonography: comparison to conventional colonoscopy for the detection of colorectal pathology. Gut 2003;52:1738–43.

[100] Albrecht T, Hohmann J, Oldenburg A, et al. Detection and characterization of liver metastases. Eur Radiol 2004;14(Suppl 8):P25–33.

[101] Jang HJ, Kim TK, Wilson SR. Imaging of malignant liver masses: characterization and detection. Ultrasound Q 2006;22:19–29.

[102] Bhattacharjya S, Bhattacharjya T, Baber S, et al. Prospective study of contrast-enhanced computed tomography, computed tomography during arterioportography, and magnetic resonance imaging for staging colorectal liver metastases for liver resection. Br J Surg 2004;91: 1361–9.

[103] Mahfouz A-E, Hamm B, Taupitz M, et al. Hypervascular liver lesions: differentiation of focal nodular hyperplasia from malignant tumors with dynamic gadolinium-enhanced MR imaging. Radiology 1993;186:133–8.

[104] Mahfouz A-E, Hamm B, Wolf K-J. Peripheral wash-out: a sign of malignancy on dynamic gadolinium-enhanced MR images of focal liver lesions. Radiology 1994;190:49–52.

[105] Titu LV, Breen DJ, Nicholson AA, et al. Is routine magnetic resonance imaging justified for the early detection of resectable liver metastases from colorectal cancer? Dis Colon Rectum 2006;49:810–5.

[106] Warburg O. On the origin of cancer cells. Science 1956;123:309–14.

[107] Weber WA, Ott K, Becker K, et al. Prediction of response to preoperative chemotherapy in adenocarcinomas of the esophagogastric junction by metabolic imaging. J Clin Oncol 2001;19: 3058–65.

[108] Wieder HA, Brucher BL, Zimmermann F, et al. Time course of tumor metabolic activity during chemoradiotherapy of esophageal squamous

cell carcinoma and response to treatment. J Clin Oncol 2004;22:900–8.

[109] Ott K, Fink U, Becker K, et al. Prediction of response to preoperative chemotherapy in gastric carcinoma by metabolic imaging: results of a prospective trial. J Clin Oncol 2003;21: 4604–10.

[110] Choi MY, Lee KM, Chung JK, et al. Correlation between serum CEA level and metabolic volume as determined by FDG PET in postoperative patients with recurrent colorectal cancer. Ann Nucl Med 2005;19:123–9.

[111] Zervos EE, Badgwell BD, Burak WE Jr, et al. Fluorodeoxyglucose positron emission tomography as an adjunct to carcinoembryonic antigen in the management of patients with presumed recurrent colorectal cancer and nondiagnostic radiologic workup. Surgery 2001;130:636–43 [discussion: 643–4].

[112] Kemeny NE, Gonen M. Hepatic arterial infusion after liver resection. N Engl J Med 2005;352: 734–5.

[113] Fong Y, Saldinger PF, Akhurst T, et al. Utility of 18F-FDG positron emission tomography scanning on selection of patients for resection of hepatic colorectal metastases. Am J Surg 1999; 178:282–7.

[114] Selzner M, Hany TF, Wildbrett P, et al. Does the novel PET/CT imaging modality impact on the treatment of patients with metastatic colorectal cancer of the liver? Ann Surg 2004;240:1027–34.

[115] Akhurst TJ, Gonen M, Tuorto S, et al. Response to neoadjuvant chemotherapy as measured by PET predicts outcome after liver resection for colorectal metastasis. J Clin Oncol 2006;24: 3056.

[116] Hixson LJ, Fennerty MB, Sampliner RE, et al. Prospective blinded trial of the colonoscopic miss-rate of large colorectal polyps. Gastrointest Endosc 1991;37:125–7.

[117] Van Dam J. Novel methods of enhanced endoscopic imaging. Gut 2003;52(Suppl 4):12–6.

[118] Quirke P, Durdey P, Dixon MF, et al. Local recurrence of rectal adenocarcinoma due to inadequate surgical resection: histopathological study of lateral tumor spread and surgical excision. Lancet 1986;2:996–9.

[119] Herbst F. Pelvic radiological imaging: a surgeon's perspective. Eur J Radiol 2003;47:135–41.

[120] Salerno G, Daniels IR, Fisher SE, et al. A comparison of digital rectal examination versus magnetic resonance imaging in the prediction of circumferential resection margin status in patients [abstract P172]. Colorectal Disease 2005; 7(Suppl 2):56.

[121] Schaffzin DM, Wong DW. Endorectal ultrasound in the preoperative evaluation of rectal cancer. Clin Colorectal Cancer 2004;4:124–32.

[122] Kwok H, Bissett IP, Hill GI. Preoperative staging of rectal cancer. Int J Colorectal Dis 2000;15: 9–20.

[123] Bipat S, Glas AS, Slors FJ, et al. Rectal cancer: local staging and assessment of lymph node involvement with endoluminal US, CT and MR imaging: a meta-analysis. Radiology 2004;232: 773–83.

[124] Kulinna C, Eibel R, Matzek W, et al. Staging of rectal cancer: diagnostic potential of multiplanar reconstructions with MDCT. AJR Am J Roentgenol 2004;183:421–7.

[125] Brown G, Richards CJ, Bourne MW, et al. Morphologic predictors of lymph node status in rectal cancer with use of high-spatial-resolution MR imaging with histopathologic comparison. Radiology 2003;227:371–7.

[126] Brown G, Daniels IR. Preoperative staging of rectal cancer: The MERCURY Research Project. Recent Results Cancer Res 2005;165:58–74.

[127] Shoup M, Guillem JG, Alektiar KM, et al. Predictors of survival in recurrent rectal cancer after resection and intraoperative radiotherapy. Dis Colon Rectum 2002;45:585–92.

[128] Beets-Tan RG, Beets GL, Borstlap AC, et al. Preoperative assessment of local tumor extent in advanced rectal cancer: CT or high-resolution MRI? Abdom Imaging 2000;25:533–41.

[129] Gearhart SL, Frassica D, Rosen R, et al. Improved staging with pretreatment positron emission tomography/computed tomography in low rectal cancer. Ann Surg Oncol 2006;13:397–404.

[130] Guillem JG, Puig-La Calle J Jr, Akhurst T, et al. Prospective assessment of primary rectal cancer response to preoperative radiation and chemotherapy using 18-fluorodeoxyglucose positron emission tomography. Dis Colon Rectum 2000;43:18–24.

[131] Guillem JG, Moore HG, Akhurst T, et al. Sequential preoperative fluorodeoxyglucose-positron emission tomography assessment of response to preoperative chemoradiation: a means for determining long term outcomes of rectal cancer. J Am Coll Surg 2004;199:1–7.

[132] Mortazavi A, Shaukat A, Othman E, et al. Postoperative computed tomography scan surveillance for patients with stage II and III colorectal cancer; worthy of further study? Am J Clin Oncol 2005;28:30–5.

[133] Pfister DG, Benson AB III, Somerfield MR. Clinical practice: surveillance strategies after curative treatment of colorectal cancer. N Engl J Med 2004;350:2375–82.

[134] Rodriguez-Moranta F, Salo J, Arcusa A, et al. Postoperative surveillance in patients with colorectal cancer who have undergone curative resection: a prospective, multicenter, randomized, controlled trial. J Clin Oncol 2006;24: 385–93.

[135] Gollub MJ, Akhurst T, Markowitz AJ, et al. Combined CT colonography and [18]FDG PET imaging of colon polyps: a potential technique for selective cancer and pre-cancerous lesion detection. Am J Roentgenol 2007;188:1–9.

ELSEVIER
SAUNDERS

RADIOLOGIC
CLINICS
OF NORTH AMERICA

Radiol Clin N Am 45 (2007) 119–147

Imaging of Kidney Cancer

Jingbo Zhang, MD*, Robert A. Lefkowitz, MD, Ariadne Bach, MD

Kidney cancers account for about 3% of all cancer cases as well as about 3% of all cancer deaths in the United States, with 38,890 new diagnoses and 12,840 deaths expected in 2006 [1]. According to the National Cancer Institute's Surveillance, Epidemiology, and End Results (SEER) Program, between 1998 and 2002, the age-adjusted incidence and death rates for kidney cancers were 12.1 and 4.2 per 100,000, and between 1995 and 2001, the overall 5-year survival rate of patients with kidney cancer was 64.6% [2]. It is estimated that approximately $1.9 billion is spent in the United States each year on treatment of kidney cancer [3]. The incidence of kidney cancers has been increasing at a rate of about 2% per year for the past 30 years [2]. The overall mortality rate from kidney cancers has increased slightly over the past 2 decades, but not as rapidly as the incidence rate. This discrepancy is due to a significant improvement in 5-year survival [4]. These trends may be at least partially attributable to improved diagnostic capabilities. Newer radiographic techniques are detecting renal tumors more frequently and at a lower disease stage, when tumors can be resected for cure [5–11].

The kidney is a retroperitoneal structure surrounded by perirenal fat and the renal (Gerota's) fascia. Most renal tumors arise from the renal parenchyma (referred to as renal cell tumors, renal cortical tumors, or renal parenchymal tumors), with a much smaller number arising from the urothelium of the renal collecting system (urothelial carcinoma or transitional cell carcinoma [TCC]) or the mesenchyma (eg, angiomyolipoma, leiomyoma, liposarcoma). Advances in molecular genetics in the last decade have expanded understanding of renal cell tumors significantly. Now it is understood that renal cortical tumors are a family of neoplasms with distinct cytogenetics and molecular defects, unique histopathologic features, and different malignant potentials [12–16]. In the conclusions of a workshop entitled "Impact of Molecular Genetics on the Classification of Renal Cell Tumours," which was held in Heidelberg in October 1996, a new classification system was proposed [14]. This classification system subdivides renal cell tumors into benign and malignant parenchymal neoplasms and, where possible, limits each subcategory to the most commonly documented

Department of Radiology, Memorial Sloan-Kettering Cancer Center, Cornell University Weill Medical College, 1275 York Avenue, C278D, New York, NY 10021, USA
* Corresponding author.
E-mail address: zhangj12@mskcc.org (J. Zhang).

0033-8389/07/$ – see front matter © 2006 Elsevier Inc. All rights reserved.
radiologic.theclinics.com

doi:10.1016/j.rcl.2006.10.011

genetic abnormalities. Historically, malignant renal cell tumors have been described as a single entity, such as hypernephroma, renal cancer, renal adenocarcinoma, and renal cell carcinoma (RCC). By the Heidelberg classification, malignant renal parenchymal tumors include common or conventional RCC (also known as the clear cell type, accounting for about 75% of renal neoplasms in surgical series), papillary RCC (accounting for 10%), chromophobe RCC (accounting for 5%), collecting duct (Bellini duct) carcinoma (accounting for 1%), and rarely unclassified tumors [14]. Medullary carcinoma of the kidney is a variant of collecting duct carcinoma and was initially described in patients who were sickle cell trait–positive [14]. Benign renal parenchymal tumors include renal oncocytoma (5%) and the rarer metanephric adenoma, metanephric adenofibroma, and papillary renal cell adenoma.

Malignant renal cell tumors occur nearly twice as often in men as in women [9]. The age at diagnosis is generally older than 40 years; the median age is in the mid-60s [9]. Past international, multicenter, population-based, case-control studies have provided insight into the environmental risk factors for development of malignant renal cell tumor [17–23]. Diet [23]; cigarette smoking [20]; unopposed estrogen exposure [17]; body mass index in women and, to a lesser extent, in men [21]; occupational exposure to petroleum products, heavy metals, or asbestos [18]; and hypertension, treatment for hypertension, or both [19] have been reported associated with malignant renal cell tumors. The risk of RCC also has been reported to be increased in patients with acquired cystic kidney disease associated with long-term hemodialysis [24]. Heredity plays a role in some cases, with the risk of the disease increasing fourfold when a first-degree relative carries the diagnosis [22], but only a small fraction of patients have an affected family member. Certain familial syndromes, such as von Hippel–Lindau disease [26], also are associated with malignant renal cell tumors. In addition, a few kindreds with familial clear cell carcinoma have been reported and were found to have chromosomal abnormalities [14,27,28]. Cytogenetic and molecular genetic analyses of tumors carried by these families have contributed substantially to understanding of renal tumor pathogenesis on a molecular level [29].

The different subtypes of renal cell tumors are associated with distinctively different disease progression and metastatic potential [30–33]. The conventional clear cell carcinomas, accounting for approximately 90% of the metastases, have the greatest metastatic potential, whereas papillary and chromophobe carcinomas (accounting for approximately 10% of metastases) are associated with less metastatic potential [33]. The overall 5-year survival rates for papillary and chromophobe subtypes (80–90%) are much higher than that for conventional RCC (50–60%) [34–36]. Among these three most common types of malignant renal cortical tumors, the chromophobe type is associated with the least metastatic potential and best prognosis [12,15,30,31,33,36,37].

In addition to histologic subtypes, other independent predictors of patient prognosis include patient age, functional status, symptomatic tumor presentation, stage (discussed in detail later in this article), and the Fuhrman nuclear grade [38–47]. Symptomatic tumor presentation, higher stage, and higher nuclear grades correlate with greater biologic aggressiveness of the tumor and increased metastatic potential.

Bilateral multifocal renal tumors are present in approximately 5% of patients with sporadic renal tumors [48,49]. As in solitary disease, conventional clear cell histology is the most common histologic subtype; concordance between histologic subtypes among tumors was found to be 76% in one study [48]. Bilateral multifocal tumors and unilateral tumors have comparable prognoses when treated with surgery [48,49].

Detection and diagnosis

Common symptoms that lead to the detection of a renal mass are hematuria, flank mass, and flank pain. The combination of these symptoms is present, however, in only 10% of cases. Less frequently, patients present with signs or symptoms resulting from metastatic disease, such as bone pain, adenopathy, and pulmonary symptoms. Other presentations include signs or symptoms such as fever, weight loss, anemia, or a varicocele.

Diagnostic imaging of renal masses has evolved dramatically over the past 2 decades. CT, MR imaging, and ultrasonography are being increasingly performed in place of traditional diagnostic imaging tests, such as intravenous urography and angiography. Among these diagnostic tools, CT is considered the modality of choice for detection and diagnosis of renal cortical tumors, with MR imaging and ultrasound frequently applied as problem-solving tools or in patients with contraindications to contrast-enhanced CT. The advent of multislice CT has led to faster acquisition times, higher spatial resolution, and the greatest number of CT examinations ever performed; this has led to a great increase in the detection and earlier diagnosis of renal cortical tumor [5–11]. Currently, up to 70% of tumors are discovered incidentally, with a median tumor size of less than 5 cm

[10,11,16,50]. Among all renal cortical tumors detected, 20% may be benign, and 25% may be relatively indolent papillary or chromophobe carcinomas [30,31,34–36].

Although it is important to make a preoperative diagnosis of the tumor type for treatment planning and patient counseling, there are no well-established imaging criteria for diagnosing the histologic subtypes without operative resection, and the role of biopsy is controversial [51,52]. It has been suggested that certain imaging features may be associated with different renal cortical tumor subtypes [53–58]. The diagnosis of renal masses, especially the incidentally detected ones, remains problematic, however [5,59,60]. The techniques and established and potential roles of imaging in the diagnosis of renal cortical tumors with solid soft tissue components are presented subsequently. A discussion of imaging of cystic renal masses follows.

CT scan

A dedicated imaging protocol is needed for optimized evaluation of the renal mass by CT. At the authors' institution, a CT scan dedicated for evaluation of a renal mass typically consists of three imaging series performed during breath hold: precontrast, corticomedullary phase, and late nephrographic/early excretory phase [61–63]. *Precontrast images* are essential for evaluation of the presence of calcifications and provide a baseline density measurement for evaluating the degree and pattern of enhancement in cystic or solid renal masses [63]. *Corticomedullary images* (typical scan delay 70–85 seconds after injection) are superior in the assessment of lesion vascularity, renal vascular anatomy, and tumor involvement of venous structures [61]. In addition, they are probably the most informative images for lesion characterization. A relatively thin slice thickness of 2.5 mm may be obtained through the kidneys. To minimize radiation exposure, a standard slice thickness of 5 mm may be obtained through the rest of the body if such imaging is to be performed in the same setting. Not all renal tumors are well delineated during the corticomedullary phase, however, and images obtained during a later phase of enhancement (ie, the nephrographic or excretory phase) must be included to facilitate the detection of renal masses, especially those of smaller size [63–70]. In addition, *excretory phase images* (these typically can be achieved with a scan delay of 3 minutes) are helpful for delineation of anatomic abnormalities or tumor involvement of the renal collecting system [61]. High accuracy (sensitivity 100%, specificity 95%) has

been reported in the detection of renal masses when proper technique is applied [70].

Solid renal tumors

In terms of differentiation of solid renal tumors, limited investigations have been performed in the past regarding whether certain imaging features may be associated with specific subtypes of renal cortical tumor [53–58]. The most consistent and valuable parameter probably is the degree of enhancement because clear cell carcinomas enhance to a greater degree than other subtypes of malignant lesions, especially papillary carcinomas. This was shown in studies from the groups of Herts, Jinzaki, Kim, and Ruppert-Kohlmayr [53–55,57,58]. In addition, Herts and colleagues [53] showed that papillary RCCs are typically homogeneous, and Sheir and associates [58] showed that cystic degeneration was more evident in the clear cell subtype than in the other subtypes. Sheir and associates [58] reported, however, that a hypervascular pattern was more prevalent in papillary than in chromophobe subtypes, a finding inconsistent with the findings of the other studies cited. Most of these studies included only malignant lesions or in some cases subgroups of malignant lesions in their analyses.

In a series of 198 solid renal tumors that were resected at the authors' institution, 55% were of the clear cell type, 15% were papillary, 12% were chromophobe, 7% were oncocytomas, and 3% were lipid-poor angiomyolipomas [71]. Almost half of all renal tumors are either benign or relatively indolent malignant tumors. *Conventional clear cell* renal carcinoma is the most vascular type among all malignant renal cortical tumors, as shown by its greater degree of enhancement after administration of intravenous contrast material [54,55,58,71]. A mixed enhancement pattern containing enhancing solid soft tissue and low-attenuation areas that may represent cystic or necrotic changes was most predictive of the clear cell type (Fig. 1) [71]. Oncocytomas may overlap, however, with clear cell RCC in terms of imaging features and degree of enhancement (Fig. 2) [54,71]. Classic angiographic findings for *oncocytoma* have been reported in the past, including a spoke-wheel pattern, a homogeneous tumor blush, and a sharp, smooth rim [72]. None of these findings is specific, however, and a RCC may have any or all of the classic findings [72]. On CT scans, the diagnosis of oncocytoma may be suggested if a central stellate scar is identified within an otherwise homogeneous tumor (Fig. 3) [73]. Oncocytoma may often manifest as a complex hypervascular mass, however, sometimes associated with adjacent neovascularity and perinephric stranding, and cannot be reliably differentiated from clear cell carcinoma (Fig. 4) [71].

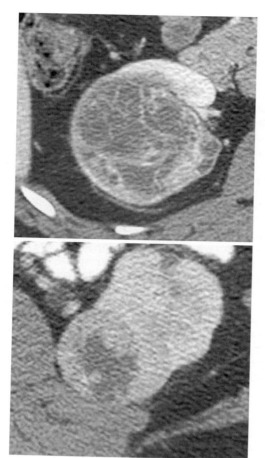

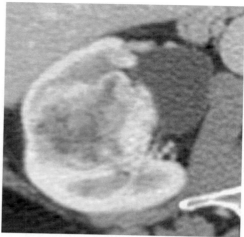

Fig. 2. A 56-year-old woman with right renal oncocytoma. Contrast-enhanced CT image during renal parenchymal phase shows a right renal mass with a mixed enhancement pattern that mimics clear cell RCC.

Homogeneously high-attenuation on unenhanced CT images and homogeneous enhancement on contrast-enhanced CT images have been reported to suggest angiomyolipoma containing abundant muscle and minimal fat [74]. Based on the authors' experience, however, these features may be shared by fat-poor angiomyolipomas and the more indolent type of RCCs (papillary and chromophobe) (Fig. 8) [71].

Generally, the presence of calcifications in a solid renal mass suggests malignancy [71,75]. Rarely,

Fig. 1. (*A*) A 50-year-old man with clear cell carcinoma in right kidney. Contrast-enhanced CT image during renal parenchymal phase shows a right renal mass with a mixed enhancement pattern containing enhancing solid soft tissue and low-attenuation areas that may represent cystic or necrotic changes. (*B*) A 63-year-old man with clear cell carcinoma in left kidney. Contrast-enhanced CT image during renal parenchymal phase shows a left renal mass with a mixed enhancement pattern with a greater amount of solid components than (*A*).

In the authors' study, *papillary* RCCs were typically less vascular compared with most other types of renal tumors and most commonly manifested as homogeneous (Fig. 5) or peripheral enhancement (Fig. 6) [71]. A low tumor-to-aorta enhancement ratio or tumor-to-normal renal parenchyma enhancement ratio was highly indicative of papillary RCC [71]. This is consistent with the finding of Herts and colleagues [53] that a high tumor-to-parenchyma enhancement ratio ≥25%) essentially excludes the possibility of a tumor being papillary RCC.

Chromophobe RCCs are more variable in their degrees and patterns of enhancement (Fig. 7) [71].

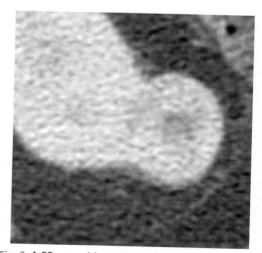

Fig. 3. A 58-year-old man with left renal oncocytoma. Contrast-enhanced CT image during renal parenchymal phase shows a left renal mass with nearly homogeneous enhancement and a small low-attenuation central scar.

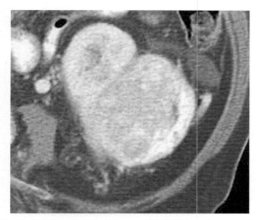

Fig. 4. A 94-year-old woman with left renal oncocytoma. Contrast-enhanced CT image during renal parenchymal phase shows a 7-cm left renal mass. The mass shows a degree of enhancement similar to that of renal parenchyma with heterogeneity and peritumoral vascularity mimicking clear cell RCC.

a malignant renal tumor may be diffusely calcified (Fig. 9).

Cystic renal tumors

Numerous articles have been published on the subject of cystic renal masses. The widely quoted Bosniak classification system grades the cystic renal masses for the likelihood of malignancy based on the complexity of these lesions [76]. When any solid enhancing component is present, the cystic renal mass is graded as a Bosniak type 4 lesion, highly suspicious for malignancy. As discussed earlier, further differentiation of this group of lesions may be possible based on the characteristics of their solid soft tissue components. Cystic tumors with thin walls and septations without solid components in an adult may represent benign cystic nephroma, multilocular cystic RCC, or, rarely, cystic hamartoma of the renal pelvis [31]. These tumors are similar in their gross appearances and cannot be differentiated by preoperative imaging studies (Fig. 10) [31]. When such a cystic mass does represent multilocular cystic RCC, however, it may be of no, or at most little, malignant potential [31] and carries a distinctly better prognosis than other forms of RCC [77]. This is probably because although these masses may contain clear cells, they generally are associated with a lower Fuhrman grade (1 or 2) on histopathology.

One common pitfall in characterizing renal lesions by CT is the presence of pseudoenhancement in renal cysts on contrast-enhanced CT images. This pseudoenhancement is thought to be due to volume averaging and beam hardening effects, and

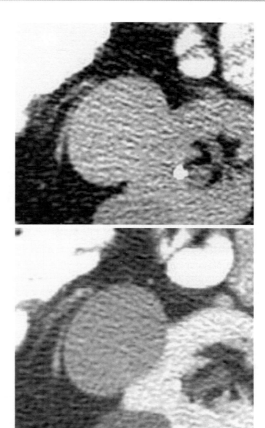

Fig. 5. A 63-year-old man with papillary carcinoma of the right kidney. (*A*) Precontrast CT image shows a mass of smooth counter and homogeneous attenuation the same as or slightly higher than that of the adjacent renal parenchyma. (*B*) Postcontrast CT image in the renal parenchymal phase shows uniform, mild enhancement of 35 HU in the renal mass.

the degree of pseudoenhancement is greater in smaller renal cysts [78–84]. In certain cases, the degree of pseudoenhancement may well surpass the 10 HU threshold commonly used to differentiate nonenhancing simple cysts from enhancing solid lesions (Fig. 11) [78–84]. In these cases, ultrasound or MR imaging may prove helpful.

MR imaging

MR imaging has many advantages over other modalities in the detection and staging of renal neoplasms, owing to its intrinsic high soft tissue contrast, direct multiplanar imaging capabilities, and availability of a non-nephrotoxic, renally excreted contrast agent [85]. State-of-the-art MR imaging of renal masses includes the following breath-hold sequences: (1) a T1-weighted in and out of phase gradient echo sequence, which is helpful in

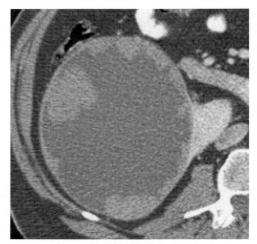

Fig. 6. A 58-year-old man with a 15-cm papillary RCC arising from the right kidney. Contrast-enhanced CT image during renal parenchymal phase shows a right renal mass with mild enhancement of 35 HU in peripherally distributed soft tissue. No enhancement is identified in the central low-attenuation region.

identification of macroscopic and microscopic fat in a renal tumor (Fig. 12) [86]; (2) a T2-weighted half-Fourier single-shot fast spin-echo sequence in axial or coronal planes, which is useful for evaluating the overall anatomy, renal collecting system, and complexity of a cystic renal lesion (Fig. 10); and (3) a dynamic contrast-enhanced T1-weighted fat-suppressed sequence [87]. For dynamic contrast-enhanced images, three-dimensional fast spoiled gradient echo sequences are typically performed [87–89] before and after contrast administration during the arterial, corticomedullary, and nephrographic phases for evaluation of the presence and pattern of enhancement in a renal mass [87,88]. Multiplanar reconstruction may be performed if necessary to delineate better the spatial relationship of the renal mass to adjacent anatomic structures. If necessary, a dedicated MR angiography sequence during the arterial phase may be performed for better visualization of accessory renal vessels and facilitation of surgical planning. Coronal T1-weighted images also may be obtained during the excretory phase with administration of diuretics, from which maximum intensity projection images can be obtained to produce intravenous pyelography–like images.

MR imaging is useful in the detection and differentiation of cystic and solid renal lesions [90], with accuracy comparable or superior to that of CT [91]. In addition, MR imaging can be performed safely in patients with renal failure and used for evaluation of renal tumors in these patients [92,93], an obvious advantage because many patients with renal

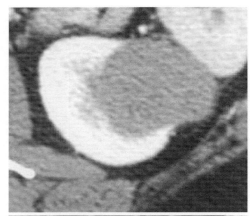

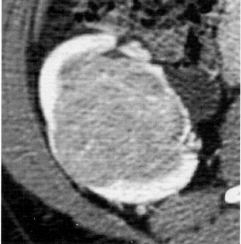

Fig. 7. (*A*) A 60-year-old woman with left chromophobe RCC. Contrast-enhanced CT image during renal parenchymal phase shows a left renal mass with homogeneous enhancement. (*B*) A 48-year-old woman with right chromophobe RCC. Contrast-enhanced CT image during renal parenchymal phase shows a right renal mass with heterogeneous enhancement.

masses are at risk of renal insufficiency at presentation or after surgical treatment. For these reasons, MR imaging may function as an excellent tool for initial diagnosis and post-treatment follow-up in these patients. It is reliable for evaluation of small renal masses [92,94] owing to its superior soft tissue contrast, whereas CT can be problematic because of pseudoenhancement (Fig. 11). In addition, because of its multiplanar capability, MR imaging may be superior to CT for determining the origin of a renal mass [71].

Solid renal tumors are typically isointense or slightly hypointense on T1-weighted images [90,95], although some renal tumors may contain hemorrhage or a lipid component and show T1

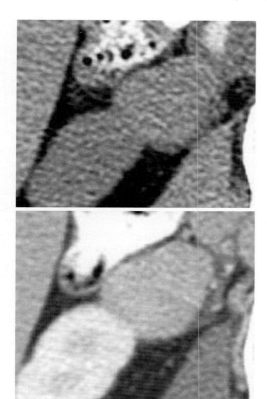

hyperintensity (Fig. 12) [93]. Clear cell carcinomas may contain intracellular lipids and show focal or diffuse signal loss on opposed-phase images, which does not always indicate angiomyolipoma (see Fig. 12) [87,96,97]. Renal cortical tumors tend to be mildly hyperintense [95] on T2-weighted images and show variable enhancement on dynamic contrast-enhanced images [90]. Simple cysts are hypointense on T1-weighted images and hyperintense on T2-weighted images. Although some complex cysts may show a higher T1 signal and lower T2 signal owing to hemorrhage, debris, or proteinaceous material, there should be no enhancement in cysts after administration of contrast. Identification of the presence of contrast enhancement is essential in diagnosing a solid renal neoplasm. It has been reported that the optimal percentage of enhancement threshold for distinguishing cysts from solid tumors on MR imaging is 15% when measurement is performed 2 to 4 minutes after administration of contrast material [98]. This threshold may be achieved with quantitative analysis of enhancement with signal intensity measurements [98]. Qualitative analysis of enhancement with image subtraction is equally accurate, particularly in the setting of masses that are hyperintense on unenhanced MR images [99]. Similar to those seen on CT, three patterns of enhancement have been observed in RCCs on MR imaging: predominantly peripheral, heterogeneous, and homogeneous [90].

CT and MR imaging perform similarly in classifying most cystic renal masses [100]. In some cases, however, MR images may depict additional septa, thickening of the wall or septa, or enhancement, which may lead to an upgraded Bosniak cyst classification and affect case management [100].

Fig. 8. A 58-year-old woman with lipid-poor right renal angiomyolipoma. (*A*) Precontrast CT image shows a homogeneous soft tissue mass that has slightly higher attenuation than the renal parenchyma. (*B*) Postcontrast parenchymal phase CT image shows homogeneous enhancement of approximately 120 HU in this mass. Note peripheral location of the mass.

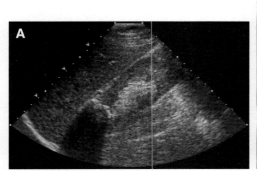

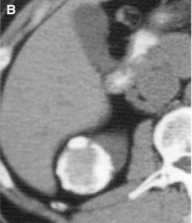

Fig. 9. A 59-year-old man with papillary renal carcinoma. (*A*) Ultrasound of the right kidney shows a 5-cm calcified mass in the upper pole. (*B*) Unenhanced CT image shows heavy calcification in the periphery of this mass.

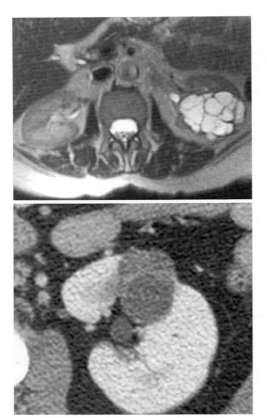

Fig. 10. (A) A 68-year-old woman with breast cancer. T2-weighted single-shot fast spin-echo MR image shows a complex cystic mass in the left kidney, which was proved to be a multilocular cystic nephroma on pathology. (B) A 52-year-old woman with multilocular cystic RCC in the left kidney. Contrast-enhanced CT image at renal parenchymal phase shows a cystic mass containing several thickened enhancing septations in the left kidney. Pathology revealed a Furhman nuclear grade of I/IV.

Ultrasonography

Ultrasound is an important problem-solving tool for evaluation of renal masses. One of the most important roles of ultrasound is in the characterization of renal lesions as cystic or solid. Because the diagnosis of a simple renal cyst denotes benignity, strict criteria need to be adhered to. The lesion must be completely anechoic, have a thin imperceptible wall, have posterior enhancement, have a round or oval shape, and be avascular. Rarely, a benign cyst can become complex in the setting of hemorrhage or infection and could mimic a solid lesion (Fig. 13). Cysts that do not fulfill all of the criteria of a simple cyst are complex, and the possibility of a cystic renal carcinoma may need to be considered depending on a cyst's radiographic features (Fig. 14). Correlation with other imaging modalities, such as CT and MR imaging, is recommended. Features on ultrasound suggesting a malignant cystic lesion include a thickened cystic wall, numerous septations, thickened or nodular septations, irregular or central calcifications, and the presence of flow in the septations or cystic wall on Doppler imaging [101].

Most RCCs on ultrasound are solid. Cystic areas and calcifications may be present (Fig. 15). Small, 3 cm or less, renal masses are more likely to be hyperechoic than larger tumors [102]. Ultrasound and cross-sectional imaging modalities (CT and MR imaging) complement each other in the characterization of renal lesions. In the subgroup of patients whose renal lesions are "indeterminate" on ultrasound, a dedicated renal protocol CT or MR imaging may help characterize the lesion further [103]. Conversely, ultrasound may prove useful for renal lesions that are considered indeterminate on CT [95].

Solid renal masses on ultrasound usually need to be evaluated with a renal protocol CT for the

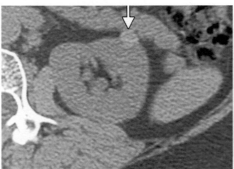
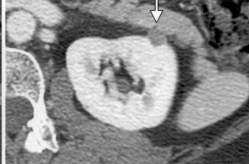

Fig. 11. A 58-year-old man with benign high-density cyst in left kidney. (A) Precontrast CT image shows a small left renal mass of 71 HU in attenuation. (B) Contrast-enhanced CT image during renal parenchymal phase shows increased attenuation to 94 HU (a pseudoenhancement of 23 HU) in this small mass.

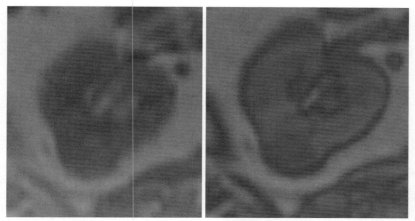

Fig. 12. A 67-year-old woman with right renal clear cell carcinoma. (*A* and *B*) T1-weighted dual-echo gradient echo MR images of the right kidney show loss of signal in right renal mass on opposed phase relative to in-phase image. (*A*) In-phase. (*B*) Opposed phase.

presence of fat. If fat is present in the lesion on CT, in most cases an angiomyolipoma can be diagnosed. Rarely, however, RCC may engulf the perirenal or sinus fat, and a liposarcoma may contain fatty components. Malignancy should be suspected on the basis of the following criteria: presence of intratumoral calcifications; large, irregular tumor invading the perirenal or sinus fat; large necrotic tumor with small foci of fat; and association with nonfatty lymph nodes or venous invasion [104–106].

Limited attempts have been made to differentiate renal cancer into the different histologic subtypes based on ultrasound characteristics. Papillary RCCs tend to be hypoechoic or isoechoic, but some also may be hyperechoic (**Fig. 16**) [56]. Work has been done in ultrasound using Doppler imaging, which allows for assessment of vascular flow [107]. Contrast-enhanced ultrasound has been found to be useful in the diagnosis of renal cortical tumors and in the detection of tumor blood flow in hypovascular renal masses [108,109]. A study from the authors' institution indicates that vascular flow within a renal mass, identified by color and power Doppler, is strongly associated with conventional clear cell carcinoma [110]. The vascular distribution at power Doppler potentially could add information in differentiation of small solid renal masses. It has been shown that peripheral or mixed penetrating and peripheral patterns are seen in all RCCs and some benign angiomyolipomas and oncocytomas, whereas intratumoral focal or penetrating patterns are characteristic of angiomyolipoma [111].

Renal ultrasound is not considered a useful screening modality because small lesions can be easily missed [112]. CT detects more and smaller renal masses than does ultrasound, but the two

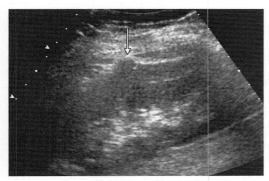

Fig. 13. A 67-year-old woman with benign epithelial cyst in left kidney. Ultrasound of the left kidney shows a small lesion (*arrow*) with internal echoes mimicking a solid lesion.

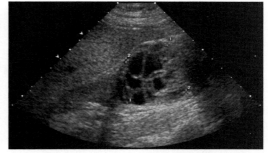

Fig. 14. A 40-year-old man with clear cell renal carcinoma of the right kidney. Ultrasound revealed a 5-cm complex cystic mass in the lower pole of the right kidney. Color Doppler documented the presence of vascularity in the septations (not shown).

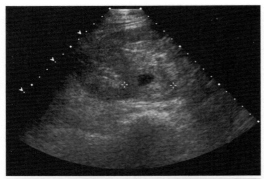

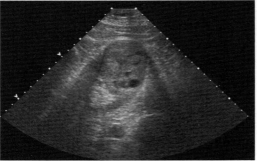

Fig. 15. (*A*) A 74-year-old man with clear cell renal carcinoma in right kidney. Ultrasound showed a 4 cm × 5 cm heterogeneous mass in the posterior medial right kidney containing solid and cystic components. (*B*) A 37-year-old man with clear cell renal carcinoma of the left kidney. Ultrasound showed a 6 cm × 7 cm mass in the interpolar region of left kidney. The mass was predominately solid with scattered cystic areas.

modalities are comparable in characterizing 1- to 3-cm lesions [113]. Although renal sonography may not be the best method for generalized primary screening, it still may be beneficial in "secondary" screening in a more selected patient population, such as in the elderly asymptomatic population [114].

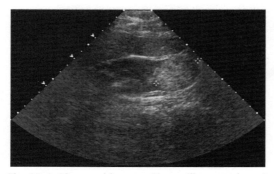

Fig. 16. A 46-year-old man with papillary renal carcinoma in right kidney. Ultrasound showed a solid 5-cm hyperechoic mass in the lower pole of the right kidney.

Nuclear scintigraphy

Although fluorodeoxyglucose (FDG) positron emission tomography (PET) has been established as an efficient imaging modality for the management of certain cancers, its role in imaging of renal cortical tumors has not yet been clearly defined. Varying sensitivity of FDG PET for the detection of renal malignancy has been reported, ranging from 40% to 94% [115–118]. Several factors may explain the false-negative results of FDG PET for detection of renal malignancy. First, normal renal excretion of FDG may have decreased the contrast between tumor and normal surrounding tissues, reducing the efficacy of PET in detecting primary renal malignancy [115]. Second, other factors, such as histologic subtypes, Fuhrman grades, or tumor vascularity, may have played a role. False-positive results by FDG PET have been reported in patients with benign inflammatory processes of the kidney or benign tumors such as oncocytomas [115,119]. A discrepancy has been observed between poor visualization of the primary renal malignancy and high uptake of FDG by metastases in the same patient [115]. FDG PET may have a potential role in evaluation of distant metastases, especially when equivocal findings are present on conventional studies, and in the differentiation between recurrence and post-treatment changes [115,117,118,120]. PET with new radiopharmaceutical agents, such as radioisotope-labeled monoclonal antibodies with specificity for RCC, may be able to provide in vivo diagnosis and determination of phenotype in the future.

Other renal tumors

Urothelial carcinoma

Urothelial tumors of the renal pelvis represent approximately 7% of primary renal neoplasms [121] and approximately 5% of urinary tract tumors [122]. Urothelial tumors of the renal pelvis are similar to those in the urinary bladder in pathologic features, epidemiologic distributions, and risk factors (which are discussed in detail in the article by Zhang and colleagues elsewhere in this issue). Urothelial carcinoma (or TCC) accounts for 90% of pelvicalyceal malignant tumors, whereas squamous cell carcinomas, which are radiologically indistinguishable from TCC, account for the other 10% [122].

TCC is often multifocal, presenting as synchronous or metachronous lesions. This known multifocality requires thorough examination of the entire urinary tract in high-risk patients, such as patients with bladder cancer or known chemical exposure [121]. Traditionally, excretory intravenous urography (IVU) has been the screening examination of choice for the detection of upper urinary tract neoplasms for patients with hematuria or for high-risk patients. IVU has been shown to miss 40% of upper tract neoplasms, however [121]. With the advent of multidetector CT enabling the rapid acquisition of thin-section images through the entire urinary tract, CT urography (CTU) has begun to supersede IVU as the imaging examination of choice to detect upper urinary tract tumors. The techniques and applications of CTU are discussed in detail in the article by Zhang and colleagues elsewhere in this issue.

On imaging, TCC of the renal pelvis manifests as a focal soft tissue mass or focal wall thickening. On noncontrast images, these tumors measure approximately 30 HU and most of the time can be differentiated from water (approximately 0 HU), blood clot (50–75 HU), and calculi (>100 HU) [123]. The enhancement pattern of urothelial neoplasms (typically mild-to-moderate early enhancement with washout on delayed images) can be similar to that of renal cortical neoplasms, although the latter are typically more vascular [123–125]. Of TCCs, 85% are early stage, superficial papillary neoplasms. In the excretory phase of CTU, early stage TCC appears as a sessile filling defect within the high-density contrast excreted into the renal collecting system; the tumor expands the collecting system with compression of the renal sinus fat (Fig. 17). Alternatively, early stage tumors can appear as focal or diffuse mural thickening, pelvicalyceal irregularity, or focally obstructed calyces (Fig. 18) [123,124]. Fifteen percent of TCCs are more aggressive, infiltrating lesions that show mural thickening and present at a more advanced stage, often with invasion into the renal parenchyma (Fig. 19) [124].

CT plays a role in staging urothelial tumors. Although CT cannot accurately distinguish T1 tumor (limited to uroepithelium and lamina propria) from T2 tumor (extending into muscularis propria,

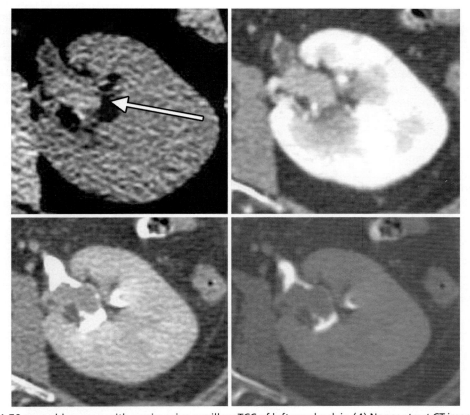

Fig. 17. A 76-year-old woman with noninvasive papillary TCC of left renal pelvis. (*A*) Noncontrast CT image shows soft tissue in left renal pelvis (*arrow*) slightly higher in attenuation than renal parenchyma. (*B*) Contrast-enhanced image during renal parenchymal phase shows uniform enhancement of approximately 80 HU in the mass. A clear fat plane is identified between the tumor and the kidney, indicating absence of renal parenchymal invasion. (*C* and *D*) Delayed, excretory phase CT images show a corresponding filling defect in the collecting system on soft tissue (*C*) and bone windows (*D*).

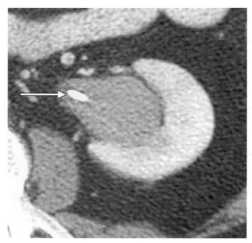

Fig. 18. A 54-year-old man with high-grade papillary urothelial carcinoma of left renal pelvis confined to mucosa of renal pelvis (stage T1). Contrast-enhanced CT shows a uniform soft tissue mass in left renal pelvis encasing a renal stent (*arrow*). A thin fat plane is maintained around the mass.

but not beyond), this modality is accurate in distinguishing early stage, T1 and T2 tumors from advanced-stage, T3 (invading peripelvic fat or renal parenchyma) and T4 (invading adjacent organs or abdominal wall or extending through renal parenchyma into perinephric fat) tumors; this distinction is important because studies have shown a significant difference in survival between stage II and III lesions [125]. Advanced stage tumor is suspected when the normally low-density renal sinus fat shows an increase in attenuation owing to tumor infiltration, or when the fat plane between the tumor and the renal parenchyma is lost; in some cases, CT may show direct invasion of tumor into

the renal parenchyma, which can appear as an infiltrating renal mass (Fig. 19) [123–125]. Occasionally, uroepithelial neoplasms invading the renal parenchyma can appear similar radiologically to centrally located renal cortical neoplasms invading the renal sinus, although in general TCC tends to be more centrally located and is more likely to expand the kidney centrifugally, while preserving the renal contour (Fig. 20) [122,125]. Although advanced TCC can invade the renal vein and inferior vena cava on rare occasions, RCC has a much greater predilection for spreading in this fashion [125]. For staging of advanced tumors, CT, superior to IVU, also allows high-quality imaging of the lymph nodes, liver, bones, and lungs, which are the most common sites of metastatic disease from urothelial neoplasms [124].

In the past, radical nephroureterectomy has been the standard treatment for renal and ureteral TCC. Newer renal-preserving techniques, such as laser ablation, endoscopic fulguration, or segmental excision, are now the preferred treatments, however, for patients who have early stage, low-grade tumors, a solitary kidney, bilateral TCC, or suboptimal renal function and for patients who are poor surgical candidates [123,124]. The clinical outcomes for these newer procedures are similar to outcomes for more radical surgery when the tumors are detected at an early stage [124]. Early detection of upper tract TCC with urine cytology and cross-sectional imaging is essential.

Metastases

Rarely, solid tumors—most commonly primary tumors of the lung, breast, stomach, or contralateral kidney—do metastasize to the kidney [87,126]. Renal metastases are often multiple and bilateral and usually are seen with metastases elsewhere in the

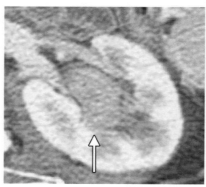
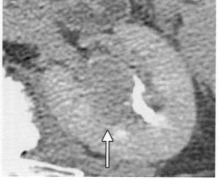

Fig. 19. A 71-year-old woman with invasive TCC of the left renal pelvis. (*A* and *B*) CT urogram shows a mass in the renal pelvis on the renal parenchymal (*A*) and excretory phase (*B*) images. The fat plane between the mass and the renal parenchyma is obliterated (*arrows*), indicating tumor invasion into renal parenchyma as confirmed by pathology.

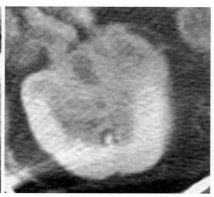

Fig. 20. A centrally located renal cortical tumor may mimic a uroepithelial tumor with renal parenchymal invasion. (*A*) A 72-year-old woman with conventional clear cell carcinoma of the right kidney. Contrast-enhanced CT shows a right renal mass invading the renal sinus, mimicking advanced stage TCC of the renal pelvis. (*B*) A 69-year-old woman with squamous cell carcinoma of renal pelvis. Contrast-enhanced CT shows a heterogeneous mass in the renal sinus with renal parenchymal invasion.

body. In patients with known primary malignancies, renal metastases are four times more common than primary renal neoplasms [127]. In the absence of metastases to other organs, however, a solitary renal mass in a patient with a known primary malignancy is more likely to represent primary RCC than metastatic disease [128]. The imaging features of renal metastases are otherwise nonspecific: Renal metastases are usually more infiltrative than RCC and less vascular, in particular, than conventional clear cell carcinoma; however, the imaging features of RCC and renal metastases often overlap, and a biopsy is frequently necessary to distinguish these entities (**Fig. 21**) [87]. Because clinical management

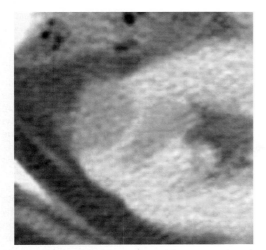

Fig. 21. A 46-year-old woman with metastatic colon cancer. Contrast-enhanced CT image shows a solid mass in the right kidney proven to represent metastasis of colorectal origin at pathology.

for a primary renal tumor and a metastatic renal lesion is completely different, it is important for a radiologist to consider this differential diagnosis.

Lymphoma

The kidney is one of the most common sites of extranodal lymphoma. Most extranodal lymphomas are non-Hodgkin lymphomas, and lymphoma is the third most common tumor, after lung and breast cancer, to involve the kidney secondarily [101,129]. Although 33% of patients with lymphoma have renal involvement in autopsy studies, the ante mortem incidence ranges from 0.5% to 8.3% [129].

Because lymphoid tissue is normally absent in the kidney, it is believed that primary renal lymphoma is extremely rare, with most cases secondarily involving the kidney by direct extension or hematogenous spread [101,129]. Direct extension of lymphoma can occur when lymphoma of the retroperitoneum invades the renal capsule (transcapsular spread) or infiltrates the renal sinus, encasing the ureter, renal pelvis, and renal vascular structures [101]. Because of the lack of associated fibrosis, lymphoma typically encases the renal hilar structures without obstruction (**Fig. 22**) [101,129]. From there, lymphoma can extend into the renal parenchyma via the medullary pyramids. When lymphoma gains access to the renal parenchyma, by direct extension or hematogenous spread, it initially involves the renal interstitium, using vessels, collecting ducts, and nephrons as scaffolding to grow.

Because the cells infiltrate between and separate, rather than destroy, these structures, lymphoma can appear subtle on imaging studies in its early stages

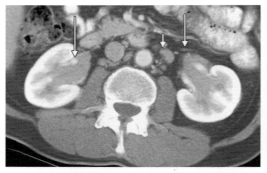

Fig. 22. A 74-year-old man with small lymphocytic lymphoma. Contrast-enhanced CT image shows homogeneous soft tissue infiltrating the renal sinuses bilaterally, encasing the renal hilar structures without urinary obstruction or vascular occlusion (*long arrows*). Note associated retroperitoneal adenopathy (*short arrow*).

[101]. Lymphomatous lesions often cause relatively little mass effect and generally do not deform the renal collecting system or renal contour. As the lesions enlarge, they may compress the calyces, but the reniform shape of the kidney usually is preserved even if the entire organ is infiltrated by tumor. Less often, these tumors may grow rapidly in a nonuniform fashion, creating a focal mass that projects beyond the contour of the kidney, mimicking a primary renal cortical neoplasm but remaining unencapsulated [101]. Renal lymphoma is typically homogeneous and shows a lower degree of enhancement than adjacent renal parenchyma on CT and MR imaging. Renal lymphoma can have several patterns on cross-sectional imaging [130]. Most cases manifest with multiple soft tissue masses in one or both kidneys. Less common imaging patterns include a solitary renal mass, direct invasion of the renal hilum or renal sinus by bulky retroperitoneal masses, and infiltration of the

perirenal space without significant renal parenchymal involvement or diffuse infiltration of the entire kidney (Fig. 23) [129,131]. Most patients also present with adjacent retroperitoneal adenopathy (see Figs. 22 and 23) [129].

Primary renal mesenchymal tumors

Primary renal mesenchymal tumors include malignant and benign lesions. Malignant renal mesenchymal sarcomas are rare, comprising less than 1% of all adult renal tumors and mostly involving patients between 40 and 70 years old [132,133]. The most common primary renal sarcoma is leiomyosarcoma followed by liposarcoma and fibrosarcoma. Less common renal sarcomas include malignant fibrous histiocytoma, rhabdomyosarcoma, osteosarcoma, chondrosarcoma, malignant peripheral nerve sheath tumor, clear cell sarcoma, and angiosarcoma [122,132,133].

Sarcomas of the kidney often arise from the renal capsule or sinus and usually can be distinguished from RCC because they lie outside the renal parenchyma [122,133]. In contrast to RCC, renal sarcomas are often extremely exophytic, displacing, distorting, or compressing the renal parenchyma without parenchymal invasion; as a result, there is often a smooth interface between the tumor and the renal parenchyma [133,134]. Renal sarcomas that do arise within the renal parenchyma are difficult to distinguish from the more common renal cortical tumors, however. On CT, renal sarcomas are typically large heterogeneous soft tissue masses with areas of necrosis (Fig. 24). A specific histologic diagnosis usually cannot be made except in most cases of liposarcoma, in which part or all of the tumor is composed of macroscopic fat. In contrast to RCC, renal sarcomas do not tend to invade the renal vein or inferior vena cava [133].

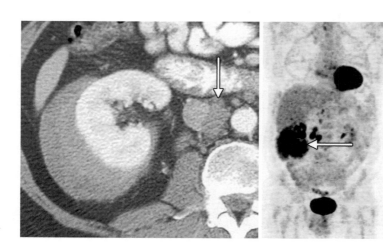

Fig. 23. A 51-year-old man with mantle cell lymphoma involving right kidney. (*A*) Contrast-enhanced CT shows homogeneous soft tissue mass infiltrating the perirenal space without gross renal parenchymal involvement or mass effect on the renal parenchyma. Note retroperitoneal adenopathy in the inter-aortocaval region (*arrow*). (*B*) FDG PET scan shows intense uptake in the region of the right kidney (*arrow*) corresponding to the lymphomatous mass on CT.

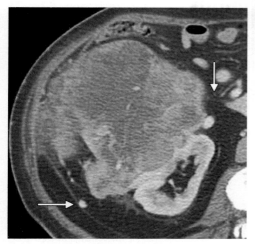

Fig. 24. A 78-year-old man with high-grade spindle cell and pleomorphic sarcoma arising from the right renal capsule on pathology. Contrast-enhanced CT shows a peripherally located large right renal mass. Note the peritumoral vascularity (*arrows*) associated with this large mass.

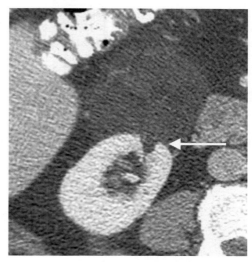

Fig. 25. A 63-year-old woman with right renal angiomyolipoma. Contrast-enhanced CT shows a large predominantly fatty mass in the right kidney. Note the defect in the renal parenchyma where the lesion arises from the kidney (*arrow*). This defect suggests the diagnosis of angiomyolipoma instead of liposarcoma.

Large exophytic angiomyolipomas are another relevant entity worthy of discussion. Angiomyolipomas, also known as renal hamartomas, are the most common benign mesenchymal tumors in the kidney. These lesions contain mature adipose tissue, smooth muscle, and blood vessels. Occasionally, they can manifest as large exophytic renal masses that contain varying degrees of fat and soft tissue, mimicking the appearance of renal capsular liposarcoma. Given the different treatments and prognoses for these two lesions, distinguishing between them radiologically is crucial. Because angiomyolipomas arise from the renal parenchyma rather than the capsule, a defect in the parenchyma is almost always visible at the site of the tumor's origin (Fig. 25), whereas liposarcomas do not cause such a defect. Angiomyolipomas also tend to be more vascular than liposarcomas and are more likely than liposarcoma to contain one or more large vessels within the lesion. Additional features that suggest the diagnosis of angiomyolipoma instead of liposarcoma are the presence of intralesional hemorrhage, the smaller overall size of the lesion, and the presence of additional angiomyolipomas within the kidney [134].

Although rare, benign mesenchymal renal neoplasms besides angiomyolipomas also can occur, including leiomyomas, lipomas, fibromas, neurogenic tumors, and hemangiomas [122]. Renal leiomyomas, which most commonly occur in middle-aged women, are the most common of these tumors, and similar to their malignant counterparts, they arise from smooth muscle cells located

in the renal capsule, pelvis, calyx, or blood vessels [135]; as a result, these tumors tend to be peripheral or parapelvic in location [136]. They have a variable radiographic pattern, which can range from an entirely solid to a purely cystic mass (Fig. 26) [136]. Although leiomyomas are generally smaller and more homogeneous than leiomyosarcomas, their appearance can be similar [127,136]. Leiomyomas and leiomyosarcomas occasionally can contain

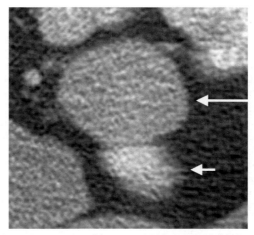

Fig. 26. A 49-year-old woman with incidental left renal leiomyoma arising from the left renal capsule on pathology. Contrast-enhanced CT image shows a homogeneous mass (*long arrow*) arising peripherally from the upper pole of the left kidney (*short arrow*).

calcifications; these two entities cannot be confidently distinguished preoperatively unless gross invasion is observed, in which case the diagnosis of leiomyoma is virtually eliminated [136].

Staging

Currently, the most commonly used staging system is the TNM system [137] of the American Joint Committee on Cancer (Table 1). The patient's overall disease stage is determined by American Joint Committee on Cancer stage groupings (Table 2) [137].

Cancer-specific survival for patients treated with surgery is highly correlated with the tumor stage (Table 3) [138]. Precise staging is crucial for preoperative planning and prognosis. An overall staging accuracy of 91% by preoperative CT has been reported in the past, with most staging errors related to the diagnosis of perinephric extension of tumor [139]. Detection of perinephric tumor extension has no significant impact on therapy, but carries prognostic significance. Currently, there is no reliable indicator for perinephric tumor spread on CT. Perinephric stranding may be present in the absence of tumor spread. One study showed that 50% of patients with tumor confined within the renal capsule showed perinephric stranding [139]. The presence of an intact pseudocapsule, composed of compressed normal renal parenchyma and fibrous tissue surrounding the renal mass, has been reported to be helpful in local staging of renal cortical tumors [140,141]. The pseudocapsule is best detected by T2-weighted imaging on MR imaging [140,141]. The presence of an intact pseudocapsule suggests a lack of perinephric fat invasion [141].

CT has been found to have a high negative predictive value for adrenal involvement from RCC [142]. It is suggested that only when the adrenal gland is not identified, not displaced or not enlarged on CT, adrenalectomy should be performed as part of radical nephrectomy, although even in this select group adrenal involvement was present in only 26% of the cases in one study [142].

Evaluation of the venous system in patients with renal malignancy is crucial for treatment planning. Previously performed with conventional venography, this evaluation is now being done with noninvasive cross-sectional imaging. A thrombus involving the renal vein or inferior vena cava in a patient with malignant renal tumor may represent tumor thrombus directly extending from the primary location or a bland blood clot or both. The presence of enhancement within the thrombus indicates tumor thrombus, whereas bland thrombus would not enhance after contrast administration (Figs. 27 and 28). In some cases, the tumor thrombus

Table 1:　**TNM staging for renal cancer**

T	Primary tumor
TX	Primary tumor cannot be assessed
T0	No evidence of primary tumor
T1	Tumor ≤7 cm in greatest dimension, limited to the kidney
T1a	Tumor ≤4 cm in greatest dimension, limited to the kidney
T1b	Tumor >4 cm but ≤7 cm in greatest dimension, limited to the kidney
T2	Tumor >7 cm in greatest dimension, limited to the kidney
T3	Tumor extends into major veins or invades adrenal gland or perinephric tissues, but not beyond Gerota's fascia
T3a	Tumor directly invades adrenal gland or perirenal and/or renal sinus fat, but not beyond Gerota's fascia
T3b	Tumor grossly extends into the renal vein or its segmental (ie, muscle-containing) branches or the vena cava below the diaphragm
T3c	Tumor grossly extends into the vena cava above the diaphragm or invades the wall of the vena cava
T4	Tumor invades beyond Gerota's fascia
N	**Regional lymph nodes**
NX	Regional lymph nodes cannot be assessed
N0	No regional lymph node metastasis
N1	Metastasis in a single regional lymph node
N2	Metastasis in >1 regional lymph node
M	**Distant metastasis**
MX	Distant metastasis cannot be assessed
M0	No distant metastasis
M1	Distant metastasis

Table 2: **Stage grouping for renal cancer**

Stage I	T1, N0, M0
Stage II	T2, N0, M0
Stage III	T1, N1, M0
	T2, N1, M0
	T3, N0, M0
	T3, N1, M0
Stage IV	T4, N0, M0
	T4, N1, M0
	Any T, N2, M0
	Any T, any N, M1

may extend beyond the margin of the inferior vena cava, indicating invasion of the wall of the inferior vena cava [143].

On cross-sectional imaging, assessment of lymph nodes relies on anatomic size criteria, and cross-sectional imaging is limited for detecting normal-sized lymph nodes that harbor low-volume metastatic disease or differentiating metastatic adenopathy from lymph node enlargement with a benign etiology. The sensitivity of CT for detection of regional lymph node metastases is reported to be 95% [144]. False-positive findings of 58% have been reported, however, when a size criterion of 1 cm is used for determining nodal metastasis, owing to reactive or other benign nodal changes [139,144]. These false-positive findings were more frequent in patients with tumor involvement of the renal vein and tumor necrosis [144].

The most common metastatic sites from malignant renal cortical tumors include lung, bone, brain, liver, and mediastinum [145]. As a general rule, small renal tumors are unlikely to present initially with metastases, although there are occasional exceptions. CT of the abdomen and pelvis and a chest radiograph are essential studies in the initial workup. A chest CT scan can be obtained if the chest radiograph is abnormal, or advanced primary disease is present. Despite advances in CT technology, the sensitivity for the detection of pulmonary metastases from extrathoracic primary

tumors ranges from 75% to 95%, but is lower (50–70%) for pulmonary metastases smaller than 6 mm [146,147]. In addition, pulmonary nodules with benign causes may lead to false-positive results. RCC is associated with hypervascular liver metastasis, particularly when the primary tumor is of the clear cell type. It has been shown that portal venous phase imaging detects 90% of liver metastases from RCC, with the addition of precontrast or hepatic arterial phase imaging increasing the sensitivity in lesion detection to almost 100% [148]. Rarely, advanced RCC also may metastasize to the mesentery (**Fig. 29**). Bone metastases from RCC are most commonly lytic (**Fig. 30**). Because 85% of patients with bone metastases from RCC present with bone pain, a bone scan is not routinely performed unless the patient complains of bone pain or has an elevated serum alkaline phosphatase. In addition, because osseous metastases from RCC are usually lytic without osteoblastic activity, bone scan may be negative in these cases. MR imaging may be considered in evaluation of symptomatic patients. Similarly, imaging of the brain with CT or MR imaging is performed when brain metastasis is suggested by history or by physical examination (**Fig. 31**).

The overall accuracy of MR imaging in staging is comparable or superior to that of CT [71,95,149]. Most likely because of its multiplanar capabilities and superior soft tissue contrast, MR imaging seems to have advantages over CT in the evaluation of tumor vascular extension, the differentiation of perihilar lymph node metastases from vessels, and the assessment of direct tumor invasion into adjacent organs [71,95,150]; MR imaging also can be used to differentiate tumor reliably from bland thrombus [150]. These capabilities make MR imaging an excellent staging modality that should be used when the CT findings are equivocal [71]. MR imaging is not accurate in indicating bowel and mesentery involvement, but technical advances and the introduction of bowel contrast medium may change this in the future [71].

Treatment planning

RCC is one of the few tumors in which well-documented cases of spontaneous tumor regression in the absence of therapy exist, and occasionally patients with locally advanced or metastatic disease may exhibit indolent courses lasting several years, but this occurs very rarely and may not lead to long-term survival. Surgical treatment is currently the only curative therapy for localized RCC and is indicated for patients with stage I, II, or III disease.

Table 3: **Survival rates for renal cancer by T stage**

T stage of renal malignancy	Cancer-specific survival	
	5-y	10-y
T1	95%	95%
T2	88%	81%
T3	59%	43%
T4	20%	14%

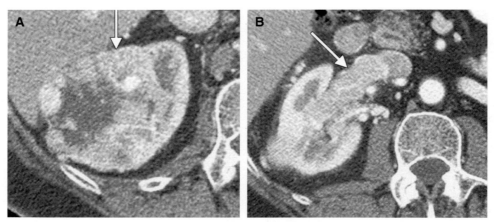

Fig. 27. A 78 year-old man with right clear cell renal carcinoma. (*A*) Contrast-enhanced CT shows a large hetero-geneous tumor (*arrow*) in the upper pole of the right kidney. (*B*) Contrast-enhanced CT at the level of the renal hilum shows a large expanding, enhancing tumor thrombus (*arrow*) in the right renal vein, bulging into the inferior vena cava.

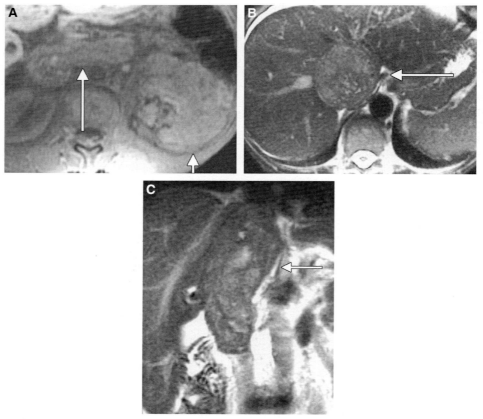

Fig. 28. MR images in a 77-year-old woman with a malignant left renal cortical tumor showing venous invasion. (*A*) Axial fat-suppressed T1-weighted image shows a left renal mass (*short arrow*) with tumor thrombus extend-ing into the left renal vein (*long arrow*). (*B* and *C*) Axial and coronal T2-weighted single-shot fast spin-echo sequences show marked expansion of the inferior vena cava from tumor thrombus (*arrows*).

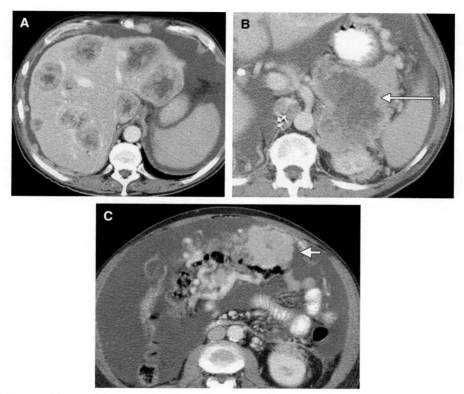

Fig. 29. A 67-year-old man with liver and peritoneal metastases from clear cell carcinoma. (*A*) Contrast-enhanced CT image shows multiple hepatic metastases. (*B*) Contrast-enhanced CT image shows a large heterogeneous metastatic lesion to pancreatic tail (*arrow*). (*C*) Contrast-enhanced CT image shows peritoneal metastases (*short arrow*).

Long-term survival can be achieved in about half of patients with tumor extension into the vena cava, but it is thought that the prognosis of these patients is primarily influenced by known adverse prognostic factors, such as capsular invasion, nodal disease, and distant metastases, rather than vena caval tumor thrombus itself [138,151,152]. Imaging, especially MR imaging, plays a crucial role in determining the extent of caval thrombus because intracardiac extension requires the assistance of

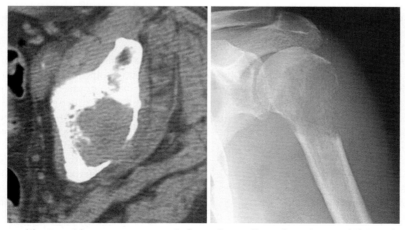

Fig. 30. A 75-year-old man with osseous metastasis from clear cell renal carcinoma. (*A*) Unenhanced CT image shows a lytic lesion in the left acetabulum. (*B*) Radiograph of left shoulder shows a lytic lesion in the proximal left humerus with associated pathologic fracture.

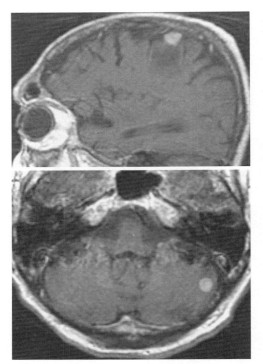

Fig. 31. A 67-year-old woman with brain metastases from clear cell renal carcinoma. (A) Sagittal T1-weighted contrast-enhanced MR image of the brain shows an enhancing mass in the cerebrum. (B) Axial T1-weighted contrast-enhanced MR image of the brain shows an enhancing mass in the cerebellum.

experienced cardiovascular surgeons for resection and may entail venovenous or cardiopulmonary bypass techniques, with or without circulatory arrest [152]. Depending on the extent of tumor thrombus, perioperative mortality is high [152].

Because disease in the regional lymph nodes and distant metastases have a great negative impact on survival, aggressive surgery in patients with gross nodal involvement or distant metastases is considered unwarranted because it contributes little to survival [151]. Most patients with nodal involvement eventually relapse with distant metastases despite lymphadenectomy [153], but regional nodal dissection does provide diagnostic and prognostic information and the only potential curative therapy. In addition, enlarged lymph nodes on imaging could have a benign etiology; patients with mild regional adenopathy on imaging still may be considered for surgery [139,144]. In highly selected cases, surgical resection of locally recurrent RCC or a solitary metastasis may be associated with long-term survival [9,154].

Radical nephrectomy, defined as removal of all the contents within the Gerota's fascia, including the kidney, perirenal fat, ipsilateral adrenal gland, and regional lymph nodes, has been the traditional mainstay of surgical resection. More recent studies have suggested, however, that in most patients adrenal-sparing nephrectomy may be considered, with resection of the ipsilateral adrenal gland restricted only to patients with large upper-pole tumors or abnormal-appearing adrenal glands on CT [142].

The long-term renal health of patients with renal tumors is an important clinical consideration for the following reasons: (1) Renal cortical tumors may be bilateral and multifocal in hereditary and nonfamilial forms; (2) a significant number of these tumors carry a low metastatic potential and good long-term prognosis [155]; and (3) as the patients age, they are at risk for development of added intrinsic renal damage from common diseases, such as diabetes, hypertension, and glomerulonephritis [156]. Partial nephrectomy should be considered a diagnostic and therapeutic surgical approach for renal cortical masses [32] whenever possible. Radical nephrectomy for renal lesions that could be removed by partial nephrectomy risk renal impairment in a substantial proportion of patients with benign or relatively indolent disease. Although it used to be reserved for patients with bilateral tumors, renal insufficiency, or an anatomically or functionally solitary kidney, partial nephrectomy is now being offered as a standard surgical option to all patients with renal lesions measuring 4 cm or smaller even in the setting of a normal contralateral kidney [157]. Evidence suggests that if technically feasible, partial nephrectomy also should be considered for tumors 7 cm in size for better renal function preservation [158]. It has been shown that disease-free survival rates are similar between renal cortical tumors treated with radical and partial nephrectomy in properly selected patients [73], but the patients treated by partial nephrectomy have a decreased risk for chronic renal insufficiency and proteinuria [73,156].

State-of-the-art multidetector CT provides thinner slices and allows for multiplanar three-dimensional image postprocessing, which may help in evaluating the anatomic relationship of the renal mass to adjacent structures, facilitating surgical planning [62,159,160]. This information is particularly crucial if nephron-sparing or laparoscopic surgery is being planned. State-of-the-art MR imaging also has been shown to be accurate for the identification and characterization of renal neoplasms amenable to partial nephrectomy [161].

Ultrasound also may assist in the preoperative evaluation of renal cortical tumors. Renal ultrasound is requested by the urologist as a template for the intraoperative ultrasound. It helps in selecting the proper surgical technique and in determining whether a partial nephrectomy can be attempted. Because of its multiplanar capability, ultrasound can show important landmarks and planes of sections.

The prognosis of patients with renal cortical tumor depends on the mode of presentation (patients with incidentally detected renal tumors have an excellent prognosis), tumor size, histology, and stage [162,163]. The likelihood of renal tumor metastases is probably associated with the size of the primary tumor [164]. With improved imaging, renal tumors are being detected incidentally in greater numbers and at smaller sizes and earlier stages [5–11]. Distant metastasis is unlikely in patients with incidentally detected small renal masses. In addition, it seems that not all malignant renal tumors undergo significant active growth [6–8], and without significant tumor growth, the risk of metastasis may be limited as well. "Watchful waiting" may be a reasonable approach in highly selected cases [6,7], especially in patients who are elderly or poor surgical candidates.

New imaging-guided therapeutic modalities, such as renal cryosurgery and radiofrequency ablation, are under active investigation [165]. It has been reported that radiofrequency ablation can completely destroy renal cancers, while transmitting minimal collateral damage to surrounding renal parenchyma [165]. The preliminary results of trials of imaging-guided radiofrequency thermal ablation or cryotherapy for treatment of primary renal tumors showed that these techniques may allow complete ablation of renal tumors with a low complication rate [165–167]. In addition, these studies showed that MR imaging is particularly useful for monitoring tumor destruction because of its excellent soft tissue contrast, high spatial resolution, multiplanar capabilities, high vascular conspicuity, and temperature sensitivity [166,167]. Untreated areas can be accurately identified on MR imaging so that the electrode can be repositioned and additional radiofrequency application performed in the same treatment session, eliminating the need for return visits for additional treatment of residual tumor, which are often required when ultrasound or CT is used for guidance [165–168]. Imaging-guided local therapy also has been used successfully for the treatment of local recurrences and isolated metastases from RCC [165,169–171]. As with the treatment of primary RCC, the long-term data on these imaging-guided therapeutic techniques is still limited, and questions remain regarding the optimal techniques and method of surveillance [172,173]. These applications should be reserved for patients who are poor surgical candidates and for whom standard therapies have been exhausted [165,169,174].

The management of patients with advanced RCC remains a clinical challenge, with systemic therapy having only limited effectiveness [29]. There is no established role for adjuvant radiation or systemic therapy in patients treated with nephrectomy, even in patients with nodal involvement or incomplete tumor resection [9,29,33,175]. No adjuvant therapy has been shown to reduce the likelihood of recurrence [176,177]. Radiation therapy with bisphosphonates may be considered for palliation of painful bone metastases.

Imaging follow-up

After surgical treatment, 20% to 30% of patients with localized renal tumors relapse. Most recurrences occur within 3 years after surgery, with the median time to relapse being 1 to 2 years [178]. Late tumor recurrence many years after initial treatment occasionally occurs. The lung is the most vulnerable site for distant recurrence, which occurs in 50% to 60% of patients (Fig. 32). Other common sites of recurrence include bone, the nephrectomy site, brain, liver, and the contralateral kidney (Figs. 33–35) [179]. Greatest tumor diameter, T stage, stage group, and nuclear grade are important factors in determining the likelihood of recurrence [179]. A long disease-free interval before recurrence and metachronous presentation of recurrence are favorable predictors of survival [154]. Efforts have been made to develop a nomogram to predict the 5-year probability of freedom from recurrence for patients with conventional clear cell RCC [180], which should be useful for patient counseling, clinical trial design, and effective patient follow-up strategies.

As discussed previously, bilateral multifocal renal tumors are present in approximately 5% of patients with sporadic renal tumors [48,49]. Although most

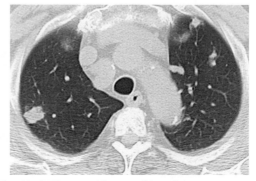

Fig. 32. A 70-year-old man with pulmonary metastases 6 months after left nephrectomy for clear cell RCC. CT image shows multiple bilateral pulmonary nodules.

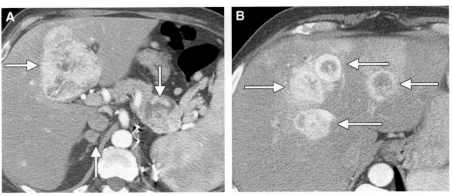

Fig. 33. A 57-year-old man with recurrence 15 years after left nephrectomy for clear cell carcinoma. (*A* and *B*) Contrast-enhanced CT images show hypervascular hepatic (*horizontal arrows*), pancreatic (*downward pointing vertical arrow*) and right adrenal (*upward pointing vertical arrow*) metastases. Note surgical clips in left nephrectomy bed in (*A*).

bilateral tumors present synchronously, asynchronous lesions may occur many years after the original nephrectomy, committing the patient to long-term follow-up [25,48,155].

For imaging surveillance, CT is the modality of choice for detection of local recurrence and distant metastases. In patients with compromised renal function or with contraindications to iodinated contrast, gadolinium-enhanced MR imaging of the abdomen and pelvis may be performed. A chest radiograph or chest CT study may be obtained for surveillance of pulmonary metastases, based on pathologic stage and as clinically indicated.

FDG PET may have a potential role in the evaluation of distant metastases, especially when findings from conventional studies are equivocal, and in the differentiation of recurrence from post-treatment changes [115,117,118,120]. Because of the high specificity and positive predictive value of FDG PET, a positive result should be considered strongly suggestive of local recurrence or metastasis, although a negative result cannot reliably rule out metastatic disease [120].

Summary

CT is the imaging modality of choice for evaluation of renal tumor. When a proper technique is used, CT provides high accuracy in detection of a renal mass. Certain imaging features and enhancement patterns on CT may help distinguish different subtypes of renal tumors. In addition, CT provides

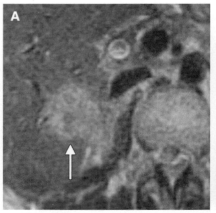
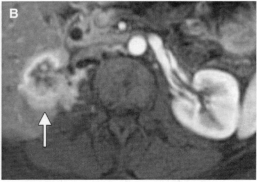

Fig. 34. A 55-year-old woman with local recurrence 3 years after right nephrectomy for clear cell carcinoma. (*A*) Axial T2-weighted single-shot fast spin-echo image shows a mass of mildly increased T2 signal extending from right nephrectomy bed into right hepatic lobe (*arrow*). (*B*) Axial contrast-enhanced T1-weighted image with fat saturation shows a heterogeneously enhancing mass extending from right nephrectomy bed into right hepatic lobe (*arrow*).

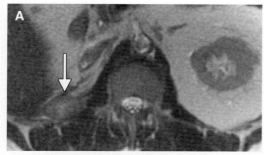

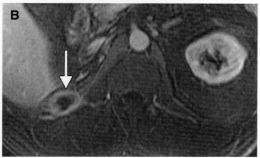

Fig. 35. A 59-year-old man with local recurrence 15 months after right nephrectomy for clear cell carcinoma. (*A*) Axial T2-weighted single-shot fast spin-echo image shows a mass of intermediate T2 signal at the right nephrectomy bed (*arrow*). (*B*) Axial contrast-enhanced T1-weighted image with fat saturation shows peripheral enhancement within this mass (*arrow*).

useful diagnostic information for treatment planning and follow-up. MR imaging and ultrasound function as valuable problem-solving tools.

References

[1] American Cancer Society. Cancer facts and figures 2006. Atlanta (GA): American Cancer Society; 2006.

[2] Ries LAG, Eisner MP, Kosary CL, et al. SEER cancer statistics review, 1975–2002. Bethesda (MD): National Cancer Institute; 2005.

[3] Provet J, Tessler A, Brown J, et al. Partial nephrectomy for renal cell carcinoma: indications, results and implications. J Urol 1991;145(3): 472–6.

[4] Kosary CL, McLaughlin JK. Kidney and renal pelvis. In: Miller BA, Ries LAG, Hankey BG, et al, editors. SEER cancer statistics review, 1973–1990. NIH publication no. 93-2789, XI.1-XI.22. Bethesda (MD): National Cancer Institute; 1993.

[5] Bosniak MA. Problems in the radiologic diagnosis of renal parenchymal tumors. Urol Clin North Am 1993;20(2):217–30.

[6] Bosniak MA. Observation of small incidentally detected renal masses. Semin Urol Oncol 1995;13(4):267–72.

[7] Bosniak MA, Birnbaum BA, Krinsky GA, et al. Small renal parenchymal neoplasms: further observations on growth. Radiology 1995; 197(3):589–97.

[8] Kassouf W, Aprikian AG, Laplante M, et al. Natural history of renal masses followed expectantly. J Urol 2004;171(1):111–3 [discussion 113].

[9] Motzer RJ, Russo P, Nanus DM, Berg WJ. Renal cell carcinoma. Curr Probl Cancer 1997;21(4): 185–232.

[10] Russo P. Renal cell carcinoma: presentation, staging, and surgical treatment. Semin Oncol 2000;27(2):160–76.

[11] Smith SJ, Bosniak MA, Megibow AJ, et al. Renal cell carcinoma: earlier discovery and increased detection. Radiology 1989;170(3 Pt 1): 699–703.

[12] Rabbani F, Reuter VE, Katz J, et al. Second primary malignancies associated with renal cell carcinoma: influence of histologic type. Urology 2000;56(3):399–403.

[13] Weiss LM, Gelb AB, Medeiros LJ. Adult renal epithelial neoplasms. Am J Clin Pathol 1995; 103(5):624–35.

[14] Kovacs G, Akhtar M, Beckwith BJ, et al. The Heidelberg classification of renal cell tumours. J Pathol 1997;183(2):131–3.

[15] Russo P. Evolving understanding and surgical management of renal cortical tumors. Mayo Clin Proc 2000;75(12):1233–5.

[16] Russo P. Localized renal cell carcinoma. Curr Treat Options Oncol 2001;2(5):447–55.

[17] Lindblad P, Mellemgaard A, Schlehofer B, et al. International renal-cell cancer study: V. reproductive factors, gynecologic operations and exogenous hormones. Int J Cancer 1995;61(2): 192–8.

[18] Mandel JS, McLaughlin JK, Schlehofer B, et al. International renal-cell cancer study: IV. occupation. Int J Cancer 1995;61(5):601–5.

[19] McLaughlin JK, Chow WH, Mandel JS, et al. International renal-cell cancer study: VIII. role of diuretics, other anti-hypertensive medications and hypertension. Int J Cancer 1995;63(2): 216–21.

[20] McLaughlin JK, Lindblad P, Mellemgaard A, et al. International renal-cell cancer study: I. tobacco use. Int J Cancer 1995;60(2):194–8.

[21] Mellemgaard A, Lindblad P, Schlehofer B, et al. International renal-cell cancer study: III. role of weight, height, physical activity, and use of amphetamines. Int J Cancer 1995;60(3):350–4.

[22] Schlehofer B, Pommer W, Mellemgaard A, et al. International renal-cell-cancer study: VI. the role of medical and family history. Int J Cancer 1996;66(6):723–6.

[23] Wolk A, Gridley G, Niwa S, et al. International renal cell cancer study: VII. Role of diet. Int J Cancer 1996;65(1):67–73.

[24] Ishikawa I, Kovacs G. High incidence of papillary renal cell tumours in patients on

chronic haemodialysis. Histopathology 1993; 22(2):135–9.

[25] Rabbani F, Herr HW, Almahmeed T, et al. Temporal change in risk of metachronous contralateral renal cell carcinoma: influence of tumor characteristics and demographic factors. J Clin Oncol 2002;20(9):2370–5.

[26] Lamiell JM, Salazar FG, Hsia YE. von Hippel-Lindau disease affecting 43 members of a single kindred. Medicine (Baltimore) 1989;68(1): 1–29.

[27] Cohen AJ, Li FP, Berg S, et al. Hereditary renal-cell carcinoma associated with a chromosomal translocation. N Engl J Med 1979;301(11):592–5.

[28] Pathak S, Strong LC, Ferrell RE, et al. Familial renal cell carcinoma with a 3;11 chromosome translocation limited to tumor cells. Science 1982;217(4563):939–41.

[29] Motzer RJ, Bander NH, Nanus DM. Renal-cell carcinoma. N Engl J Med 1996;335(12): 865–75.

[30] Beck SD, Patel MI, Snyder ME, et al. Effect of papillary and chromophobe cell type on disease-free survival after nephrectomy for renal cell carcinoma. Ann Surg Oncol 2004;11(1): 71–7.

[31] Eble JN, Bonsib SM. Extensively cystic renal neoplasms: cystic nephroma, cystic partially differentiated nephroblastoma, multilocular cystic renal cell carcinoma, and cystic hamartoma of renal pelvis. Semin Diagn Pathol 1998;15(1): 2–20.

[32] McKiernan J, Yossepowitch O, Kattan MW, et al. Partial nephrectomy for renal cortical tumors: pathologic findings and impact on outcome. Urology 2002;60(6):1003–9.

[33] Motzer RJ, Bacik J, Mariani T, et al. Treatment outcome and survival associated with metastatic renal cell carcinoma of non-clear-cell histology. J Clin Oncol 2002;20(9): 2376–81.

[34] Amin MB, Corless CL, Renshaw AA, et al. Papillary (chromophil) renal cell carcinoma: histomorphologic characteristics and evaluation of conventional pathologic prognostic parameters in 62 cases. Am J Surg Pathol 1997; 21(6):621–35.

[35] Renshaw AA, Henske EP, Loughlin KR, et al. Aggressive variants of chromophobe renal cell carcinoma. Cancer 1996;78(8):1756–61.

[36] Crotty TB, Farrow GM, Lieber MM. Chromophobe cell renal carcinoma: clinicopathological features of 50 cases. J Urol 1995;154(3): 964–7.

[37] Kondagunta GV, Drucker B, Schwartz L, et al. Phase II trial of bortezomib for patients with advanced renal cell carcinoma. J Clin Oncol 2004;22(18):3720–5.

[38] Ficarra V, Righetti R, Pilloni S, et al. Prognostic factors in patients with renal cell carcinoma: retrospective analysis of 675 cases. Eur Urol 2002;41(2):190–8.

[39] Frank I, Blute ML, Cheville JC, et al. An outcome prediction model for patients with clear cell renal cell carcinoma treated with radical nephrectomy based on tumor stage, size, grade and necrosis: the SSIGN score. J Urol 2002; 168(6):2395–400.

[40] Gettman MT, Blute ML, Spotts B, et al. Pathologic staging of renal cell carcinoma: significance of tumor classification with the 1997 TNM staging system. Cancer 2001;91(2): 354–61.

[41] Bretheau D, Lechevallier E, de Fromont M, et al. Prognostic value of nuclear grade of renal cell carcinoma. Cancer 1995;76(12):2543–9.

[42] Ficarra V, Righetti R, Martignoni G, et al. Prognostic value of renal cell carcinoma nuclear grading: multivariate analysis of 333 cases. Urol Int 2001;67(2):130–4.

[43] Fiori E, De Cesare A, Galati G, et al. Prognostic significance of primary-tumor extension, stage and grade of nuclear differentiation in patients with renal cell carcinoma. J Exp Clin Cancer Res 2002;21(2):229–32.

[44] Fuhrman SA, Lasky LC, Limas C. Prognostic significance of morphologic parameters in renal cell carcinoma. Am J Surg Pathol 1982;6(7): 655–63.

[45] Lohse CM, Blute ML, Zincke H, et al. Comparison of standardized and nonstandardized nuclear grade of renal cell carcinoma to predict outcome among 2,042 patients. Am J Clin Pathol 2002;118(6):877–86.

[46] Ficarra V, Guille F, Schips L, et al. Proposal for revision of the TNM classification system for renal cell carcinoma. Cancer 2005;104(10):2116–23.

[47] Gudbjartsson T, Hardarson S, Petursdottir V, et al. Histological subtyping and nuclear grading of renal cell carcinoma and their implications for survival: a retrospective nation-wide study of 629 patients. Eur Urol 2005;48: 593–600.

[48] Patel MI, Simmons R, Kattan MW, et al. Long-term follow-up of bilateral sporadic renal tumors. Urology 2003;61(5):921–5.

[49] Richstone L, Scherr DS, Reuter VR, et al. Multifocal renal cortical tumors: frequency, associated clinicopathological features and impact on survival. J Urol 2004;171(2 Pt 1):615–20.

[50] Silver DA, Morash C, Brenner P, et al. Pathologic findings at the time of nephrectomy for renal mass. Ann Surg Oncol 1997;4(7):570–4.

[51] Dechet CB, Zincke H, Sebo TJ, et al. Prospective analysis of computerized tomography and needle biopsy with permanent sectioning to determine the nature of solid renal masses in adults. J Urol 2003;169(1):71–4.

[52] Lechevallier E, Andre M, Barriol D, et al. Fine-needle percutaneous biopsy of renal masses with helical CT guidance. Radiology 2000; 216(2):506–10.

[53] Herts BR, Coll DM, Novick AC, et al. Enhancement characteristics of papillary renal

neoplasms revealed on triphasic helical CT of the kidneys. AJR Am J Roentgenol 2002; 178(2):367–72.

[54] Jinzaki M, Tanimoto A, Mukai M, et al. Double-phase helical CT of small renal parenchymal neoplasms: correlation with pathologic findings and tumor angiogenesis. J Comput Assist Tomogr 2000;24(6):835–42.

[55] Kim JK, Kim TK, Ahn HJ, et al. Differentiation of subtypes of renal cell carcinoma on helical CT scans. AJR Am J Roentgenol 2002;178(6): 1499–506.

[56] Press GA, McClennan BL, Melson GL, et al. Papillary renal cell carcinoma: CT and sonographic evaluation. AJR Am J Roentgenol 1984;143(5): 1005–9.

[57] Ruppert-Kohlmayr AJ, Uggowitzer M, Meissnitzer T, et al. Differentiation of renal clear cell carcinoma and renal papillary carcinoma using quantitative CT enhancement parameters. AJR Am J Roentgenol 2004;183(5): 1387–91.

[58] Sheir KZ, El-Azab M, Mosbah A, et al. Differentiation of renal cell carcinoma subtypes by multislice computerized tomography. J Urol 2005; 174(2):451–5 [discussion 455].

[59] Israel GM, Bosniak MA. Renal imaging for diagnosis and staging of renal cell carcinoma. Urol Clin North Am 2003;30(3):499–514.

[60] Silverman SG, Lee BY, Seltzer SE, et al. Small (< or = 3 cm) renal masses: correlation of spiral CT features and pathologic findings. AJR Am J Roentgenol 1994;163(3):597–605.

[61] Kauczor HU, Schwickert HC, Schweden F, et al. Bolus-enhanced renal spiral CT: technique, diagnostic value and drawbacks. Eur J Radiol 1994;18(3):153–7.

[62] Sheth S, Scatarige JC, Horton KM, et al. Current concepts in the diagnosis and management of renal cell carcinoma: role of multidetector ct and three-dimensional CT. Radiographics 2001;21(Spec No):S237–54.

[63] Schreyer HH, Uggowitzer MM, Ruppert-Kohlmayr A. Helical CT of the urinary organs. Eur Radiol 2002;12(3):575–91.

[64] Yuh BI, Cohan RH, Francis IR, et al. Comparison of nephrographic with excretory phase helical computed tomography for detecting and characterizing renal masses. Can Assoc Radiol J 2000;51(3):170–6.

[65] Yuh BI, Cohan RH. Different phases of renal enhancement: role in detecting and characterizing renal masses during helical CT. AJR Am J Roentgenol 1999;173(3):747–55.

[66] Yuh BI, Cohan RH. Helical CT for detection and characterization of renal masses. Semin Ultrasound CT MR 1997;18(2):82–90.

[67] Szolar DH, Kammerhuber F, Altziebler S, et al. Multiphasic helical CT of the kidney: increased conspicuity for detection and characterization of small (<3-cm) renal masses. Radiology 1997;202(1):211–7.

[68] Cohan RH, Sherman LS, Korobkin M, et al. Renal masses: assessment of corticomedullary-phase and nephrographic-phase CT scans. Radiology 1995;196(2):445–51.

[69] Birnbaum BA, Jacobs JE, Ramchandani P. Multiphasic renal CT: comparison of renal mass enhancement during the corticomedullary and nephrographic phases. Radiology 1996; 200(3):753–8.

[70] Kopka L, Fischer U, Zoeller G, et al. Dual-phase helical CT of the kidney: value of the corticomedullary and nephrographic phase for evaluation of renal lesions and preoperative staging of renal cell carcinoma. AJR Am J Roentgenol 1997;169(6):1573–8.

[71] Zhang J, Lefkowitz R, Ishill N, et al. Differentiation of solid renal cortical tumors by CT. Radiology, in press.

[72] Ambos MA, Bosniak MA, Valensi QJ, et al. Angiographic patterns in renal oncocytomas. Radiology 1978;129(3):615–22.

[73] Quinn MJ, Hartman DS, Friedman AC, et al. Renal oncocytoma: new observations. Radiology 1984;153(1):49–53.

[74] Jinzaki M, Tanimoto A, Narimatsu Y, et al. Angiomyolipoma: imaging findings in lesions with minimal fat. Radiology 1997;205(2): 497–502.

[75] Daniel WW, Hartman GW, Witten DM, et al. Calcified renal mass: a review of ten years experience at the Mayo Clinic. Radiology 1972;103: 503–8.

[76] Bosniak MA. The current radiological approach to renal cysts. Radiology 1986;158(1):1–10.

[77] Brinker DA, Amin MB, de Peralta-Venturina M, et al. Extensively necrotic cystic renal cell carcinoma: a clinicopathologic study with comparison to other cystic and necrotic renal cancers. Am J Surg Pathol 2000;24(7):988–95.

[78] Birnbaum BA, Maki DD, Chakraborty DP, et al. Renal cyst pseudoenhancement: evaluation with an anthropomorphic body CT phantom. Radiology 2002;225(1):83–90.

[79] Maki DD, Birnbaum BA, Chakraborty DP, et al. Renal cyst pseudoenhancement: beam-hardening effects on CT numbers. Radiology 1999; 213(2):468–72.

[80] Coulam CH, Sheafor DH, Leder RA, et al. Evaluation of pseudoenhancement of renal cysts during contrast-enhanced CT. AJR Am J Roentgenol 2000;174(2):493–8.

[81] Bae KT, Heiken JP, Siegel CL, et al. Renal cysts: is attenuation artifactually increased on contrast-enhanced CT images? Radiology 2000;216(3): 792–6.

[82] Heneghan JP, Spielmann AL, Sheafor DH, et al. Pseudoenhancement of simple renal cysts: a comparison of single and multidetector helical CT. J Comput Assist Tomogr 2002;26(1): 90–4.

[83] Gokan T, Ohgiya Y, Munechika H, et al. Renal cyst pseudoenhancement with beam hardening

effect on CT attenuation. Radiat Med 2002; 20(4):187–90.

[84] Abdulla C, Kalra MK, Saini S, et al. Pseudoenhancement of simulated renal cysts in a phantom using different multidetector CT scanners. AJR Am J Roentgenol 2002;179(6):1473–6.

[85] Pretorius ES, Wickstrom ML, Siegelman ES. MR imaging of renal neoplasms. Magn Reson Imaging Clin N Am 2000;8(4):813–36.

[86] Israel GM, Hindman N, Hecht E, et al. The use of opposed-phase chemical shift MRI in the diagnosis of renal angiomyolipomas. AJR Am J Roentgenol 2005;184(6):1868–72.

[87] Zhang J, Israel GM, Krinsky GA, et al. Masses and pseudomasses of the kidney: imaging spectrum on MR. J Comput Assist Tomogr 2004; 28(5):588–95.

[88] Heiss SG, Shifrin RY, Sommer FG. Contrast-enhanced three-dimensional fast spoiled gradient-echo renal MR imaging: evaluation of vascular and nonvascular disease. Radiographics 2000; 20(5):1341–52 [discussion 1353–4].

[89] Semelka RC, Hricak H, Stevens SK, et al. Combined gadolinium-enhanced and fat-saturation MR imaging of renal masses. Radiology 1991; 178(3):803–9.

[90] Eilenberg SS, Lee JK, Brown J, et al. Renal masses: evaluation with gradient-echo Gd-DTPA-enhanced dynamic MR imaging. Radiology 1990;176(2):333–8.

[91] Semelka RC, Shoenut JP, Kroeker MA, et al. Renal lesions: controlled comparison between CT and 1.5-T MR imaging with nonenhanced and gadolinium-enhanced fat-suppressed spin-echo and breath-hold FLASH techniques. Radiology 1992;182(2):425–30.

[92] Bosniak MA, Rofsky NM. Problems in the detection and characterization of small renal masses. Radiology 1996;198(3):638–41.

[93] John G, Semelka RC, Burdeny DA, et al. Renal cell cancer: incidence of hemorrhage on MR images in patients with chronic renal insufficiency. J Magn Reson Imaging 1997;7(1): 157–60.

[94] Scialpi M, Di Maggio A, Midiri M, et al. Small renal masses: assessment of lesion characterization and vascularity on dynamic contrast-enhanced MR imaging with fat suppression. AJR Am J Roentgenol 2000;175(3):751–7.

[95] Fein AB, Lee JK, Balfe DM, et al. Diagnosis and staging of renal cell carcinoma: a comparison of MR imaging and CT. AJR Am J Roentgenol 1987;148(4):749–53.

[96] Outwater EK, Bhatia M, Siegelman ES, et al. Lipid in renal clear cell carcinoma: detection on opposed-phase gradient-echo MR images. Radiology 1997;205(1):103–7.

[97] Outwater EK, Blasbalg R, Siegelman ES, et al. Detection of lipid in abdominal tissues with opposed-phase gradient-echo images at 1.5 T: techniques and diagnostic importance. Radiographics 1998;18(6):1465–80.

[98] Ho VB, Allen SF, Hood MN, et al. Renal masses: quantitative assessment of enhancement with dynamic MR imaging. Radiology 2002;224(3): 695–700.

[99] Hecht EM, Israel GM, Krinsky GA, et al. Renal masses: quantitative analysis of enhancement with signal intensity measurements versus qualitative analysis of enhancement with image subtraction for diagnosing malignancy at MR imaging. Radiology 2004; 232(2):373–8.

[100] Israel GM, Hindman N, Bosniak MA. Evaluation of cystic renal masses: comparison of CT and MR imaging by using the Bosniak classification system. Radiology 2004;231(2):365–71.

[101] Hartman DS, David CJ Jr, Goldman SM, et al. Renal lymphoma: radiologic-pathologic correlation of 21 cases. Radiology 1982;144(4): 759–66.

[102] Forman HP, Middleton WD, Melson GL, et al. Hyperechoic renal cell carcinomas: increase in detection at US. Radiology 1993;188(2):431–4.

[103] Prasad SR, Saini S, Stewart S, et al. CT characterization of "indeterminate" renal masses: targeted or comprehensive scanning? J Comput Assist Tomogr 2002;26(5):725–7.

[104] Helenon O, Chretien Y, Paraf F, et al. Renal cell carcinoma containing fat: demonstration with CT. Radiology 1993;188(2):429–30.

[105] Helenon O, Merran S, Paraf F, et al. Unusual fat-containing tumors of the kidney: a diagnostic dilemma. Radiographics 1997;17(1):129–44.

[106] Strotzer M, Lehner KB, Becker K. Detection of fat in a renal cell carcinoma mimicking angiomyolipoma. Radiology 1993;188(2):427–8.

[107] Taylor KJ, Ramos I, Carter D, et al. Correlation of Doppler US tumor signals with neovascular morphologic features. Radiology 1988;166 (1 Pt 1):57–62.

[108] Tamai H, Takiguchi Y, Oka M, et al. Contrast-enhanced ultrasonography in the diagnosis of solid renal tumors. J Ultrasound Med 2005; 24(12):1635–40.

[109] Kim JK, Kim SH, Jang YJ, et al. Renal angiomyolipoma with minimal fat: differentiation from other neoplasms at double-echo chemical shift FLASH MR imaging. Radiology 2006;239(1): 174–80.

[110] Raj GV, Bach A, Iasonos A, et al. Utility of preoperative color Doppler ultrasonography in predicting the histology of renal lesions. J Urol 2007;177:53–8.

[111] Jinzaki M, Ohkuma K, Tanimoto A, et al. Small solid renal lesions: usefulness of power Doppler US. Radiology 1998;209(2):543–50.

[112] Warshauer DM, McCarthy SM, Street L, et al. Detection of renal masses: sensitivities and specificities of excretory urography/linear tomography, US, and CT. Radiology 1988; 169(2):363–5.

[113] Jamis-Dow CA, Choyke PL, Jennings SB, et al. Small (< or = 3-cm) renal masses: detection

[114] Malaeb BS, Martin DJ, Littooy FN, et al. The utility of screening renal ultrasonography: identifying renal cell carcinoma in an elderly asymptomatic population. BJU Int 2005;95(7): 977–81.

[115] Aide N, Cappele O, Bottet P, et al. Efficiency of [(18)F]FDG PET in characterising renal cancer and detecting distant metastases: a comparison with CT. Eur J Nucl Med Mol Imaging 2003; 30(9):1236–45.

[116] Goldberg MA, Mayo-Smith WW, Papanicolaou N, et al. FDG PET characterization of renal masses: preliminary experience. Clin Radiol 1997;52(7):510–5.

[117] Montravers F, Grahek D, Kerrou K, et al. Evaluation of FDG uptake by renal malignancies (primary tumor or metastases) using a coincidence detection gamma camera. J Nucl Med 2000; 41(1):78–84.

[118] Ramdave S, Thomas GW, Berlangieri SU, et al. Clinical role of F-18 fluorodeoxyglucose positron emission tomography for detection and management of renal cell carcinoma. J Urol 2001;166(3):825–30.

[119] Blake MA, McKernan M, Setty B, et al. Renal oncocytoma displaying intense activity on 18F-FDG PET. AJR Am J Roentgenol 2006;186(1): 269–70.

[120] Schoder H, Larson SM. Positron emission tomography for prostate, bladder, and renal cancer. Semin Nucl Med 2004;34(4):274–92.

[121] Caoili EM, Cohan RH, Inampudi P, et al. MDCT urography of upper tract urothelial neoplasms. AJR Am J Roentgenol 2005;184(6):1873–81.

[122] Rha SE, Byun JY, Jung SE, et al. The renal sinus: pathologic spectrum and multimodality imaging approach. Radiographics 2004;24(Suppl 1):S117–31.

[123] Urban BA, Buckley J, Soyer P, et al. CT appearance of transitional cell carcinoma of the renal pelvis: Part 1. early-stage disease. AJR Am J Roentgenol 1997;169(1):157–61.

[124] Browne RF, Meehan CP, Colville J, et al. Transitional cell carcinoma of the upper urinary tract: spectrum of imaging findings. Radiographics 2005;25(6):1609–27.

[125] Urban BA, Buckley J, Soyer P, et al. CT appearance of transitional cell carcinoma of the renal pelvis: Part 2. advanced-stage disease. AJR Am J Roentgenol 1997;169(1):163–8.

[126] Wagle DG, Moore RH, Murphy GP. Secondary carcinomas of the kidney. J Urol 1975;114(1): 30–2.

[127] Curry NS. Small renal masses (lesions smaller than 3 cm): imaging evaluation and management. AJR Am J Roentgenol 1995;164(2): 355–62.

[128] Israel GM, Krinsky GA. MR imaging of the kidneys and adrenal glands. Radiol Clin North Am 2003;41(1):145–59.

[129] Cohan RH, Dunnick NR, Leder RA, et al. Computed tomography of renal lymphoma. J Comput Assist Tomogr 1990;14(6):933–8.

[130] Urban BA, Fishman EK. Renal lymphoma: CT patterns with emphasis on helical CT. Radiographics 2000;20(1):197–212.

[131] Heiken JP, Gold RP, Schnur MJ, et al. Computed tomography of renal lymphoma with ultrasound correlation. J Comput Assist Tomogr 1983;7(2):245–50.

[132] Vogelzang NJ, Fremgen AM, Guinan PD, et al. Primary renal sarcoma in adults: a natural history and management study by the American Cancer Society, Illinois Division. Cancer 1993; 71(3):804–10.

[133] Shirkhoda A, Lewis E. Renal sarcoma and sarcomatoid renal cell carcinoma: CT and angiographic features. Radiology 1987;162(2): 353–7.

[134] Israel GM, Bosniak MA, Slywotzky CM, et al. CT differentiation of large exophytic renal angiomyolipomas and perirenal liposarcomas. AJR Am J Roentgenol 2002;179(3):769–73.

[135] Nagar AM, Raut AA, Narlawar RS, et al. Giant renal capsular leiomyoma: study of two cases. Br J Radiol 2004;77(923):957–8.

[136] Steiner M, Quinlan D, Goldman SM, et al. Leiomyoma of the kidney: presentation of 4 new cases and the role of computerized tomography. J Urol 1990;143(5):994–8.

[137] Kidney. In: American Joint Committee on Cancer. AJCC Cancer Staging Manual. 6th edition. New York: Springer; 2002. p. 323–5.

[138] Javidan J, Stricker HJ, Tamboli P, et al. Prognostic significance of the 1997 TNM classification of renal cell carcinoma. J Urol 1999;162(4): 1277–81.

[139] Johnson CD, Dunnick NR, Cohan RH, et al. Renal adenocarcinoma: CT staging of 100 tumors. AJR Am J Roentgenol 1987;148(1):59–63.

[140] Yamashita Y, Honda S, Nishiharu T, et al. Detection of pseudocapsule of renal cell carcinoma with MR imaging and CT. AJR Am J Roentgenol 1996;166(5):1151–5.

[141] Roy C Sr, El Ghali S, Buy X, et al. Significance of the pseudocapsule on MRI of renal neoplasms and its potential application for local staging: a retrospective study. AJR Am J Roentgenol 2005;184(1):113–20.

[142] Gill IS, McClennan BL, Kerbl K, et al. Adrenal involvement from renal cell carcinoma: predictive value of computerized tomography. J Urol 1994;152(4):1082–5.

[143] Didier D, Racle A, Etievent JP, et al. Tumor thrombus of the inferior vena cava secondary to malignant abdominal neoplasms: US and CT evaluation. Radiology 1987;162(1 Pt 1): 83–9.

[144] Studer UE, Scherz S, Scheidegger J, et al. Enlargement of regional lymph nodes in renal cell carcinoma is often not due to metastases. J Urol 1990;144(2 Pt 1):243–5.

[145] Hilton S. Imaging of renal cell carcinoma. Semin Oncol 2000;27(2):150–9.

[146] Diederich S, Semik M, Lentschig MG, et al. Helical CT of pulmonary nodules in patients with extrathoracic malignancy: CT-surgical correlation. AJR Am J Roentgenol 1999;172(2): 353–60.

[147] Margaritora S, Porziella V, D'Andrilli A, et al. Pulmonary metastases: can accurate radiological evaluation avoid thoracotomic approach? Eur J Cardiothorac Surg 2002;21(6):1111–4.

[148] Raptopoulos VD, Blake SP, Weisinger K, et al. Multiphase contrast-enhanced helical CT of liver metastases from renal cell carcinoma. Eur Radiol 2001;11(12):2504–9.

[149] Semelka RC, Shoenut JP, Magro CM, et al. Renal cancer staging: comparison of contrast-enhanced CT and gadolinium-enhanced fat-suppressed spin-echo and gradient-echo MR imaging. J Magn Reson Imaging 1993;3(4): 597–602.

[150] Myneni L, Hricak H, Carroll PR. Magnetic resonance imaging of renal carcinoma with extension into the vena cava: staging accuracy and recent advances. Br J Urol 1991;68(6):571–8.

[151] Cherrie RJ, Goldman DG, Lindner A, et al. Prognostic implications of vena caval extension of renal cell carcinoma. J Urol 1982;128(5): 910–2.

[152] Bissada NK, Yakout HH, Babanouri A, et al. Long-term experience with management of renal cell carcinoma involving the inferior vena cava. Urology 2003;61(1):89–92.

[153] Phillips E, Messing EM. Role of lymphadenectomy in the treatment of renal cell carcinoma. Urology 1993;41(1):9–15.

[154] Kavolius JP, Mastorakos DP, Pavlovich C, et al. Resection of metastatic renal cell carcinoma. J Clin Oncol 1998;16(6):2261–6.

[155] Grimaldi G, Reuter V, Russo P. Bilateral non-familial renal cell carcinoma. Ann Surg Oncol 1998;5(6):548–52.

[156] McKiernan J, Simmons R, Katz J, et al. Natural history of chronic renal insufficiency after partial and radical nephrectomy. Urology 2002; 59(6):816–20.

[157] Gilbert SM, Russo P, Benson MC, et al. The evolving role of partial nephrectomy in the management of renal cell carcinoma. Curr Oncol Rep 2003;5(3):239–44.

[158] Dash A, Vickers AJ, Schachter LR, et al. Comparison of outcomes in elective partial vs radical nephrectomy for clear cell renal cell carcinoma of 4–7 cm. BJU Int 2006;97(5): 939–45.

[159] Chernoff DM, Silverman SG, Kikinis R, et al. Three-dimensional imaging and display of renal tumors using spiral CT: a potential aid to partial nephrectomy. Urology 1994;43(1): 125–9.

[160] Lee CT, Hilton S, Russo P. Renal mass within a horseshoe kidney: preoperative evaluation with three-dimensional helical computed tomography. Urology 2001;57(1):168.

[161] Pretorius ES, Siegelman ES, Ramchandani P, et al. Renal neoplasms amenable to partial nephrectomy: MR imaging. Radiology 1999; 212(1):28–34.

[162] Lee CT, Katz J, Fearn PA, et al. Mode of presentation of renal cell carcinoma provides prognostic information. Urol Oncol 2002;7(4): 135–40.

[163] Kattan MW, Reuter V, Motzer RJ, et al. A postoperative prognostic nomogram for renal cell carcinoma. J Urol 2001;166(1):63–7.

[164] Duffey BG, Choyke PL, Glenn G, et al. The relationship between renal tumor size and metastases in patients with von Hippel-Lindau disease. J Urol 2004;172(1):63–5.

[165] Zagoria RJ, Hawkins AD, Clark PE, et al. Percutaneous CT-guided radiofrequency ablation of renal neoplasms: factors influencing success. AJR Am J Roentgenol 2004;183(1):201–7.

[166] Lewin JS, Nour SG, Connell CF, et al. Phase II clinical trial of interactive MR imaging-guided interstitial radiofrequency thermal ablation of primary kidney tumors: initial experience. Radiology 2004;232(3):835–45.

[167] Silverman SG, Tuncali K, vanSonnenberg E, et al. Renal tumors: MR imaging-guided percutaneous cryotherapy—initial experience in 23 patients. Radiology 2005;236(2):716–24.

[168] Gervais DA, McGovern FJ, Wood BJ, et al. Radio-frequency ablation of renal cell carcinoma: early clinical experience. Radiology 2000; 217(3):665–72.

[169] Zagoria RJ. Percutaneous image-guided radiofrequency ablation of renal malignancies. Radiol Clin North Am 2003;41(5):1067–75.

[170] McLaughlin CA, Chen MY, Torti FM, et al. Radiofrequency ablation of isolated local recurrence of renal cell carcinoma after radical nephrectomy. AJR Am J Roentgenol 2003; 181(1):93–4.

[171] Zagoria RJ, Chen MY, Kavanagh PV, et al. Radio frequency ablation of lung metastases from renal cell carcinoma. J Urol 2001;166(5):1827–8.

[172] Wagner AA, Solomon SB, Su LM. Treatment of renal tumors with radiofrequency ablation. J Endourol 2005;19(6):643–52 [discussion 652–3].

[173] Varkarakis IM, Allaf ME, Inagaki T, et al. Percutaneous radio frequency ablation of renal masses: results at a 2-year mean followup. J Urol 2005;174(2):456–60 [discussion 460].

[174] Su LM, Jarrett TW, Chan DY, et al. Percutaneous computed tomography-guided radiofrequency ablation of renal masses in high surgical risk patients: preliminary results. Urology 2003; 61(4, Suppl 1):26–33.

[175] Motzer RJ, Russo P. Systemic therapy for renal cell carcinoma. J Urol 2000;163(2):408–17.

[176] Messing EM, Manola J, Wilding G, et al. Phase III study of interferon alfa-NL as adjuvant

treatment for resectable renal cell carcinoma: an Eastern Cooperative Oncology Group/Intergroup trial. J Clin Oncol 2003;21(7): 1214–22.

[177] Clark JI, Atkins MB, Urba WJ, et al. Adjuvant high-dose bolus interleukin-2 for patients with high-risk renal cell carcinoma: a cytokine working group randomized trial. J Clin Oncol 2003;21(16):3133–40.

[178] Sandock DS, Seftel AD, Resnick MI. A new protocol for the followup of renal cell carcinoma based on pathological stage. J Urol 1995; 154(1):28–31.

[179] Chae EJ, Kim JK, Kim SH, et al. Renal cell carcinoma: analysis of postoperative recurrence patterns. Radiology 2005;234(1): 189–96.

[180] Sorbellini M, Kattan MW, Snyder ME, et al. A postoperative prognostic nomogram predicting recurrence for patients with conventional clear cell renal cell carcinoma. J Urol 2005;173(1): 48–51.

ELSEVIER
SAUNDERS

RADIOLOGIC
CLINICS
OF NORTH AMERICA

Radiol Clin N Am 45 (2007) 149–166

Ovarian Cancer

Svetlana Mironov, MD*, Oguz Akin, MD, Neeta Pandit-Taskar, MD,
Lucy E. Hann, MD

- Epidemiology
- Relevant histopathology
- Ovarian cancer screening
- Lesion characterization
- Staging
- Posttreatment follow-up
- Recurrent ovarian tumor resectability
- Summary
- References

Epidemiology

Ovarian cancer is a leading cause of death from gynecologic malignancy and the fifth most common cause of cancer death in women. It is estimated that in 2006, 20,180 new cases of ovarian cancer will be diagnosed, and 15,310 women will die of this disease in the United States [1]. Detection of stage I disease can have a significant impact on 5-year survival, which approaches 80% to 90% in patients with stage I disease, but ranges from 5% to 50% in women with stage III–IV disease. Currently, almost 60% to 65% of patients present with stage III at the time of diagnosis, making ovarian cancer one of the most lethal malignancies.

Relevant histopathology

Primary ovarian neoplasms are differentiated by the cell origin, such as surface epithelium, germ cell, and stromal cells. Approximately 90% of primary ovarian cancers are epithelial tumors, arising from the surface epithelium. Based on the degree of differentiation, epithelial tumors are divided into three major categories: well differentiated (10%), moderately differentiated (25%), and poorly differentiated (65%). Less differentiated tumors are associated with worse prognosis. Epithelial neoplasms are separated into two major categories: invasive (80%) and noninvasive (borderline) tumors (20%), which are associated with different prognostic characteristics. Epithelial invasive tumors are subdivided further into five histopathologic groups: serous tumor (50%), mucinous neoplasm (20%), endometrioid carcinoma (20%), clear cell carcinoma (10%), and undifferentiated tumor (<5%). Another subtype of epithelial tumor is Brenner tumor, which is almost invariably benign.

The primary goal of radiologic assessment is differentiation of malignant tumors from benign tumors, rather than determination of histologic subtype. Sometimes it is possible, however, to suggest the histologic subtype of an epithelial neoplasm based on particular imaging features [2].

For the most common epithelial neoplasms, serous cystadenocarcinomas are bilateral in more than 50% of cases, with peak age of presentation 70 to 75 years old. The typical imaging finding is a large-volume ascites out of proportion to the size of bilateral complex adnexal masses of irregular shape with polypoid excrescences on the surface. Widespread peritoneal carcinomatosis with omental infiltration by the tumor (so-called omental caking) is invariably present in cases of serous papillary carcinoma.

Department of Radiology, Cornell University Weill Medical College, Memorial Sloan-Kettering Cancer Center, 1275 York Avenue, C278, New York, NY 10021, USA
* Corresponding author.
E-mail address: mironovs@mskcc.org (S. Mironov).

doi:10.1016/j.rcl.2006.10.012

Mucinous neoplasms are seen in older patients with a later peak age of 75 to 80 years. These tumors manifest as large, unilateral, multiseptated masses with a variable ratio of solid to cystic components. The presence of an enhancing solid component within a multicystic mass is a strong indicator of malignant etiology. A benign counterpart of mucinous cystadenocarcinoma, mucinous cystadenoma, typically has the appearance of a multiloculated cystic mass with thin septations (Fig. 1). Different compartments or locules within the mass have different densities of mucin on CT and different signal intensities on MR imaging.

Endometrioid cancers are usually bilateral mixed solid and cystic masses, which can be associated with endometrial hyperplasia and even concomitant endometrial carcinoma. Clear cell tumor

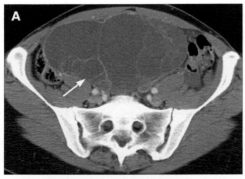

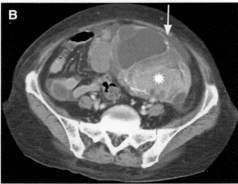

Fig. 1. Two different patients with mucinous ovarian neoplasms. (*A*) Mucinous borderline tumor of the ovary. Contrast-enhanced axial section through the pelvis shows a large multiloculated cystic mass (*arrow*) with thin internal septations, suggesting a relatively benign process. No ancillary findings, such as ascites or peritoneal carcinomatosis, are evident. (*B*) Malignant counterpart of mucinous ovarian tumor—mucinous cystadenocarcinoma (*arrow*). The mass is more complex than cystadenoma and contains a considerable enhancing heterogeneous solid component (*asterisk*), characteristic of malignant neoplasms.

manifests at the younger age of 55 to 59 years and has the typical appearance of a solitary complex cystic mass with a vascular solid mural nodule. It is associated with endometriosis and occasionally may arise within endometriomas [3]. Finally, undifferentiated tumors are solid, usually bilateral masses with varying degrees of necrosis. They are generally associated with poor prognosis.

Approximately 20% of all epithelial neoplasms are borderline tumors, also referred to as "tumors of low malignant potential." These neoplasms are associated with better prognosis. The patients (>90% of whom present with stage I disease) are 10 to 15 years younger than women with invasive epithelial carcinoma. Borderline tumors can be serous or mucinous. The risk of contralateral involvement in serous borderline tumor is 25% to 60%. Patients with serous borderline tumors, which express micropapillary features, have increased risk of relapse compared with patients without micropapillary features. The tumor can recur as a low-grade serous carcinoma years after initial treatment. Mucinous borderline tumors often manifest as large unilateral cystic masses with thin septations. The risk of bilateral involvement is low, and peritoneal involvement and ascites are rare. A woman with a borderline mucinous neoplasm should undergo appendectomy along with thorough gastrointestinal investigation to rule out a primary gastrointestinal neoplasm. Imaging features of borderline tumors are similar to those of malignant masses, and there are no specific features that allow confident differentiation of borderline neoplasms from stage I disease [4,5]. Borderline tumors are treated with surgical excision and staging. Patients with borderline tumors treated with conservative unilateral oophorectomy or cystectomy to preserve fertility require close monitoring and prolonged imaging follow-up because they have an increased recurrence rate compared with women treated with complete total abdominal hysterectomy and bilateral salpingo-oophorectomy.

Nonepithelial ovarian neoplasms include malignant germ cell tumors and malignant sex cord tumors. Malignant germ cell and sex cord tumors account for approximately 10% of primary ovarian cancers.

Malignant germ cell tumors are more frequent in young patients. The most common subtypes are dysgerminoma, immature teratoma, and endodermal sinus tumor. Dysgerminoma is an equivalent of seminoma in male patients. Patients present with a unilateral, predominantly solid mass with varying degrees of necrosis and hemorrhage. Nodal metastases are more frequent than peritoneal disease. The patients are treated with unilateral salpingo-oophorectomy and chemotherapy. Immature ovarian teratoma is usually a unilateral solid mass with coarse calcifications and occasionally a small amount of fat within the mass. Mature elements may coexist within the same ovary and within the contralateral ovary in 10% of cases. Immature teratoma metastasizes via peritoneal surfaces.

Sex cord tumors derive from ovarian stroma and account for only 1% to 2% of all ovarian malignancies. Of the different subtypes of sex cord tumors, only granulosa cell tumors are seen with considerable frequency. These tumors are predominantly solid and are hormonally active, contributing to early detection. Granulosa cell tumors are divided into juvenile and adult types. Adult granulosa cell tumors present in perimenopausal women with uterine bleeding secondary to estrogen-induced endometrial hyperplasia. Untreated endometrial hyperplasia can progress to endometrial carcinoma in 5% to 25% of patients. Granulosa cell tumors can be androgenic and present with virilization. The typical imaging findings are solid, usually unilateral masses. They can have a typical spongelike appearance on MR imaging owing to multiple cystic components. Granulosa cell tumors have a predisposition to hemorrhage; 15% patients can present with hemoperitoneum resulting from occasional tumor rupture. These tumors are treated with surgical resection and generally have a good prognosis. They can recur as peritoneal implants many years after surgery, however, and prolonged follow-up is required. Care should be exercised in evaluation of patients treated for granulosa cell cancer. Recurrent peritoneal implants may appear as well-circumscribed, round and oval homogeneous intraperitoneal masses, which are difficult to differentiate from unopacified bowel loops on CT [6,7].

Secondary neoplasms of the ovary (metastases) are relatively rare, accounting for only 5% of cases. The most frequent offenders are gastric carcinoma (particularly adenocarcinoma with signet features, so-called Krukenberg's tumors), colon cancer, pancreatic cancer, breast cancer, and melanoma. Metastases are frequently bilateral and at imaging range from solid enhancing lesions with different degrees of necrosis to complex cystic masses of various sizes. Although multilocularity at ultrasound or MR imaging favors the diagnosis of primary rather than secondary neoplasm, accurate distinction between primary and secondary ovarian tumor is difficult [8].

Lymphoma of the ovaries is extremely rare and usually is a manifestation of non-Hodgkin disease. Lymphoma should be suspected in the presence of bilateral solid homogeneous ovarian masses with little contrast enhancement [9].

Primary peritoneal carcinoma may arise years after oophorectomy and may resemble the pattern of spread of ovarian carcinoma with ascites and peritoneal tumor implants. Relevant clinical and surgical history is essential for differential diagnosis.

Ovarian cancer screening

The goal of ovarian cancer screening is to reduce mortality by detection of potentially curable stage I invasive epithelial ovarian cancers. Serum CA-125 measurements and ultrasound are used either singly or in combination [10–18]. Criteria for an abnormal ultrasound screening are ovary enlarged for age, persistent ovarian mass, or cyst with nodularity and septations. Because physiologic changes such as hemorrhagic cysts may give false-positive results, it is important that only persistent abnormalities be considered abnormal. The glycoprotein serum CA-125 marker is elevated in 80% of ovarian cancers, most of which are advanced at presentation, but CA-125 is elevated in only 50% of stage I ovarian tumors. CA-125 also is insensitive for mucinous and germ cell tumors, but these tumors with good prognosis are less significant for screening.

Radiologists should be aware of the current literature regarding ovarian cancer screening to respond appropriately to patients' concerns about disease prevention and screening strategies. Results of large screening trials vary according to the screening methods and study design [10–18]. Studies that use CA-125 alone report a higher percentage of advanced tumors with fewer stage I tumors; however, more recent studies that use serial CA-125 measurements have shown improved results [19]. When ultrasound is used primarily, more stage I tumors are detected, but because ultrasound lacks specificity, many women with abnormal screening results may undergo unnecessary surgery for benign disease.

Another issue is that screening, particularly the initial prevalent screen, may identify borderline, germ cell tumors or granulosa cell tumors that are biologically less aggressive. Alternatively, high-grade serous tumors may develop and reach an advanced stage in the interval between screens (**Fig. 2**) [20], and primary peritoneal cancers may develop without any evident ovarian mass.

Results for any screening test are improved if the prevalence of disease is high in the screened population. Lifetime risk of ovarian cancer is only 1.3% in the general population, but it is increased to 12% in women with genetic predisposition. Women with Lynch II hereditary nonpolyposis colon cancer syndrome have an approximately 10% lifetime risk of developing ovarian cancer [21,22]. Lifetime risk of invasive epithelial cancer is even higher (15–65%) for women with *BRCA* mutations. *BRCA* mutations often are associated with high-grade serous

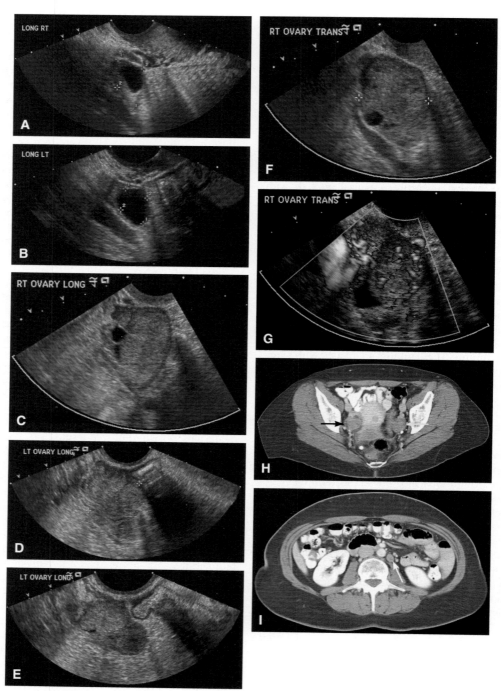

Fig. 2. A 53-year-old woman with family history of ovarian and breast cancer developed bilateral stage III high-grade papillary serous ovarian cancer within a 6-month interval between screening ultrasounds. (*A* and *B*) Ultrasound revealed bilateral simple follicles, normal-sized ovaries with volume of 6 mL bilaterally; CA-125 was normal at 16 U/mL. (*C–G*) Ultrasound 6 months later; right ovarian volume increased to 19 mL, and left ovarian volume was 16 mL. The ovaries contained solid hypervascular masses and had lobulated contours. CA-125 was elevated to 67 U/mL. (*H* and *I*) CT scan revealed bilateral ovarian enlargement (*black arrow*) and leiomyomatous uterus. Left para-aortic adenopathy (*white arrows*) and small pelvic ascites also were present.

ovarian cancers or peritoneal cancers that are less frequently detected at an early stage by screening [20,23–26]. A report of 1100 women at moderate or high risk found 13 ovarian cancers; 10 were found at screening, but only 2 of these were stage I tumors [16]. Three ovarian tumors, all of an advanced stage, were undetected by screening. In addition, 29 women with benign disease underwent diagnostic surgery [16]. These results illustrate the difficulties of ovarian cancer screening even in women at high risk.

To date, there is no evidence that screening reduces mortality from ovarian cancer. Current guidelines state that screening is not recommended in premenopausal or postmenopausal women with or without a family history of ovarian cancer [16]. For women at high risk because of *BRCA* mutations or other hereditary factors suggesting genetic predisposition, screening may be performed until prophylactic oophorectomy after childbearing years [20,27,28].

Lesion characterization

In patients with a known or suspected adnexal mass, ultrasound is highly accurate in the assessment of tumor location (eg, differentiation of uterine from adnexal masses) and in distinguishing between a benign and malignant adnexal lesion. The optimal use of ultrasound requires the analysis of morphologic features and Doppler findings [29–32].

Ovarian masses with septations greater than 3 mm, mural nodularity, and papillary projections suggest the diagnosis of malignant ovarian neoplasm [33–35]. The most significant feature is the presence of solid components within an ovarian mass [36]. Some benign lesions, most commonly endometriomas and hemorrhagic cysts, may have similar appearance to malignant ovarian tumors. For premenopausal women, it is important that ovarian lesions have follow-up to exclude transient physiologic changes that may mimic ovarian carcinoma. Morphologic scoring systems are used to standardize diagnosis of ovarian cancer by assigning numerical scores for various ultrasound features, such as size, wall thickness, solid components, and number and thickness of septations [37–40], but similar excellent interobserver variability is reported when subjective criteria are used [41].

Color and pulsed Doppler techniques may aid diagnosis of ovarian cancer. Central color Doppler flow within solid components of an ovarian mass has been shown to be an accurate predictor of malignancy [36,42,43]. Brown and colleagues [36] studied 211 adnexal masses including 28 malignancies to determine the best discrimination between benignity and malignancy by gray-scale and Doppler. A nonhyperechoic solid component within a mass, central blood flow on color Doppler imaging, free intraperitoneal fluid, and septations within a mass had 93% sensitivity and 93% specificity for diagnosis of malignancy.

On spectral Doppler, ovarian cancers generally have low-resistance waveforms because tumor neovasculature lacks smooth muscle, and arteriovenous shunting may occur [35]. Although initial reports suggested high sensitivity and specificity for resistance index cutoff value of 0.4 and pulsatility index of 1, subsequent studies found specific values less reliable because many benign lesions, including corpora lutea, may have similar waveforms [35,40,44–48]. These benign lesions are more common in premenopausal women; when low-resistance ovarian flow is seen in a postmenopausal woman, the finding should be considered highly suspicious for malignant ovarian neoplasm.

Current evidence is that the combination of ovarian morphology and Doppler perform best for characterization of adnexal masses. Buy and coworkers [49] used gray-scale ultrasound and duplex and color Doppler to evaluate 132 adnexal masses, including 98 benign, 3 borderline, and 31 malignant masses. Adding color Doppler to gray-scale morphologic information increased specificity from 82% to 97% and increased positive predictive value from 63% to 97%, but there was no added information from duplex Doppler indices. A large meta-analysis comparing morphologic assessment, Doppler ultrasound, color Doppler flow imaging, and combined techniques for characterization of adnexal masses using summary receiver operator curves found the best diagnostic performance for combined techniques (0.92), followed in decreasing order by morphologic assessment alone (0.85), Doppler indices (0.82), and color Doppler flow (0.73) [30].

It is impossible to differentiate histologic subtypes of primary ovarian tumors by ultrasound appearance, but there are some features that should be considered. Epithelial ovarian tumors are typically cystic, but endometrioid tumors may be solid. Mucinous cystadenocarcinomas are more septated than serous cystadenocarcinomas and may have fluid with low-level echoes. Malignant germ cell tumors are predominately solid, as are stromal tumors. Primary ovarian carcinomas are frequently bilateral, varying with subtype; approximately 50% of serous cystadenocarcinomas and 30% of endometrioid cancers are bilateral, whereas clear cell and mucinous tumors are bilateral in 20% of cases [8,35,50].

Despite advances in ultrasound technology, many adnexal lesions are still classified as indeterminate, particularly in cases of endometriomas and cystic teratomas. In a setting of sonographically indeterminate adnexal masses, MR imaging is used as a problem-solving tool. The main advantage of MR imaging is that it can provide tissue characterization based on signal properties [51].

For adequate evaluation of adnexal masses on MR imaging, T1-weighted and T2-weighted images are fundamental in the delineation of pelvic anatomy and tumor. Fat-saturated T1-weighted images help distinguish between fat and hemorrhage. Gadolinium-enhanced T1-weighted images help characterize the internal architecture of cystic lesions and improve detection of solid components [52,53].

Although signal intensity characteristics can be used to narrow the differential diagnosis of an adnexal mass, no MR signal characteristics specific for ovarian cancer are recognized. Distinction of malignant from benign lesions is based mainly on morphologic criteria. The presence of papillary projections in a cystic mass is highly suggestive of ovarian cancer. Sonographically, fibrinous debris and occasionally a clot adherent to the cyst wall may mimic the papillary projections. The neoplastic papillary projections enhance with gadolinium administration, however, and clot and debris do not. Other features suggesting malignant etiology include vascular septations thicker than 3 mm, septal nodularity, and single or multiple enhancing solid components within a cystic mass [33,54,55]. Necrosis within a solid lesion is also a strong indicator of malignancy.

A study showed that the presence of enhancing solid tissue was 91% sensitive and 88% specific for malignancy (Fig. 3) [53]. Another study showed that necrosis within a solid lesion and vegetations within a cystic lesion were the features most predictive for malignancy, with an accuracy of 93% on gadolinium-enhanced MR imaging [56]. In patients with clinically or sonographically detected complex adnexal masses, MR imaging was shown to have 91% accuracy for the diagnosis of malignancy. In this study, the imaging features associated with malignancy were solid-cystic complex mass, wall irregularity, vegetations on the wall and septations in a cystic lesion, large size of the lesion, and early enhancement on dynamic contrast-enhanced MR images. On multiple logistic regression analysis, ancillary findings, such as ascites, peritoneal disease, or adenopathy, were the factors most significantly indicative of malignancy [57]. MR imaging has been shown to be superior to Doppler ultrasound and conventional CT in diagnosis of malignant ovarian masses (the estimated area under receiver operating characteristic curve [AUC] was 0.78 for ultrasound, 0.87 for CT, and 0.91 for MR imaging) [58].

A study using meta-analysis and bayesian analysis showed that in women with an indeterminate ovarian mass detected by gray-scale ultrasound, MR imaging contributed to change in probability of ovarian cancer in premenopausal and postmenopausal women more than did CT or combined gray-scale and Doppler ultrasound [59]. In the characterization of an ovarian lesion, the cost-benefit study and the net cost analysis have shown that the use of MR imaging in the evaluation of sonographically indeterminate adnexal lesions resulted in fewer surgical procedures, better patient triage, and net cost savings [60].

Although CT has not traditionally been used in the characterization of an adnexal mass, studies have shown that the utility of thin-section multislice CT is equivalent to that of ultrasound. CT characterization of an adnexal mass relies on the depiction of morphologic features of enhancing mural nodularity or heterogeneity and necrosis within a solid lesion (Fig. 4). Ancillary findings, such as ascites and peritoneal carcinomatosis, on ultrasound, CT, or MR imaging are strong indicators of a malignant etiology for an adnexal mass.

The use of positron emission tomography (PET) has been investigated for the detection and characterization of primary ovarian masses. PET scanning with fluorodeoxyglucose (FDG) is based on uptake in functionally active tissue that uses glucose. Physiologic uptake of FDG in ovaries during different phases of the menstrual cycle [61] may prove to be a limitation for detection of primary ovarian cancer. In addition, a variety of benign lesions, such as serous and mucinous cystadenomas, corpus luteum cysts, and dermoid cysts, are known to accumulate FDG and may contribute to false-positive results [62,63]. Differentiation of benign from malignant lesions using PET scans alone is impossible. The distinction generally requires correlation with a detailed clinical history and morphologic imaging such as ultrasound, CT, or MR imaging. PET imaging with current FDG radiotracers can be applied to the characterization of adnexal masses, but its efficacy is not contributory after ultrasound and MR imaging findings are evaluated [62].

Staging

Traditionally, ovarian cancer was staged surgically with pathologic confirmation. Surgical staging is based on the International Federation of Obstetrics and Gynecology (FIGO) classification system, first introduced in 1964 and revised in 1985. FIGO/TNM staging is summarized in Table 1 [64]. Stage

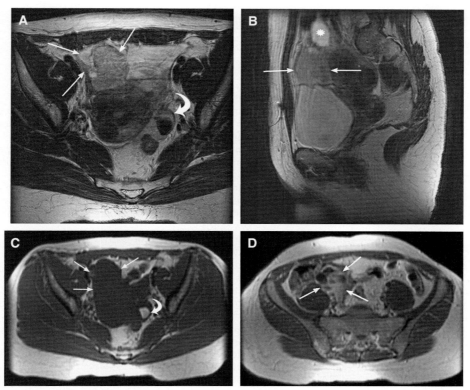

Fig. 3. A 46-year-old woman with endometriosis and poorly differentiated papillary serous carcinoma of the right ovary. (A and B) T2-weighted axial and sagittal images show a complex, predominantly solid right adnexal mass (arrows); the small cystic component is marked by an asterisk. (C) The left ovary contains a small endometrioma (curved arrow on axial image), bright on T1-weighted image and "shaded" on T2-weighted image. (D) Postgadolinium T1-weighted image shows heterogeneous enhancement of a solid component of the right ovarian mass (arrows), characteristic of malignancy.

FIGO I/T1 ovarian cancer refers to tumor confined to the ovaries. Stage FIGO II/T2 corresponds to ovarian cancer with metastases confined to the true pelvis. Stage FIGO III/T3 indicates ovarian cancer with extrapelvic peritoneal metastases and regional nodal disease. The size of peritoneal metastases (whether they are <2 cm or >2 cm) determines differentiation between stage T3B and stage T3C disease. Stage FIGO IV/TNM any T1, any N, M1 consists of ovarian cancer with pleural, distant nodal disease, or hematogenous spread. The management of ovarian cancer depends on staging. Comprehensive staging laparotomy includes total abdominal hysterectomy, bilateral salpingo-oophorectomy, omentectomy, peritoneal washings, random sampling of multiple peritoneal sites (including pelvic sidewall, paracolic gutters, cul-de-sac, surface of bladder, rectum, and diaphragm), and pelvic and retroperitoneal lymphadenectomy.

Understanding of the typical pattern of ovarian cancer spread assists in tumor detection and localization, making preoperative cross-sectional imaging a road map for a surgeon. Ovarian cancer primarily spreads locally in the pelvis to the opposite ovary (6–13%) and to the uterus (5–25%). Intraperitoneal dissemination is the most common route of ovarian cancer spread, which can be

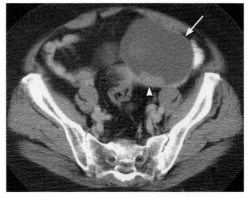

Fig. 4. Axial CT contrast-enhanced image of the pelvis in a 50-year-old woman with ovarian clear cell carcinoma. An enhancing mural nodule (arrowhead) within a complex cystic mass (arrow) is a characteristic feature of cystic malignant lesions.

Table 1: FIGO and TNM staging systems for ovarian cancer

TNM categories			FIGO stages	
Primary tumor (T)				
TX				Primary tumor cannot be assessed
T0				No evidence of primary tumor
T1			I	Tumor limited to ovaries (one or both)
T1a			IA	Tumor limited to one ovary; capsule intact, no tumor on ovarian surface. No malignant cells in ascites or peritoneal washing*
T1b			IB	Tumor limited to both ovaries; capsules intact, no tumor on ovarian surface. No malignant cells in ascites or peritoneal washings*
T1c			IC	Tumor limited to one or both ovaries with any of the following: capsule ruptured, tumor on ovarian surface, malignant cells in ascites or peritoneal washings
T2			II	Tumor involves one or both ovaries with pelvic extension and/or implants
T2a			IIA	Extension and/or implants on uterus and/or tube(s). No malignant cells in ascites or peritoneal washings
T2b			IIB	Extension to and/or implants on other pelvic tissues. No malignant cells in ascites or peritoneal washings
T2c			IIC	Pelvic extension and/or implants (T2a or T2b) with malignant cells in ascites or peritoneal washings
T3			III	Tumor involves one or both ovaries with microscopically confirmed peritoneal metastasis outside the pelvis
T3a			IIIA	Microscopic peritoneal metastasis beyond pelvis (no macroscopic tumor)
T3b			IIIB	Macroscopic peritoneal metastasis beyond pelvis ≤ 2 cm in greatest dimension
T3c			IIIC	Peritoneal metastasis beyond pelvis >2 cm in greatest dimension and/or regional lymph node metastasis
Regional lymph nodes (N)				
NX				Regional lymph nodes cannot be assessed
N0				No regional lymph node metastasis
N1			IIIC	Regional lymph node metastasis
Distant metastasis (M)				
MX				Distant metastasis cannot be assessed
M0				No distant metastasis
M1			IV	Distant metastasis (excludes peritoneal metastasis)
Stage grouping				
I	T1	N0	M0	
IA	T1a	N0	M0	
IB	T1b	N0	M0	
IC	T1c	N0	M0	
II	T2	N0	M0	
IIA	T2a	N0	M0	
IIB	T2b	N0	M0	
IIC	T2c	N0	M0	
III	T3	N0	M0	
IIIA	T3a	N0	M0	
IIIB	T3b	N0	M0	
IIIC	T3c	N0	M0	
	Any T	N1	M0	
Stage IV	Any T	Any N	M1	

* The presence of nonmalignant ascites is not classified. The presence of ascites does not affect staging unless malignant cells are present.

explained by ovarian anatomy. The ovary is covered by a single layer of surface epithelium. The tumor cells exfoliate from the affected epithelium, which frequently has macroscopic and microscopic polypoid excrescences and spread with peritoneal fluid. Peritoneal metastases follow the direction of clockwise flow of peritoneal fluid throughout the peritoneal cavity, facilitated by the normal bowel peristasis. The normal peritoneal fluid circulates preferentially upward from the right paracolic gutter to the right subdiaphragmatic space and crosses the midline and circulates downward to the left paracolic gutter and pelvis. Peritoneal metastases appear as nodular or plaquelike enhancing soft tissue masses of varying sizes. The most common locations are the peritoneal reflections, where the peritoneal fluid tends to stay longer. Peritoneal nodules are frequently present in the cul-de-sac, paracolic gutters, subdiaphragmatic space, splenic hilum, porta hepatis, and along the falciform ligament. Other common locations are the ileocecal valve and rectosigmoid junction, where the sigmoid colon makes a turn (Fig. 5). Diffuse infiltration of the omentum by the tumor is called omental caking.

The presence of lymph node metastases in ovarian cancer is an important prognostic feature. Knowledge of the anatomy of the ovarian lymphatic drainage is crucial in understanding the pathways of ovarian cancer nodal dissemination. Most commonly, nodal metastasis ascends along the gonadal vessels to the retroperitoneum. Dissemination along the broad ligament can result in internal iliac, obturator, and external iliac adenopathy. Lymphadenopathy can reach the superficial and deep inguinal nodes via the round ligaments. This mechanism explains the occasional presence of ovarian cancer nodal metastases in the groin (Fig. 6). The frequency of nodal metastases in a patient with T1 or T2 disease is close to 15% and increases to 65% in M1 disease. In ovarian cancer patients, a threshold of short-axis measurements of 1 cm or larger is used to define malignant adenopathy; however, it showed a disappointing low sensitivity of only 50%. The specificity with that threshold was 95%. Superior diaphragmatic adenopathy is detected in approximately 15% of patients with advanced ovarian cancer and is usually associated with grave prognosis (Fig. 7) [65].

Although distant metastasis is rare at the time of diagnosis, the common sites of distant spread at autopsy include the liver (45–48%), lung (34–39%), pleura (25%), adrenal gland (21%), and spleen (20%); bone and brain metastases are seen in less than 10% (Fig. 8). Knowledge of the frequency of distant metastasis in ovarian cancer guides the imaging algorithm for patient surveillance.

Optimal debulking refers to the reduction of all tumor deposits to a maximal diameter of less than 1 cm. Patients who are optimally debulked show better response to chemotherapy and subsequently have a better prognosis. Staging of ovarian cancer can be effectively accomplished with preoperative CT scanning. Multidetector CT is highly accurate in the depiction of tumor implants larger than 1 cm throughout the abdomen and pelvis. Implants measuring 1 cm or less are difficult to detect, however, and CT sensitivity decreases to 25% to 50% for such small-volume disease [66]. The efficacy of nonhelical CT in the diagnosis of peritoneal metastases in ovarian cancer has a sensitivity of 63% to 79% and a specificity of 100% [66]. Helical CT improves performance, showing sensitivity of 85% to 93% and specificity of 91% to 96%. This improved accuracy likely reflects the increasing use of thinner sections and multiplanar review of the data, which aid in the detection of small implants and help in the distinction of peritoneal tumor deposits from unopacified bowel loops [67].

Although CT is the primary imaging modality for staging ovarian cancer, a Radiologic Diagnostic Oncology Group (RDOG) study showed that MR imaging may be equal to CT [68]. One advantage of MR imaging is that it provides better soft tissue contrast than does CT. In patients with advanced disease, MR imaging and CT perform similarly in determination of the location, distribution, and size of peritoneal implants. A study comparing ultrasound, MR imaging, and CT for diagnosing and staging advanced ovarian cancer showed that for the detection of peritoneal metastases, MR imaging and CT (AUC = 0.96 for both) were more accurate than ultrasound (AUC = 0.86), especially in the subdiaphragmatic spaces and hepatic surfaces [68,69]. The use of MR imaging is currently limited, however, by expense, lack of availability, prolonged scanning time, and a relative shortage of radiologists with adequate reading experience.

In the evaluation of nodal disease, using a size threshold of equal or greater than 1 cm in short axis to define adenopathy, MR imaging was slightly more accurate than CT in the evaluation of nodal metastasis (sensitivity and specificity were 43% and 89% for CT and 38% and 84% for MR imaging) [68]. Although enlarged nodes are likely to be metastatic, CT and MR imaging are unable to exclude disease in nonenlarged nodes.

Differentiation between stage III and stage IV disease has a direct impact on patient management. The management of FIGO stage III disease is primary surgical debulking, whereas patients with stage IV disease are treated with chemotherapy and cytoreduction.

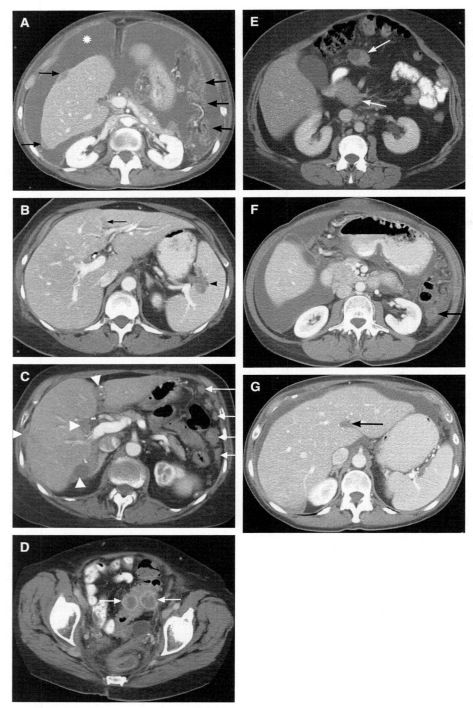

Fig. 5. Axial contrast-enhanced images of the abdomen and pelvis in three different patients illustrate the typical pattern of peritoneal spread of tumor, characteristic of stage III ovarian cancer. The tumor follows the flow of peritoneal fluid and tends to deposit in peritoneal recesses. (*A*) Massive ascites (*asterisk*) with perihepatic capsular implants (*arrows on the left*) and diffuse omental infiltration, known as omental caking (*arrows on the right*). (*B*) Tumor deposit along the falciform ligament (*arrow*) and in the splenic hilum (*arrowhead*). (C) Capsular-based perihepatic implants (*arrowheads*) and tumor deposits in the left paracolic gutter (*arrows*). (*D*) Serosal tumor implants on the surface of the sigmoid colon (*arrows*). (*E*) Peritoneal tumor implants in the root of the mesentery (*arrows*). (*F*) Implant in the left paracolic gutter (*arrow*). (*G*) Tumor deposit along the fissure of the ligamentum teres (*arrow*).

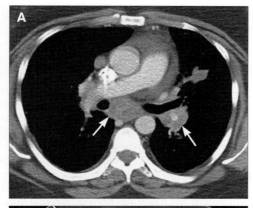

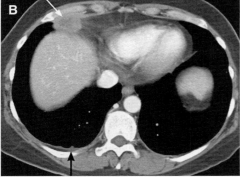

Fig. 6. Axial contrast-enhanced CT section in a patient with stage IV ovarian cancer manifested with disease in the chest. (*A*) Malignant mediastinal and bilateral hilar adenopathy (*arrows*). (*B*) Superior diaphragmatic adenopathy (*white arrow*) and right pleural thickening (*black arrow*).

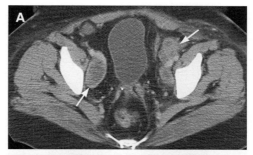

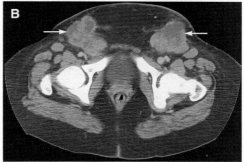

Fig. 7. Moderately differentiated papillary serous ovarian carcinoma. (*A* and *B*) Bilateral pelvic and inguinal lymphadenopathy (*arrows*) develops as a result of tumor spread along the iliac vessels and round ligament.

There are two potential pitfalls in assigning FIGO stage IV disease:

1. Pleural effusion in a patient with ovarian cancer can be benign or malignant. Pleural thickening or nodularity in addition to pleural effusion indicates the malignant nature of effusion. In the absence of those imaging findings, thoracentesis is indicated.
2. When only axial sections of either CT or MR imaging are evaluated, there is a potential pitfall in differentiating between liver surface implants (stage III with peritoneal spread) and true intraparenchymal metastases (as a result of hematogenous spread and so stage IV disease). Sagittal or coronal reformatted images may assist in differentiating the two types. Multislice CT allows reformatting the images and can be as accurate as MR imaging.

In the evaluation of liver parenchymal metastases CT and MR imaging perform similarly, although in the diagnosis of liver lesions in the setting of preexisting liver disease MR imaging may be superior [68].

The role of FDG PET has been explored for ovarian cancer staging. Numerous studies have been performed, although most of them have been limited by small numbers of patients and use of a PET scanner alone. More recent studies have been performed with PET/CT hybrid cameras that allow more accurate detection and localization of the lesions. In the primary staging of ovarian cancer, FDG PET may be helpful (especially when used in addition to CT [70] to evaluate equivocal or indeterminate lesions further and to establish distant metastatic sites. Prior studies using FDG PET have reported a positive predictive value of 86% and accuracy of 90% with sensitivity of 96% and negative predictive value of 75% [71,72].

Disseminated peritoneal tumor deposits may be microscopic or very small in size. FDG PET is limited in resolution and is not optimal for detecting lesions less than 0.5 cm in size. Detection of microscopic disease is difficult on most other imaging modalities as well. Rose and colleagues [73] studied 17 patients before second-look surgery and reported very low sensitivity (10%) and specificity (42%). The study was conducted in patients with

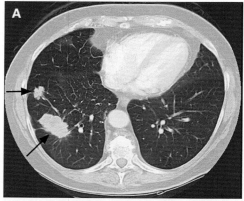

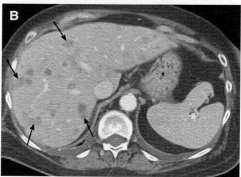

Fig. 8. A patient with stage IV poorly differentiated papillary serous carcinoma of the ovary. (*A*) Axial CT image of the chest shows metastases in the right lung (*arrows*). (*B*) Section through the liver shows multiple intraparenchymal metastases (*arrows*).

optimal primary cytoreduction who had complete clinical response to prior treatment; however, it used a PET scanner only. All missed lesions were small (<6 mm). Later studies have reported better results, with sensitivity and specificity of 66% and 94%, after primary debulking [74]. Positive predictive value was 93% for peritoneal disease measuring 5 mm for various cancers [75].

The imaging observations that are crucial to management may be divided into observation related to characterization of the primary tumor, identification of metastatic disease to prevent understaging, and identification of patients who would benefit from neoadjuvant chemotherapy before the primary debulking procedure. Preoperative CT and MR imaging were found to be highly accurate in the detection of inoperable tumor and the prediction of suboptimal debulking (sensitivity, specificity, positive predictive value, and negative predictive value were 76%, 92%, 94% and 96%). The two modalities were equally effective (*P*=1.0) in the detection of inoperable tumor. This study suggests that imaging may help triage inoperable

patients to more appropriate neoadjuvant chemotherapy group [76–78].

Posttreatment follow-up

Patients treated for ovarian cancer are followed up with serial measurements of CA-125 and either CT scan or MR imaging of the abdomen and pelvis. CT of the chest should not be performed routinely, unless no sites of recurrence are detected on CT of the abdomen and pelvis, and tumor markers are elevated [79,80].

Serum CA-125 is a strong indicator of epithelial tumor activity [81,82]. It has been shown that in patients with complete response to therapy, three consecutive elevations in CA-125 values even within the normal range of 0 to 35 U/mL at 1- to 3-month intervals are associated with a significant risk of recurrence and may occur before the imaging findings become positive. In one study, the mean time from the third early increase in serum CA-125 to clinical or radiologic confirmation of recurrence was 189 days [83]. The role of imaging is crucial, however, for localizing the anatomic sites of suspected recurrent tumor. Familiarity with the spectrum of imaging findings of recurrent ovarian cancer facilitates accurate diagnosis and ensures prompt treatment. Recurrent ovarian malignancies manifest as pelvic masses, peritoneal tumor implants (commonly in paracolic gutters, cul-de-sac, root of the mesentery, serosal surface of the bowel), malignant ascites, or lymphadenopathy. Occasionally, recurrent disease may present as pleuroparenchymal lesions or liver metastasis [84].

Knowledge of medical terminology used during different stages of ovarian cancer after the initial treatment and its relationship to patient management is essential in understanding the potential role of imaging. Specific terms are used to define the behavior patterns of ovarian cancer after initial treatment as follows:

- *Persistent disease* **is present when, after a tumor partially responds to initial therapy, there is an immediate elevation in CA-125 or clinical evidence of disease. The role of imaging in persistent disease is limited, unless the patient develops acute clinical symptoms (eg, bowel or urinary obstruction).**
- *Chemotherapy-resistant disease* **is defined as tumor recurrence detected less than 6 months after completion of initial treatment. CT can be used to document the extent of tumor recurrence and monitor response to treatment.**
- *Refractory, unresponsive, or progressive tumors* **are tumors that progress during initial**

therapy. Imaging is rarely used in this patient category, unless clinical symptoms develop (eg, bowel or urinary obstruction). Imaging can be used to document disease progression and assists in future development of different treatment regimens.

- *Recurrent ovarian cancer* is defined as tumor recurrence after a complete initial response to first-line therapy, a negative second-look operation (if performed), and a disease-free interval greater than 6 months.

The treatment of recurrent ovarian cancer depends on tumor bulk and location and ranges from surgical debulking to medical palliation. In this patient group, an increase in survival is seen only when the secondary cytoreduction is optimal [85]. Identification of unresectable recurrent cancer is clinically relevant, assists in patient management, and directly affects the outcome. The survival rate after secondary cytoreduction varies from 17% to 62%. An attempt should be made to predict resectability with preoperative imaging to spare the patient unnecessary surgery. Few studies describe the utility of helical CT and MR imaging in the evaluation of recurrent cancer. In a longitudinal study comparing MR imaging with CA-125 and physical examination, sensitivity, specificity, accuracy, and positive predictive value were 91%, 87%, 90%, and 72% for gadolinium-enhanced MR imaging and 53%, 94%, 63%, and 38% for CA-125. The corresponding values for physical examination were 26%, 94%, 43%, and 29% [86].

FDG PET also has been used to evaluate the presence of disease in patients before second-look laparotomy (SLL) or laparoscopy. SLL is the most accurate way of assessing the presence of microscopic and macroscopic disease; however, it is an invasive procedure. Use of FDG PET imaging instead of SLL is reported to be feasible and cost-effective [87]. FDG PET has high predictive value (93%) and provides prognostic information. Kim and associates [88] compared the prognostic value of FDG PET with that of SLL in 55 patients with advanced ovarian cancer treated with chemotherapy and found no significant differences in disease-free intervals between patients who were evaluated with PET and patients who were evaluated with SLL.

Most studies using FDG PET in ovarian cancer have been conducted to assess the utility of PET in early detection of recurrent disease. In a direct comparison with CT or MR imaging, Delbeke and colleagues reported sensitivity and specificity of 83% to 91% and 66% to 93% for FDG PET and 45% to 91% and 46% to 84% for CT or MR imaging [89].

More recent studies also have shown a high sensitivity of FDG PET for detection of recurrent disease [90]. The sensitivity remains low for lesions less than 5 to 10 mm. Detection may be better, however, with newer cameras and PET/CT fusion units that have better resolution and anatomic correlation allowing detection of lesions measuring 5 mm [91]. The exact magnitude of the clinical impact of detection of microscopic disease has yet to be properly studied. FDG PET helps localize the sites of disease so that surgery or biopsy can be directed better. This is useful in cases where conventional imaging fails to detect recurrent disease [92].

FDG PET may be more useful in detecting recurrence in the setting of negative conventional imaging studies and an increasing CA-125 [93–95]. In a study by Murakami and colleagues [93] in which 90 patients were evaluated, PET alone identified recurrence in 17 (37%), including in 50% of these 17 patients, normal-sized retroperitoneal nodal metastases. In patients with an asymptomatic increase of CA-125, PET had a sensitivity of 87.5%. The combined sensitivity of PET and CA-125 was 97.8%. PET/CT is of incremental value to CT alone in detecting viable disease in equivocal cases, when interfering and unopacified bowel or postsurgical changes may mimic recurrent disease [96]. PET/CT also can help localize the sites of recurrent tumor in such patients so that surgery or biopsy can be better directed (Fig. 9) [97].

Overall, FDG PET imaging holds promise in the evaluation of recurrent or residual disease where other radiographic findings are equivocal and uncertain. Newer tracers are being evaluated to improve detection; however, the sensitivity to microscopic disease is still limited.

Recurrent ovarian tumor resectability

In patients selected for secondary cytoreduction, the bulk of the tumor burden is usually present in the pelvis. Two types of pelvic recurrence are described: central recurrence at the vaginal cuff and pelvic sidewall recurrence. The size of a pelvic mass is not an indicator of surgical outcome; however, the extension of a mass to the pelvic sidewall is. In cases of small-volume recurrent disease in the pelvis, multiplanar MR imaging is superior to CT in the assessment of pelvic tumor resectability because MR imaging can better outline the fat plane separating the tumor from the pelvic sidewall. The presence of a fat plane at least 3 mm in thickness is considered adequate for resection. The important consideration is that tumor invasion of the bladder and rectum is not a contraindication to definitive

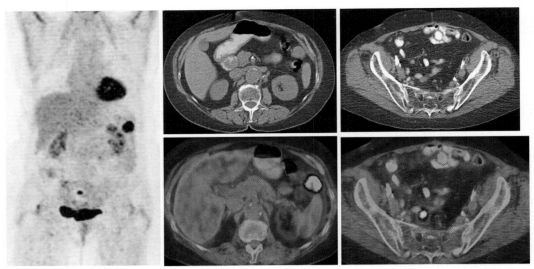

Fig. 9. PET/CT of a 63-year-old woman with recurrent ovarian cancer. Intense uptake is seen in the region of peritoneal implants in left upper quadrant and presacral region.

surgery. These patients can be treated with pelvic exenteration (Fig. 10). In the past, the presence of hydronephrosis was considered to indicate unresectable disease. With development of new surgical techniques and involvement of urologists, these patients are no longer considered inoperable. They may undergo a urinary diversion procedure as long as the pelvic sidewall is free of tumor. Preoperative PET/CT is an essential part of curative pelvic exenteration planning to document the absence of tumor elsewhere.

In patients undergoing secondary cytoreduction, pelvic sidewall invasion and large bowel obstruction are significant indicators of tumor nonresectability. Similar to primary ovarian cancer, bulky upper abdominal disease, such as tumor in the gastrohepatic ligament, gallbladder fossa, porta hepatis, and root of the mesentery, precludes optimal surgical debulking (Fig. 11). The presence of large bowel obstruction is a strong indication of tumor nonresectability. In the presence of large bowel obstruction, secondary cytoreductive surgery is usually replaced by palliative approaches.

In patients with recurrent ovarian cancer considered for secondary cytoreductive surgery, preoperative CT identifies sites of disease and points out indicators of nonresectability; this may allow tailoring of the surgical approach and can have a direct impact on patient survival. The role of radiologist is not to point out unresectable disease, but to alert the clinician about potential complications during surgery. Depending on the institution, pattern of practice, and personal experience of a surgeon, patients with recurrent ovarian cancer ordinarily considered

unresectable can be triaged to surgery, whereas other patients with unresectable disease can benefit from neoadjuvant chemotherapy or radiation.

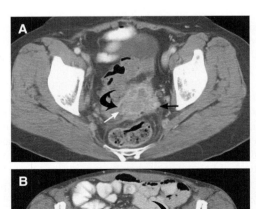

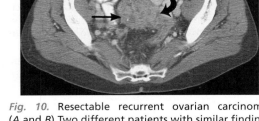

Fig. 10. Resectable recurrent ovarian carcinoma. (*A* and *B*) Two different patients with similar findings of recurrent ovarian cancer, manifested as a solitary mass in the pelvis. In both cases, the central pelvic mass (*arrows*) appears inseparable from the sigmoid colon, requiring sigmoid resection. Bilateral pelvic sidewalls are free of tumor, however, and the disease is considered surgically resectable.

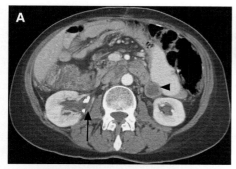

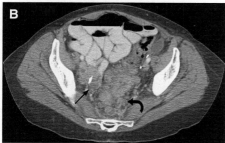

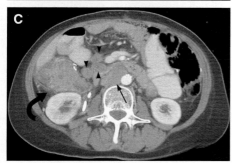

Fig. 11. Unresectable recurrent ovarian carcinoma. (*A*) Multilevel obstruction of the right ureter by tumor implants anterior to the right kidney encasing the proximal and distal right ureter with stent in place (*arrows*). Tumor deposit anterior to left kidney (*arrowhead*). (*B*) Tumor encasing the distal right ureter is inseparable from the pelvic sidewall, indicative of unresectable disease. Multiple pelvic nodules (*curved arrow*) are also evident. (*C*) Multiple tumor deposits within the root of the mesentry (*arrowheads*) in the proximity of mesenteric vessels also indicate respectability. Bulky retroperitoneal adenopathy is shown (*black arrow*). Tumor deposit anterior to the right kidney and proximal ureter (*curved arrow*).

Summary

Transvaginal ultrasound is a primary modality for adnexal mass detection and characterization. The current combined technique, which includes assessment of morphologic features and Doppler characteristics, gives the most accurate prediction of malignancy. Gadolinium-enhanced MR imaging serves as a problem-solving modality in cases of indeterminate adnexal masses. A combination of T1-weighted images and T1-weighted images with fatsaturation helps to differentiate most common benign adnexal masses, such as endometrioma and teratoma, from malignant ones. Contrast-enhanced CT of the abdomen and pelvis is the primary modality for preoperative staging and treatment follow-up. In cases of pelvic recurrence, MR imaging is a preferred modality to assess tumor resectability. In equivocal cases when tumor recurrence is suggested by an increase in the tumor marker CA-125, but tumor implants are too small to be detected by conventional CT, combined PET/CT may be valuable for determining tumor activity.

References

[1] Stat bite: Age-specific incidence and mortality rates for ovarian cancer, 1998–2002. J Natl Cancer Inst 2006;98(8):511.

[2] Jung SE, Lee JM, Rha SE, et al. CT and MR imaging of ovarian tumors with emphasis on differential diagnosis. Radiographics 2002;22(6): 1305–25.

[3] Wu TT, Coakley FV, Qayyum A, et al. Magnetic resonance imaging of ovarian cancer arising in endometriomas. J Comput Assist Tomogr 2004; 28(6):836–8.

[4] deSouza NM, O'Neill R, McIndoe GA, et al. Borderline tumors of the ovary: CT and MRI features and tumor markers in differentiation from stage I disease. AJR Am J Roentgenol 2005;184(3): 999–1003.

[5] Exacoustos C, Romanini ME, Rinaldo D, et al. Preoperative sonographic features of borderline ovarian tumors. Ultrasound Obstet Gynecol 2005;25(1):50–9.

[6] Jung SE, Rha SE, Lee JM, et al. CT and MRI findings of sex cord-stromal tumor of the ovary. AJR Am J Roentgenol 2005;185(1):207–15.

[7] Kim SH, Kim SH. Granulosa cell tumor of the ovary: common findings and unusual appearances on CT and MR. J Comput Assist Tomogr 2002;26(5):756–61.

[8] Brown DL, Zou KH, Tempany CM, et al. Primary versus secondary ovarian malignancy: imaging findings of adnexal masses in the radiology diagnostic oncology group study. Radiology 2001; 219(1):213–8.

[9] Ferrozzi F, Tognini G, Bova D, et al. Non-Hodgkin lymphomas of the ovaries: MR findings. J Comput Assist Tomogr 2000;24(3):416–20.

[10] Bourne TH, Campbell S, Reynolds KM, et al. Screening for early familial ovarian cancer with transvaginal ultrasonography and colour blood flow imaging. BMJ 1993;306:1025–9.

[11] Buys SS, Partridge E, Greene MH, et al. Ovarian cancer screening in the prostate, lung colorectal and ovarian (PLCO) cancer screening trial: findings from the initial screen of a randomized trial. Am J Obstet Gynecol 2005;193:1630–9.

[12] Campbell S, Royston P, Bhan V, et al. Novel screening strategies for early ovarian cancer by transabdominal ultrasonography. Br J Obstet Gynaecol 1990;97(4):304–11.

[13] Einhorn N, Bast R, Knapp R, et al. Long-term follow-up of the Stockholm screening study on ovarian cancer. Gynecol Oncol 2000;79:466–70.

[14] Jacobs IJ, Skates SJ, MacDonald N, et al. Screening for ovarian cancer: a pilot randomised controlled trial. Lancet 1999;353(9160):1207–10.

[15] Sato S, Yokoyama Y, Sakamoto T, et al. Usefulness of mass screening for ovarian carcinoma using transvaginal sonography. Cancer 2000;89: 582–8.

[16] Stirling D, Evans GR, Pichert G, et al. Screening for familial ovarian cancer: failure of current protocols to detect ovarian cancer at an early stage according to the International Federation of Gynecology and Obstetrics system. J Clin Oncol 2005;23:5588–96.

[17] Tailor A, Bourne TH, Campbell S, et al. Results from an ultrasound-based familial ovarian cancer screening clinic: a 10-year observational study. Ultrasound Obstet Gynecol 2003;21(4): 378–85.

[18] Van Nagell JR Jr, DePriest PD, Reedy MB, et al. The efficacy of transvaginal sonographic screening in asymptomatic women at risk for ovarian cancer. Gynecol Oncol 2000;77:350–6.

[19] Duffy MJ, Bonfrer JM, Kulpa J, et al. CA125 in ovarian cancer: European Group on Tumor Markers guidelines for clinical use. Int J Gynecol Cancer 2005;15(5):679–91.

[20] Hogg R, Friedlander M. Biology of epithelial ovarian cancer: implications for screening women at high genetic risk. J Clin Oncol 2004; 22(7):1315–27.

[21] Schmeler KM, Lynch HT, Chen LM, et al. Prophylactic surgery to reduce the risk of gynecologic cancers in the Lynch syndrome. N Engl J Med 2006;354(3):261–9.

[22] Taylor K, Schwartz PE. Cancer screening in a high risk population: a clinical trial. Ultrasound Med Biol 2001;27(4):461–6.

[23] Karlan B, Baldwin RL, Lopez-Luevanos E, et al. Peritoneal serous papillary carcinoma, a phenotypic variant of familial ovarian cancer: implications for ovarian cancer screening. Am J Obstet Gynecol 1999;180(4):917–28.

[24] King MC, Marks JH, Mandell JB. New York Breast Cancer Study Group. Breast and ovarian cancer risks due to inherited mutations in BRCA1 and BRCA2. Science 2003;302(5645):643–6.

[25] Liede A, Karlan BY, Baldwin R, et al. Cancer incidence in a population of Jewish women at risk of ovarian cancer. J Clin Oncol 2002;20(6):1570–7.

[26] Struewing JP, Hartge P, Wacholder S, et al. The risk of cancer associated with specific mutations of BRCA1 and BRCA2 among Ashkenazi Jews. N Engl J Med 1997;336(20):1401–8.

[27] Dorum A, Heimdal K, Lovslett K, et al. Prospectively detected cancer in familial breast/ovarian cancer screening. Acta Obstet Gynecol Scand 1999;78(10):906–11.

[28] Kauff ND, Satagopan JM, Robson ME, et al. Risk-reducing salpingo-oophorectomy in women with a BRCA1 or BRCA2 mutation. N Engl J Med 2002;346(21):1609–15.

[29] Cohen LS, Escobar PF, Scharm C, et al. Three-dimensional power Doppler ultrasound improves the diagnostic accuracy for ovarian cancer prediction. Gynecol Oncol 2001;82:40–8.

[30] Kinkel K, Hricak H, Ying Lu, et al. US characterization of ovarian masses: a meta-analysis. Radiology 2000;217:803–11.

[31] Kurjak A, Kupesic S, Sparac V, et al. Preoperative evaluation of pelvic tumors by Doppler and three-dimensional sonography. J Ultrasound Med 2001;20:829–40.

[32] Kurjak A, Kupesic S, Sparac V, et al. The detection of stage I ovarian cancer by three-dimensional sonography and power Doppler. Gynecol Oncol 2003;90(2):258–64.

[33] Funt SA, Hann LE. Detection and characterization of adnexal masses. Radiol Clin North Am 2002;40(3):591–608.

[34] Jain KA. Prospective evaluation of adnexal masses with endovaginal gray-scale and duplex and color Doppler US: Correlation with pathologic findings. Radiology 1994;191(1): 63–7.

[35] Salem S, Wilson SR. Gynecologic ultrasound. In: Rumack CM, Wilson SR, Charboneau JW, et al, editors. Diagnostic Ultrasound. 2nd edition. Philadelphia: Mosby; 2005.

[36] Brown DL, Doubilet PM, Miller FH, et al. Benign and malignant ovarian masses: selection of the most discriminating gray-scale and Doppler sonographic features. Radiology 1998;208: 103–10.

[37] DiSantis DJ, Scatarige JC, Kemp G, et al. A prospective evaluation of transvaginal sonography for detection of ovarian disease. AJR Am J Roentgenol 1993;161:91–4.

[38] Ferrazzi E, Zanetta G, Dordoni D, et al. Transvaginal ultrasonographic characterization of ovarian masses: comparison of five scoring systems in a multicenter study. Ultrasound Obstet Gynecol 1997;10:192–7.

[39] Kurjak A, Predanic M. New scoring system for prediction of ovarian malignancy based on transvaginal color Doppler sonography. J Ultrasound Med 1992;11:631–8.

[40] Timor-Tritsch IE, Lerner JP, Monteagudo A, et al. Transvaginal ultrasonographic characterization of ovarian masses by means of color flow-directed Doppler measurements and a morphologic scoring system. Am J Obstet Gynecol 1993;168(3 Pt 1):909–13.

[41] Timmerman D, Schwarzler P, Collins WP, et al. Subjective assessment of adnexal masses with the use of ultrasonography: an analysis of interobserver variability and experience. Ultrasound Obstet Gynecol 1999;13(1):11–6.

[42] Schelling M, Braun M, Kuhn W, et al. Combined transvaginal B-mode and color Doppler sonography for differential diagnosis of ovarian tumors: results of a multivariate logistic regression analysis. Gynecol Oncol 2000;77:78–86.

[43] Guerriero S, Alcazar JL, Coccia ME, et al. Complex pelvic mass as a target of evaluation of vessel distribution by color Doppler sonography for the diagnosis of adnexal malignancies: results of a mulitcenter European study. J Ultrasound Med 2002;21:1105–11.

[44] Brown DL, Frates MC, Laing FC, et al. Ovarian masses: can benign and malignant lesions be differentiated with color and pulsed Doppler US? Radiology 1994;190(2):333–6.

[45] Hamper UM, Sheth S, Abbas FM, et al. Transvaginal color Doppler sonography of adnexal masses: differences in blood flow impedance in benign and malignant lesions. AJR Am J Roentgenol 1993;160(6):1225–8.

[46] Levine D, Feldstein VA, Babcook CJ, et al. Sonography of ovarian masses: poor sensitivity of resistive index for identifying malignant lesions. AJR Am J Roentgenol 1994;162(6):1355–9.

[47] Salem S, White LM, Lai J. Doppler sonography of adnexal masses: the predictive value of the pulsatility index in benign and malignant disease. AJR Am J Roentgenol 1994;163(5):1147–50.

[48] Valentin L. Prospective cross-validation of Doppler ultrasound examination and gray-scale ultrasound imaging for discrimination of benign and malignant pelvic masses. Ultrasound Obstet Gynecol 1999;14(4):273–83.

[49] Buy JN, Ghossain MA, Hugol D, et al. Characterization of adnexal masses: combination of color Doppler and conventional sonography compared with spectral Doppler analysis alone and conventional sonography alone. AJR Am J Roentgenol 1996;166(2):385–93.

[50] Wagner B, Buck J, Seidman JD, et al. Ovarian epithelial neoplasms: radiologic-pathologic correlation. Radiographics 1994;14:1351–74.

[51] Rieber A, Nussle K, Stohr I, et al. Preoperative diagnosis of ovarian tumors with MR imaging: comparison with transvaginal sonography, positron emission tomography, and histological findings. AJR Am J Roentgenol 2001;177(1):123–9.

[52] Halvorsen RA Jr, Panushka C, Oakley GJ, et al. Intraperitoneal contrast material improves the CT detection of peritoneal metastases. AJR Am J Roentgenol 1991;157(1):37–40.

[53] Komatsu T, Konishi I, Madai M, et al. Adnexal masses: Transvaginal US and gadolinium-enhanced MRI assessment of intratumoral structure. Radiology 1996;198:109–15.

[54] Funt SA, Hricak H. Ovarian malignancies. Top Magn Reson Imaging 2003;14(4):329–37.

[55] Jeong YY, Outwater EK, Kang HK. Imaging evaluation of ovarian masses. Radiographics 2000;20(5):1445–70.

[56] Hricak H, Chen M, Coakley FV, et al. Complex adnexal masses: detection and characterization with MR imaging–multivariate analysis. Radiology 2000;214(1):39–46.

[57] Sohaib SA, Sahdev A, Van Trappen P, et al. Characterization of adnexal mass lesions on MR imaging. AJR Am J Roentgenol 2003;180(5):1297–304.

[58] Kurtz AB, Tsimikas JV, Tempany CM, et al. Diagnosis and staging of ovarian cancer: comparative values of Doppler and conventional US, CT, and MR imaging correlated with surgery and histopathologic analysis—report of the Radiology Diagnostic Oncology Group. Radiology 1999;212(1):19–27.

[59] Kinkel K, Lu Y, Mehdizade A, et al. Indeterminate ovarian mass at US: incremental value of second imaging test for characterization—meta-analysis and Bayesian analysis. Radiology 2005;236:85–94.

[60] Schwartz PE. Cytoreductive surgery for the management of stage IV ovarian cancer. Gynecol Oncol 1997;64(1):1–3.

[61] Subhas N, Patel PV, Pannu HK, et al. Imaging of pelvic malignancies with in-line FDG PET-CT: case examples and common pitfalls of FDG PET. Radiographics 2005;25(4):1031–43.

[62] Fenchel S, Grab D, Nuessle K, et al. Asymptomatic adnexal masses: correlation of FDG PET and histopathologic findings. Radiology 2002;223(3):780–8.

[63] Grab D, Flock F, Stöhr I, et al. Classification of asymptomatic adnexal masses by ultrasound, magnetic resonance imaging, and positron emission tomography. Gynecol Oncol 2000;77(3):454–9.

[64] Greene F, Page D, Fleming I, et al. AJCC cancer staging handbook. 6th edition. New York: Springer-Verlag; 2002.

[65] Holloway BJ, Gore PH, A'Hern RP, et al. The significance of paracardiac lymph nodes enlargement in ovarian cancer. Clin Radiol 1997;52:692–7.

[66] Coakley FV, Choi PH, Gougoutas CA, et al. Peritoneal metastases: detection with spiral CT in patients with ovarian cancer. Radiology 2002;223(2):495–9.

[67] Pannu HK, Horton KM, Fishman EK. Thin section dual-phase multidetector-row computed tomography detection of peritoneal metastases in gynecologic cancers. J Comput Assist Tomogr 2003;27(3):333–40.

[68] Tempany CM, Zou KH, Silverman SG, et al. Staging of advanced ovarian cancer: comparison of imaging modalities—report from the Radiological Diagnostic Oncology Group. Radiology 2000;215(3):761–7.

[69] Ricke J, Sehouli J, Hach C, et al. Prospective evaluation of contrast-enhanced MRI in the depiction of peritoneal spread in primary or recurrent ovarian cancer. Eur Radiol 2003;13(5):943–9.

[70] Yoshida Y, Kurokawa T, Kawahara K, et al. Incremental benefits of FDG positron emission

tomography over CT alone for the preoperative staging of ovarian cancer. AJR Am J Roentgenol 2004;182(1):227–33.

[71] Hubner KF, McDonald TW, Niethammer JG, et al. Assessment of primary and metastatic ovarian cancer by positron emission tomography (PET) using 2-[18F]deoxyglucose (2-[18F]FDG). Gynecol Oncol 1993;51:197–204.

[72] Schroder W, Zimny M, Rudlowski C, et al. The role of 18-F-fluorodeoxyglucose position imaging tomography 18-F-FGD PET in ovarian carcinoma. Int J Gynecol Cancer 1999;9(2):117–22.

[73] Rose PG, Faulhaber P, Miraldi F, et al. Positive emission tomography for evaluating a complete clinical response in patients with ovarian or peritoneal carcinoma: correlation with second-look laparotomy. Gynecol Oncol 2001;82(1):17–21.

[74] Drieskens O, Stroobants S, Gysen M, et al. Positron emission tomography with FDG in the detection of peritoneal and retroperitoneal metastases of ovarian cancer. Gynecol Obstet Invest 2003;55(3):130–4.

[75] Turlakow A, Yeung HW, Salmon AS, et al. Peritoneal carcinomatosis: role of (18)F-FDG PET. J Nucl Med 2003;44(9):1407–12.

[76] Byrom J, Widjaja E, Redman CW, et al. Can pre-operative computed tomography predict resectability of ovarian carcinoma at primary laparotomy? Br J Obstet Gynaecol 2002;109(4):369–75.

[77] Qayyum A, Coakley FV, Westphalen AC, et al. Role of CT and MR imaging in predicting optimal cytoreduction of newly diagnosed primary epithelial ovarian cancer. Gynecol Oncol 2005;96(2):301–6.

[78] Woodward PJ, Hosseinzadeh K, Saenger JS. From the archives of the AFIP: radiologic staging of ovarian carcinoma with pathologic correlation. Radiographics 2004;24(1):225–46.

[79] Dachman AH, Visweswaran A, Battula R, et al. Role of chest CT in the follow-up of ovarian adenocarcinoma. AJR Am J Roentgenol 2001;176:701–5.

[80] Sella T, Rosenbaum E, Edelmann DZ, et al. Value of chest CT scans in routine ovarian carcinoma follow-up. AJR Am J Roentgenol 2001;177:857–9.

[81] Bast RC, Xu FJ, Yu YH, et al. CA 125: the past and the future. Int J Biol Markers 1998;13(4):179–87.

[82] Santillan A, Garg R, Zahurak ML, et al. Risk of epithelial ovarian cancer recurrence in patients with rising serum CA-125 levels within the normal range. J Clin Oncol 2005;23(36):9338–43.

[83] Wilder JL, Pavlik E, Straughn JM, et al. Clinical implications of a rising serum CA-125 within the normal range in patients with epithelial ovarian cancer: a preliminary investigation. Gynecol Oncol 2003;89(2):233–5.

[84] Park CM, Kim SH, Kim SH, et al. Recurrent ovarian malignancy: patterns and spectrum of imaging findings. Abdom Imaging 2003;28(3):404–15.

[85] Chen LM, Karlan BY. Recurrent ovarian carcinoma: is there a place for surgery? Semin Surg Oncol 2000;19(1):62–8.

[86] Low RN, Duggan B, Barone RM, et al. Treated ovarian cancer: MR imaging, laparotomy reassessment, and serum CA-125 values compared with clinical outcome at 1 year. Radiology 2005;235(3):918–26.

[87] Smith GT, Hubner KF, McDonald T, et al. Cost analysis of FDG PET for managing patients with ovarian cancer. Clin Positron Imaging 1999;2(2):63–70.

[88] Kim S, Chung JK, Kang SB, et al. [18F]FDG PET as a substitute for second-look laparotomy in patients with advanced ovarian carcinoma. Eur J Nucl Med Mol Imaging 2004;31(2):196–201.

[89] Delbeke D, Martin WH. Positron emission tomography imaging in oncology. Radiol Clin North Am 2001;39(5):883–917.

[90] Nanni C, Rubello D, Farsad M, et al. (18)F-FDG PET/CT in the evaluation of recurrent ovarian cancer: a prospective study on forty-one patients. Eur J Surg Oncol 2005;31(7):792–7.

[91] Sironi S, Messa C, Mangili G, et al. Integrated FDG PET/CT in patients with persistent ovarian cancer: correlation with histologic findings. Radiology 2004;233(2):433–40.

[92] Kubik-Huch RA, Dorffler W, von Schulthess GK, et al. Value of (18F)-FDG positron emission tomography, computed tomography, and magnetic resonance imaging in diagnosing primary and recurrent ovarian carcinoma. Eur Radiol 2000;10(5):761–7.

[93] Murakami M, Miyamoto T, Lida T, et al. Whole-body positron emission tomography and tumor marker CA125 for detection of recurrence in epithelial ovarian cancer. Int J Gynecol Cancer 2006;16(Suppl 1):99–107.

[94] Pannu HK, Bristow RE, Cohade C, et al. PET-CT in recurrent ovarian cancer: initial observations. Radiographics 2004;24(1):209–23.

[95] Torizuka T, Nobezawa S, Kanno T, et al. Ovarian cancer recurrence: role of whole-body positron emission tomography using 2-[fluorine-18]-fluoro-2-deoxy- D-glucose. Eur J Nucl Med Mol Imaging 2002;29(6):797–803.

[96] Picchio M, Sironi S, Messa C, et al. Advanced ovarian carcinoma: usefulness of [(18)F]FDG-PET in combination with CT for lesion detection after primary treatment. Q J Nucl Med 2003;47(2):77–84.

[97] Barranger E, Kerrou K, Petegnief Y, et al. Laparoscopic resection of occult metastasis using the combination of FDG-positron emission tomography/computed tomography image fusion with intraoperative probe guidance in a woman with recurrent ovarian cancer. Gynecol Oncol 2005;96(1):241–4.

RADIOLOGIC
CLINICS
OF NORTH AMERICA

Radiol Clin N Am 45 (2007) 167–182

ELSEVIER
SAUNDERS

Imaging of Uterine Cancer

Oguz Akin, MD[a,b,*], Svetlana Mironov, MD[a,b],
Neeta Pandit-Taskar, MD[a,b], Lucy E. Hann, MD[a,b]

Endometrial cancer

The American Cancer Society estimates that in 2006, 41,200 new cases of cancer of the uterine corpus, mostly endometrial, will be diagnosed and 7350 women will die from this disease in the United States [1].

Endometrial cancer may develop from endometrial hyperplasia caused by unopposed estrogen stimulation; it also may develop spontaneously. Risk factors for developing endometrial cancer include conditions leading to increased estrogen exposure, such as estrogen replacement therapy (without progestin), obesity, tamoxifen use, early menarche, late menopause, nulliparity, and history of polycystic ovary disease. Pregnancy and use of oral contraceptives reduce the risk of endometrial cancer.

Up to 90% of endometrial cancers are adenocarcinomas. Depending on the glandular pattern, they are classified as well-differentiated (grade 1) to anaplastic (grade 3) tumors. Prognostic factors include tumor grade and stage, depth of myometrial invasion, and lymph node status.

Most endometrial cancers are detected at an early stage because of clinical assessment for postmenopausal bleeding. Treatment options include surgery, radiation, hormones, and chemotherapy, depending on the stage of the disease.

The 1-year relative survival rate for uterine corpus cancer is 94%. The 5-year survival rate is 96% for local disease, but it decreases to 66% for disease with regional spread and 25% for disease with distant spread.

Cervical cancer

The American Cancer Society estimates that in 2006, 9716 new cases of invasive cervical cancer will be diagnosed and 3700 women will die from this disease in the United States [1]. As Papanicolaou (Pap) smearing has become more common, incidence rates of cervical cancer have decreased and preinvasive lesions of the cervix are far more

[a] Weill Medical College of Cornell University, New York, NY, USA
[b] Department of Radiology, Memorial Sloan-Kettering Cancer Center, 1275 York Avenue, New York, NY 10021, USA
* Corresponding author. Department of Radiology, Memorial Sloan-Kettering Cancer Center, 1275 York Avenue, New York, NY 10021.
E-mail address: akino@mskcc.org (O. Akin).

0033-8389/07/$ – see front matter © 2006 Elsevier Inc. All rights reserved.
radiologic.theclinics.com

doi:10.1016/j.rcl.2006.10.009

commonly diagnosed than invasive cervical cancer. Mortality rates also have declined as a result of prevention and early detection.

Risk factors for developing cervical cancer include infection with certain types of human papillomavirus, early age at first sexual intercourse, multiple sexual partners, multiparity, history of sexually transmitted diseases, and low socioeconomic status.

Cervical intraepithelial neoplasia (CIN) is considered a precursor lesion of cervical cancer. CIN is characterized in three groups depending on cellular dysplasia: CIN 1, minor dysplasia; CIN 2, moderate dysplasia; and CIN 3, severe dysplasia or carcinoma in situ. Up to 40% of CIN 3 lesions could develop into invasive cervical cancer if left untreated. Squamous cell carcinoma accounts for 80% to 90% of cases of cervical cancer. Adenocarcinomas are rare but have a worse prognosis.

Preinvasive lesions (ie, lesions that have not yet transgressed the basement membrane) can be treated with electrocoagulation, cryotherapy, laser ablation, or local surgery. Invasive cervical cancers are treated with surgery, radiation, or chemotherapy or a combination of these three methods.

Relative 1-year and 5-year survival rates for cervical cancer patients are 88% and 73%, respectively. The 5-year survival rate is approximately 92% for localized cervical cancer [1].

Imaging has become an important adjunct to the clinical assessment of uterine cancer. When integrated with clinical findings, imaging findings can optimize cancer care and aid in the development of a treatment plan tailored to the individual patient. Traditionally, the pretreatment evaluation of uterine cancer consisted of clinical evaluation, laboratory tests, and conventional radiographic studies. The conventional imaging studies for clinical staging are being replaced by cross-sectional imaging studies, namely ultrasound (US), CT, MR imaging, and positron emission tomography (PET). This article focuses on the role of cross-sectional imaging in the management of endometrial cancer and cervical cancer.

Endometrial cancer

Screening and diagnosis

Endometrial cancer is most commonly seen in elderly women with dysfunctional uterine bleeding [1]. Approximately 12% of endometrial cancers occur in premenopausal women, however [2]. The American Cancer Society recommends that all postmenopausal women be informed about the risks and symptoms of endometrial cancer and encouraged to report any bleeding or spotting. Annual screening with endometrial biopsy beginning at age 35 should be offered to women with or at risk for hereditary nonpolyposis colon cancer [1].

Definitive diagnosis of endometrial cancer is made with endometrial sampling with endometrial biopsy or dilatation and curettage. The tissue obtained by endometrial sampling is examined under a microscope and evaluated for cancerous or precancerous abnormalities.

Transvaginal US may be used in the initial evaluation of women with postmenopausal bleeding [3–5]. US diagnosis is based on endometrial thickness measurements in the anteroposterior dimension. The Society of Radiologists in Ultrasound Consensus Panel recommends a cut-off value of 5 mm [3], but others have reported optimal results using 4 mm as the upper limit for normal endometrial thickness [6,7]. With normal endometrial thickness on transvaginal US, the risk of cancer is in the range of 1% to 5.5% [7,8]. Transvaginal US is reported to be useful for diagnosis of endometrial abnormalities and carcinoma in women with abnormal bleeding even when endometrial biopsy and hysteroscopy produce negative results [9,10].

Abnormal uterine bleeding is an early symptom of endometrial carcinoma, and there is no evidence that screening asymptomatic women is of any benefit, even in high-risk groups [11,12]. Women who undergo tamoxifen treatment for breast carcinoma have a 7.5% relative risk of endometrial cancer, but routine screening is not recommended [13]. Women with hereditary nonpolyposis colon cancer have a 40% to 60% lifetime risk of endometrial cancer, but US surveillance in the absence of symptomatic bleeding does not offer any prognostic advantage [14].

Tumor detection and staging

Staging of endometrial cancer is based on surgicopathologic International Federation of Gynecology and Obstetrics (FIGO) criteria. The TNM staging system is based on the same criteria as the FIGO system (Table 1) [15,16]. The FIGO staging system uses findings from exploratory laparotomy, total abdominal hysterectomy, bilateral salpingo-oophorectomy, peritoneal washings, sampling, and lymphadenectomy.

Surgical staging, however, is not suitable for women who are not good surgical candidates because of older age, obesity, and other medical problems. Noninvasive cross-sectional imaging is particularly helpful in such cases to depict the depth of myometrial invasion, tumor extent, and presence of lymphadenopathy. Pretreatment imaging improves patient care by assisting in determining the type and extent of surgery or radiation treatment.

Table 1: TNM and International Federation of Gynecology and Obstetrics staging systems for endometrial cancer

TNM	FIGO	T - Primary Tumor
TX		Primary tumor cannot be assessed
T0		No evidence of primary tumor
Tis	0	Carcinoma in situ
T1	I	Tumor confined to corpus uteri
T1a	IA	Tumor limited to endometrium
T1b	IB	Tumor invades less than one half of the myometrium
T1c	IC	Tumor invades one half or more of the myometrium
T2	II	Tumor invades cervix but does not extend beyond uterus
T2a	IIA	Endocervical glandular involvement only
T2b	IIB	Cervical stromal invasion
T3	III	Local and/or regional spread as specified in T3a, b, and/or N1 and FIGO IIIA, B, and C below
T3a	IIIA	Tumor involves serosa and/or adnexa (direct extension or metastasis) and/or cancer cells in ascites or peritoneal washings
T3b	IIIB	Vaginal involvement (direct extension or metastasis)
N1	IIIC	Metastasis to the pelvic and/or para-aortic lymph nodes
T4	IVA	Tumor invades bladder mucosa and/or bowel mucosa (bullous edema is not sufficient to classify a tumor as T4)
N—Regional Lymph Nodes		
NX		Regional nodes cannot be assessed
N0		No regional nodal metastasis
N1		Regional nodal metastasis
M—Distant Metastasis		
MX		Distant metastasis cannot be assessed
M0		No distant metastasis
M1	IVB	Distant metastasis (includes metastasis to intra-abdominal lymph nodes other than para-aortic, and/or inguinal lymph nodes; excludes metastasis to vagina pelvic serosa, or adnexa)

Ultrasonography

Ultrasonography, especially with a transvaginal approach, is the initial imaging modality in patients with suspected endometrial cancer. Endometrial cancer most often appears as thickened endometrium that is more than 5 mm in a postmenopausal woman or 15 mm in a premenopausal woman (Fig. 1). Echogenicity varies, but alteration of endometrial texture or focal increased echogenicity may be seen [17]. These appearances are not specific and can be observed in endometrial hyperplasia and polyps [18]. Saline infusion sonohysterography improves diagnosis for endometrial cancer with reported 89% sensitivity, 46% specificity, 16% positive predictive value, and 97% negative predictive value [19,20]. Risk of disseminating malignant cells by saline infusion sonohysterography is small, approximately 7% [21].

Color Doppler US often reveals increased vascularity with a multivessel pattern, in contrast to the pedicle artery sign seen in endometrial polyps [22–24]. Spectral Doppler indices may have low-impedance flow, but there is significant overlap in Doppler indices of benign and malignant conditions of the endometrium [25].

Myometrial invasion is depicted as irregularity of the endometrium-myometrium border and disruption of the subendometrial halo. The accuracy of US for diagnosing the depth of invasion is approximately 73% to 93%, but US is better for grade 2-3 tumors and should not be used as the sole criterion for the decision to perform extensive surgery [26–28]. Although US can be used to estimate depth of invasion, a recent meta-analysis has shown that contrast-enhanced MR imaging has better overall performance [29].

CT

On CT, endometrial cancer remains relatively low attenuation compared with myometrium after contrast administration (Fig. 1).

Early studies with conventional CT reported 84% to 88% staging accuracy for endometrial cancer [30,31]. A more recent study with helical CT reported a sensitivity of 83% and a specificity of 42% for the assessment of depth of myometrial

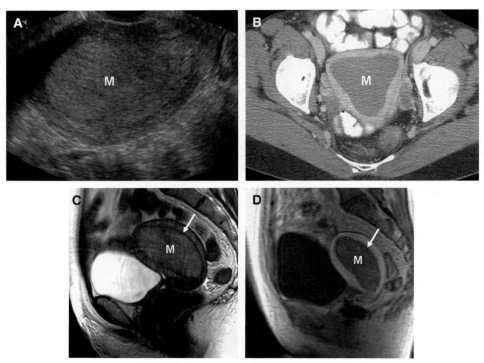

Fig. 1. A 57-year-old woman with endometrial cancer. Transvaginal US (*A*), contrast-enhanced CT (*B*), and sagittal T2-weighted (*C*) and postcontrast T1-weighted MR imaging (*D*) show a large endometrial mass (*M*). Note that the low signal intensity junctional zone is intact (*arrow*) (*C*) and there is a smooth interface between the mass and the myometrium (*arrow*) (*D*). These findings rule out myometrial invasion.

invasion and a sensitivity of 25% and a specificity of 70% for the depiction of cervical invasion [32]. CT is limited for the evaluation of cervical extension and depth of myometrial invasion. CT is most commonly used in the assessment of advanced disease. CT can demonstrate invasion to the adjacent organs, such as bladder and rectum. Distant metastases from endometrial cancer are most often seen in the extrapelvic lymph nodes and peritoneum. CT is a reliable method in the assessment of enlarged lymph nodes. Peritoneal metastases on CT appear as peritoneal thickening, soft-tissue masses, and ascites. Detection of small lymph node metastases and peritoneal implants is difficult not only with CT but also with other imaging methods, however.

MR imaging

MR imaging is the most accurate modality for the pretreatment evaluation of endometrial cancer. Endometrial carcinoma is usually seen as a mass that is hypo- to isointense on T1-weighted images and hyperintense or heterogeneous on T2-weighted images compared with myometrium. On T2-weighted images if the normal low signal intensity junctional zone is intact, myometrial invasion can be excluded. If the junctional zone is not well seen because of atrophy or distention caused by a mass, the

presence of myometrial invasion is suspected if there is an irregular endometrium-myometrium interface. Dynamic postcontrast images are especially valuable in demonstrating myometrial invasion because endometrial cancer enhances less than myometrium (**Figs. 1 and 2**).

Determining the presence of myometrial invasion is a critical factor because in patients with deep myometrial invasion (invasion >50% thickness of myometrium), there is a six- to sevenfold increased prevalence of pelvic and lumboaortic lymph node metastases compared with patients with myometrial invasion that is absent or less than 50% [33]. The preoperative determination of myometrial invasion helps in planning the extent of lymphadenectomy.

Conditions that may render MR imaging evaluation of endometrial cancer difficult include the presence of an indistinct junctional zone in a postmenopausal woman, an irregular and thickened junctional zone in adenomyosis, myometrial thinning by a large tumor, and myometrial distortion by a large leiomyoma.

In the early 1990s, the overall staging accuracy of MR imaging was reported to be 83% to 92% [34–36]. A more recent study confirmed these early reports and showed that MR imaging had 87%

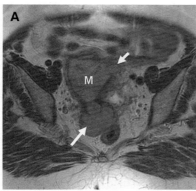 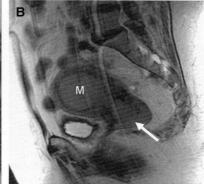

Fig. 2. A 76-year-old woman with endometrial cancer. Transverse (*A*) and sagittal (*B*) T2-weighted MR imaging show a large endometrial mass (*M*) that extends to the cervix (*arrows*). Note that the junctional zone is disrupted and the mass extends to the uterine serosa (*short arrow*) (*A*).

sensitivity and 91% specificity in assessing myometrial infiltration, 80% sensitivity and 96% specificity for cervical invasion, and 50% sensitivity and 95% specificity for lymph node assessment. There was significant agreement between MR imaging and surgicopathologic findings in assessment of myometrial invasion ($P < 0.001$) [37]. Like all other cross-sectional imaging methods, MR imaging is limited in the assessment of lymph node status because it does not allow clear differentiation between metastatic and nonmetastatic lymph nodes of similar size.

A study using meta-analysis and bayesian analysis showed that findings from contrast-enhanced MR imaging significantly affected the posttest probability of deep myometrial invasion in patients with endometrial cancer. In this study, the mean weighted pretest probabilities of deep myometrial invasion in patients with tumor grades 1, 2, and 3 were 13%, 35%, and 54%, respectively. Posttest probabilities of deep myometrial invasion for grades 1, 2, and 3 increased to 60%, 84%, and 92%, respectively, with positive MR imaging findings and decreased to 1%, 5%, and 10%, respectively, with negative MR imaging findings [38].

The role of imaging in treatment planning

Morphologic prognostic factors, including depth of myometrial invasion, cervical extension, and lymph node metastasis, influence the prognosis and treatment options in endometrial cancer [39]. Lymphadenectomy and pre- or postoperative radiation therapy are indicated in patients at high risk of extrauterine disease or lymph node metastasis. Because the probability of extrauterine disease and lymph node metastasis correlates with the depth of myometrial invasion, preoperative knowledge

of myometrial invasion is important. Tumor extension into the cervix affects the type of surgery, and parametrial invasion requires radiation as the initial treatment or a more radical surgical approach.

The value of US, CT, and MR imaging for diagnosis of myometrial invasion and cervical extension has been assessed. Several reports have indicated that MR imaging, being more accurate than CT and US, is the most advantageous technique for the evaluation of endometrial cancer [40–42]. A meta-analysis showed no significant differences in the overall performance of CT, US, and MR imaging. For the assessment of myometrial invasion, however, contrast-enhanced MR imaging performed significantly better than did non-enhanced MR imaging or US ($P < 0.002$) and demonstrated a trend toward better results, as compared with CT. The lack of data on the assessment of cervical invasion at CT or US prevented meta-analytic comparison with data obtained at MR imaging [43].

The following guidelines can be used for staging endometrial cancer [43]:

1. No imaging is required for a patient with grade 1 tumor and a non-enlarged uterus at physical examination because the pretest probability of myometrial, cervical, or nodal involvement is low. If results from the physical examination are inconclusive or if there is concomitant pelvic disease, US, CT, or MR imaging can be used for the initial radiologic investigation.
2. Patients with high-grade papillary or clear cell tumors should undergo CT or MR imaging because there is a high pretest probability of nodal involvement.
3. Patients with possible cervical involvement at physical examination or with positive or inconclusive results from endocervical curettage should undergo MR imaging, because this is

the only modality that has been shown to accurately depict cervical invasion.

4. In patients who require multifactorial assessment, contrast-enhanced MR imaging is the only modality that can be used to evaluate myometrial, cervical, and nodal involvement accurately.

Posttreatment follow-up

Recurrent endometrial cancer most commonly occurs in the vaginal cuff or pelvic sidewall. Early detection and accurate characterization of the extent of recurrent disease are important in identifying patients who might be candidates for local resection, pelvic exenteration, or radiotherapy for nonresectable disease. CT and MR imaging can demonstrate the site and extent of recurrence after surgery (Figs. 3 and 4). CT is widely available, but the superior soft-tissue contrast of MR imaging allows for better assessment of the local extent of recurrent tumor. For the evaluation of widespread recurrence CT is preferred.

A few studies have reported that PET can be useful for the detection of suspected and asymptomatic recurrent endometrial cancer (Fig. 4). One study found that in the posttherapy surveillance of endometrial carcinomas, FDG-PET had sensitivity of 96%, specificity of 78%, diagnostic accuracy of 90%, positive predictive value of 89%, and negative predictive value of 91% [44]. Another study reported that in detecting recurrent lesions and evaluating treatment responses, FDG-PET, used in conjunction with anatomic information from CT or MR imaging, showed better diagnostic ability (sensitivity 100.0%, specificity 88.2%, accuracy 93.3%) than conventional imaging (sensitivity 84.6%, specificity 85.7%, accuracy 85.0%) and

tumor markers (sensitivity 100.0%, specificity 70.6%, accuracy 83.3%) [45].

Cervical cancer

Screening and diagnosis

The Pap test is a simple procedure in which a small sample of cells is collected from the cervix and examined under a microscope. The American Cancer Society recommends screening for cervical cancer to begin approximately 3 years after a woman begins having vaginal intercourse but no later than 21 years of age [1]. Screening should be done every year with a regular Pap test or every 2 years using liquid-based tests. At or after age 30, women who have had three normal test results in a row may be screened every 2 to 3 years. Alternatively, cervical cancer screening with human papillomavirus DNA testing and conventional or liquid-based cytology can be performed every 3 years. Women with certain risk factors, such as HIV infection or a weak immune system, may be screened more often. Women aged 70 years and older who have had three or more consecutive normal Pap tests in the last 10 years may choose to stop cervical cancer screening. Screening after total hysterectomy is not necessary unless the surgery was done for cervical cancer.

Patients with suspicious findings on Pap smear or patients with high-risk human papillomavirus strains should be evaluated further with colposcopy, colposcopy-directed biopsies of the suspicious areas, and— if necessary—conization to establish the diagnosis.

Tumor detection and staging

Staging of cervical cancer is based on clinical FIGO criteria. The TNM staging system is based on the same criteria as the FIGO system (Table 2)

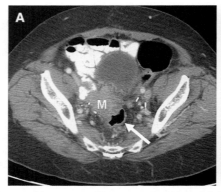
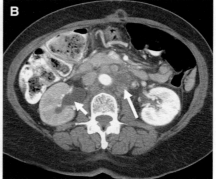

Fig. 3. A 77-year-old woman with recurrent endometrial cancer. Contrast-enhanced CT demonstrates a recurrent mass (*M*) that is inseparable from the sigmoid colon (*arrow*) in the right pelvis (*A*). Right delayed nephrogram and hydronephrosis (*short arrow*) caused by obstruction of the right ureter by the pelvic mass and extensive retroperitoneal lymphadenopathy (*arrow*) are also seen (*B*).

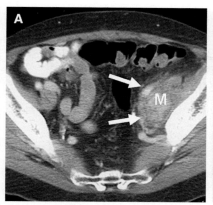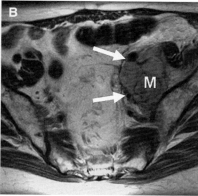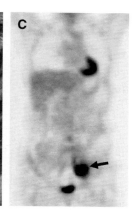

Fig. 4. A 63-year-old woman with recurrent endometrial cancer. Contrast-enhanced CT (*A*) and transverse T2-weighted MR imaging (*B*) show a left pelvic mass (*M*) that abuts the left iliac bone and partially encases the left internal and external iliac vessels (*arrow*). Coronal PET (*C*) shows intense uptake in the recurrent mass (*arrow*).

[15,16]. The FIGO staging system uses findings from physical examination, colposcopy, lesion biopsy, radiologic studies (ie, chest radiography, intravenous urography, and barium enema), and endoscopic studies (ie, cystoscopy, sigmoidoscopy) [46]. Compared with surgical staging, FIGO clinical staging causes understaging in 20% to 30% of cases in stage IB disease, 23% in stage IIB, and almost 40% in stage IIIB and overstaging in 64% of cases in stage IIIB disease [47–50]. The major limitations of clinical evaluation are in the assessment of parametrial and pelvic sidewall invasion, the estimation of tumor size (especially if the tumor is primarily endocervical in location), and the evaluation of lymph node and distant metastases.

Evidence shows that cross-sectional imaging is superior to clinical staging [51–54]. Tumor size, parametrial invasion, and lymph node status, which are all critical prognostic factors in staging and treatment planning, are well evaluated with CT and MR imaging [55]. Modern cross-sectional imaging has not been incorporated into the FIGO guidelines for routine pretreatment diagnostic evaluation of cervical cancer, however, mainly because of the principle that staging should use universally available methods and serve as a standardized means of communication among institutions around the world. There is also a lack of consensus concerning the choice of the appropriate cross-sectional imaging modality.

Ultrasonography

US plays a limited role in the staging of cervical cancer. Transabdominal sonography can be used to reveal the presence of hydronephrosis, but otherwise this modality is not recommended for the staging of cervical cancer. Endorectal and transvaginal US can be used in the assessment of extent of local disease but are inadequate for detection of pelvic sidewall involvement and lymph node metastases [56,57].

CT

CT is often used in preoperative staging and treatment planning for cervical cancer. In the evaluation of cervical cancer, oral and intravenous contrast administration is necessary. The advantages of CT are rapid acquisition time, lack of bowel motion artifact, and the ability to image organs during the peak of vascular enhancement, which allows differentiation between blood vessels and lymph nodes. The limitations of CT include difficulties in direct tumor visualization and differentiation between the tumor and normal cervical tissue. Advances in CT technology, such as multidetector scanners, are improving tumor assessment by CT. Multidetector CT uses thinner section collimation and higher table speed per rotation, which allows better spatial and contrast resolution than single-detector helical CT. Reconstruction of axial data in the coronal and sagittal planes is helpful in depicting local spread of disease. The potential role of multidetector CT with optimized scanning protocols for cervical cancer should be studied further. Currently, CT is used mainly in the detection of lymphadenopathy and advanced disease (such as distant metastasis) and in guiding percutaneous biopsies and planning radiation treatment.

CT is limited in the depiction of cervical cancer because 50% of tumors are isodense to cervical stroma on contrast-enhanced CT (Fig. 5) [58]. When the primary tumor is visible, it is hypoattenuated relative to normal cervical stroma because of necrosis, ulceration, or lower vascularity in the tumor [59].

Table 2:   **TNM and International Federation of Gynecology and Obstetrics staging systems for cervical cancer**

TNM	FIGO	T - Primary Tumor
TX		Primary tumor cannot be assessed
T0		No evidence of primary tumor
Tis	0	Carcinoma in situ
T1	I	Cervical carcinoma confined to uterus (extension to corpus should be disregarded)
T1a	IA	Invasive carcinoma diagnosed only by microscopy
T1a1	IA1	Measured stromal invasion ≤3 mm in depth and ≤7 mm in horizontal spread
T1a2	IA2	Measured stromal invasion >3 mm and not more than 5 mm with a horizontal spread ≤7 mm
T1b	IB	Clinically visible lesion confined to cervix or microscopic lesion >T1a/IA2
T1b1	IB1	Clinically visible lesion ≤4 cm in greatest dimension
T1b2	IB2	Clinically visible lesion >4 cm in greatest dimension
T2	II	Cervical carcinoma invades beyond uterus but not to pelvic wall or lower third of vagina
T2a	IIA	Tumor without parametrial invasion
T2b	IIB	Tumor with parametrial invasion
T3	III	Tumor extends to pelvic wall and/or involves lower third of vagina and/or causes hydronephrosis or nonfunctioning kidney
T3a	IIIA	Tumor involves lower third of vagina, no extension to pelvic wall
T3b	IIIB	Tumor extends to pelvic wall and/or causes hydronephrosis or nonfunctioning kidney
T4	IVA	Tumor invades mucosa of bladder or rectum, and/or extends beyond true pelvis (bullous edema is not sufficient to classify a tumor as T4)
N—Regional Lymph Nodes		
NX		Regional nodes cannot be assessed
N0		No regional nodal metastasis
N1		Regional nodal metastasis
M—Distant Metastasis		
MX		Distant metastasis cannot be assessed
M0		No distant metastasis
M1	IVB	Distant metastasis

The cervix usually has a smooth, well-defined margin if the tumor is confined within it. The major limitation of CT in the local staging of cervical cancer is that CT is not reliable for distinguishing tumor from the normal parametrial structures. Signs of early parametrial invasion on CT include increased attenuation and stranding of the parametrial fat and an ill-defined cervical margin. These findings are not specific, however, and can be caused by inflammatory or reactive changes in the parametrium without tumor extension. Advanced parametrial invasion is more easily assessed on CT when a soft-tissue mass within parametrial fat, encasement of the ureter and periuterine vessels by the tumor, or thickening and nodularity of the uterosacral ligaments are depicted. CT criteria for pelvic sidewall invasion include tumor extension to less than 3 mm from the sidewall, encasement of iliac vessels, direct invasion into pelvic sidewall muscles, and destruction of the pelvic bones [59].

The reported accuracy of contrast-enhanced CT in the detection of parametrial invasion is 76% to 80% [53,58,60]. In advanced disease with hydronephrosis and pelvic sidewall invasion, the accuracy of CT increases [61].

Involvement of the bladder and rectum can be depicted on CT; the signs include obliteration of the perivesical or perirectal fat plane by tumor, irregular thickening of the bladder or rectal wall, and an intraluminal mass. Early involvement of the bladder and the rectum is not reliably seen on CT, however, and invasion can be confirmed with cystoscopy or proctoscopy and biopsy [59].

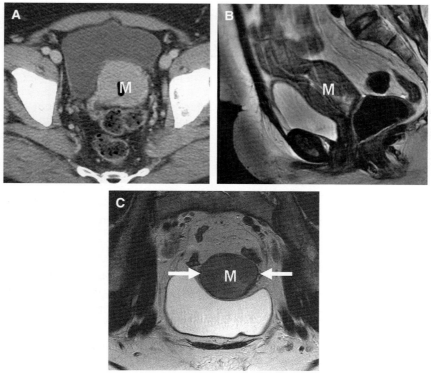

Fig. 5. A 55-year-old woman with cervical cancer. Contrast-enhanced CT (*A*), sagittal (*B*) and coronal oblique (*C*) T2-weighted MR imaging show a large cervical mass (*M*). Note that intact cervical stromal ring and smooth tumor-parametrial interface rule out parametrial invasion (*arrows*) (*C*).

For detecting lymph node involvement, CT has accuracy similar to that of MR imaging (83%–85% for CT and 88%–89% for MR imaging) [58,62,63]. Both techniques have low sensitivity (24%–70%), however, because of their inability to detect metastasis in normal-sized lymph nodes or differentiate enlarged inflammatory nodes from malignant nodes.

Distant metastases from cervical cancer are most often seen in the extrapelvic lymph nodes, peritoneum, liver, lung, and bone. Peritoneal metastases on CT appear as peritoneal thickening, soft-tissue masses and ascites. Liver can be involved, with intrahepatic metastases or surface lesions from peritoneal dissemination. Thoracic metastases manifest most commonly as multiple pulmonary nodules, mediastinal or hilar lymphadenopathy, or pleural and pericardial nodules or effusions. Bone metastases are seen as osseous destruction, which may have an associated soft-tissue component.

MR imaging

MR imaging is considered the most accurate imaging modality for the evaluation of cervical cancer because of its superb soft-tissue resolution. MR imaging is also a cost-effective study because it can substitute for several other imaging modalities. The two types of coils most commonly used in pelvic imaging are the standard gradient body coil and the phased-array surface coil. Compared with body coils, phased-array coils provide better spatial resolution by improving the signal-to-noise ratio and contributing to field homogeneity. The use of endoluminal coils (either transvaginal or transrectal) improves visualization of small tumors of the cervix; however, it does not significantly improve the accuracy of assessment of parametrial invasion. The role of MR imaging in the evaluation of cervical cancer includes pretreatment assessment of local tumor extent and nodal involvement, monitoring of treatment response, and detection of recurrent disease.

MR imaging is advantageous in the local staging of cervical cancer. T2-weighted images are especially useful for depiction of the local extent of the disease. Although cervical cancer demonstrates variable contrast enhancement, dynamic postcontrast MR imaging may improve assessment of small tumors. Contrast-enhanced T1-weighted images also may help in the detection of bladder or rectal wall invasion or delineation of fistulas.

Cervical cancer appears as a high signal intensity mass within low signal intensity cervical stroma on

T2-weighted images. In cervical cancers confined to the stroma, the low signal intensity stromal ring surrounding the high signal intensity tumor on T2-weighted images is completely intact. In the case of full-thickness stromal invasion, the low signal intensity stroma is completely replaced by high signal intensity tumor, and a smooth tumor–parametrial interface excludes parametrial invasion. Disruption of the stromal ring with nodular or irregular tumor signal intensity extending into the parametrium indicates parametrial invasion. In advanced cases, encasement of the ureter and periuterine vessels by the tumor and thickening and nodularity of the uterosacral ligaments can be depicted. In the case of vaginal invasion, disruption of the low signal intensity vaginal wall with high signal intensity tumor is seen. Tumor extending within 3 mm of the pelvic sidewall, encasement of iliac vessels, direct invasion into pelvic sidewall muscles, and destruction of the pelvic bones are signs of pelvic sidewall invasion. Disruption of the normal low signal intensity walls of the rectum or bladder indicates invasion to these adjacent organs (Figs. 5–7).

MR imaging is superior to clinical evaluation in the assessment of tumor size (one of the prognostic factors in cervical cancer) and provides measurements comparable to surgical measurements in most cases [51,53,64,65]. The reported accuracy of MR imaging in the detection of parametrial invasion ranges from 77% to 96% [51,54,66–68].

Because of its excellent soft-tissue resolution, MR imaging is advantageous in the depiction of vaginal involvement and rectal and bladder invasion. The reported accuracy of MR imaging for vaginal invasion is 86% to 93% [51,54]. MR imaging also has high accuracy (99%) in the detection of urinary bladder invasion [58].

In detecting lymph node metastases, MR imaging has accuracy similar to that of CT (88%–89% for MR imaging versus 83%–85% for CT) [63,64].

Positron emission tomography
Metabolic information from PET can supplement morphologic information obtained with cross-sectional imaging methods. Although the current use of PET in the initial evaluation of cervical cancer is still under investigation, PET imaging is an effective adjunct to CT and MR imaging in evaluating lymph node involvement, detecting distant metastases, and evaluating treatment response (Fig. 8) [69,70].

In a recent study that evaluated the usefulness of PET in nodal staging of early cervical cancers, investigators found overall node-based sensitivity and specificity of 72% and 99.7% and overall accuracy of 99.3% [71]. All undetected metastatic lymph nodes were smaller than 0.5 cm in diameter. For lymph nodes larger than 0.5 cm in diameter, sensitivity was 100% and specificity was 99.6% [71]. Another study reported that PET had overall sensitivity of 91% and specificity of 100% in the detection of metastatic lymph nodes in patients with cervical cancer [72]. In advanced cervical cancer, PET has been reported to have high sensitivity in the detection of lymph node metastases. A study in patients with cervical cancer of stages IB to IVA reported that PET had a sensitivity of 86% for the detection of pelvic and para-aortic lymph node metastasis, whereas CT had a sensitivity of only 57% [72]. Another study in advanced cervical cancer patients showed that

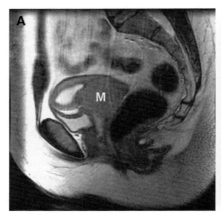
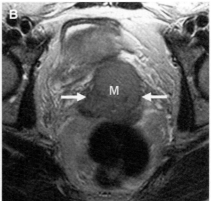

Fig. 6. A 39-year-old woman with cervical cancer. Sagittal (*A*) and transverse (*B*) T2-weighted MR imaging show a large cervical mass (*M*) that invades the lower uterine segment. Disruption of cervical stromal ring and irregular tumor-parametrial interface indicate parametrial invasion (*arrows*) (*B*).

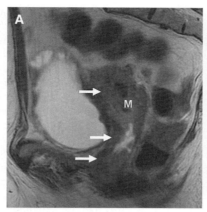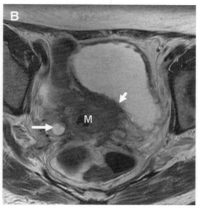

Fig. 7. A 77-year-old woman with cervical cancer. Sagittal T2-weighted MR image (*A*) shows a large cervical mass (*M*) that extends to the uterus and vagina (*arrows*). Transverse T2-weighted MR imaging (*B*) shows bilateral parametrial invasion, dilated right ureter (*arrow*), and invasion to the urinary bladder wall (*short arrow*) by the mass (*M*).

PET had a sensitivity of 75% and specificity of 92% in detecting para-aortic lymph node metastasis [73]. A meta-analysis of data from 15 studies on FDG-PET in cervical cancer reported combined pooled sensitivity and specificity of 84% and 95%, respectively, for detection of aortic lymph node metastasis and 79% and 99%, respectively, for detection of pelvic lymph node metastasis [74].

The role of imaging in treatment planning

The role of imaging in the pretreatment evaluation of cervical cancer is to help distinguish patients with stage IIA or lower who can be treated with surgery, combined radiation-chemotherapy, or—in some cases—radiation therapy alone from those with advanced disease (ie, parametrial invasion, stage $\geq$ IIB) that are best treated with radiation alone or combined with chemotherapy.

Advances in cross-sectional imaging have improved the accuracy of cervical cancer staging. In a study comparing clinical staging to staging by cross-sectional imaging, the accuracies of CT and MR imaging (53% and 86%, respectively) were higher than that of clinical staging (47%) [75]. As the value of cross-sectional imaging for tumor staging has come to be recognized, extended clinical staging incorporating findings from CT or MR imaging has become common practice without changes in the FIGO staging criteria. Meanwhile, the use of conventional radiologic examinations (intravenous urography, barium enema and lymphangiography) has become rare. A multicenter, interdisciplinary American College of Radiology Imaging Network/ Gynecologic Oncology Group prospective study conducted from 2000 to 2002 found that in the pretreatment evaluation of invasive cervical cancer, only 26.9% of patients had examination under anesthesia for FIGO clinical staging, 8.1% had cystoscopy, 8.6% had sigmoidoscopy or proctoscopy; 1% had intravenous urography, and none had barium enema or lymphangiography [76]. The large

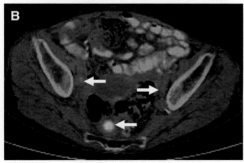

Fig. 8. An 84-year-old woman with cervical cancer. Enlarged bilateral external iliac and presacral lymph nodes (arrows) are seen on CT image (*A*). FDG uptake is seen in the same lymph nodes (*arrows*) consistent with lymph node involvement on fused PET-CT image (*B*).

discrepancy between the diagnostic tests recommended by FIGO for cervical cancer staging and the tests used in clinical practice suggests a need to reassess the FIGO guidelines.

A meta-analysis of 57 studies (38 on MR imaging, 11 on CT, and eight on MR imaging and CT) found that sensitivities for parametrial invasion were 74% (95% confidence index, 68%–79%) for MR imaging and 55% (95% confidence index, 44%–66%) for CT [77]. In the recent American College of Radiology Imaging Network/Gynecologic Oncology Group prospective multicenter clinical study, sensitivities for parametrial invasion were low for MR imaging (53%) and CT (42%) but were higher than the sensitivity of FIGO clinical staging, which was just 29% [78].

Posttreatment follow-up

After radical hysterectomy, 74% of cervical cancer recurrences are within the pelvis [79]. The most common sites of recurrent disease are the vaginal cuff, parametrium, and pelvic sidewall. Early detection and accurate characterization of the extent of recurrent disease are important to identify patients who may be candidates for local resection, pelvic exenteration, or radiotherapy for nonresectable disease. CT and MR imaging can demonstrate the site and extent of recurrence after surgery, but the superior soft-tissue contrast of MR imaging enables better assessment of the local extent of recurrent tumor. For the evaluation of widespread recurrence CT is preferred.

After radiation treatment, it is important to distinguish postradiation changes from recurrent tumor. CT remains limited in this regard [80]. T2-weighted MR imaging has high sensitivity (90%–91%) but low specificity (22%–38%) for recurrent disease in the cervix [81,82]. After radiation treatment, the tumor and the uterus decrease in size, and the cervical stroma displays low signal intensity on T2-weighted images (Fig. 9). The low specificity of T2-weighted MR imaging is caused by the fact that benign conditions such as edema, inflammation, and necrosis also may cause increased T2 signal mimicking residual tumor. The use of dynamic MR imaging with T2-weighted images improved specificity from 22% to 38% to 67% [81,83]. Early radiation change may show early enhancement, however, which mimics tumor.

In two studies on the detection of cervical cancer recurrence, PET had sensitivities of 85.7% and 90.3% and specificities of 76.1% to 86.7% [84,85]. Another study found that the sensitivity of PET for detecting recurrence was 80% in asymptomatic women and 100% in symptomatic women [86]. FDG-PET also can be useful in women who present with elevated markers but negative conventional imaging. A study reported that PET detected recurrence in 94% of patients with negative conventional imaging findings [87].

Summary

Imaging has become an important adjunct to the assessment of endometrial and cervical cancer. When integrated with clinical findings, imaging findings can optimize treatment planning. Imaging continually evolves in response to changes in clinical practice and technologic improvements. The choice of imaging modality is not only case specific but also depends on local gynecologic practice, radiologic expertise, and equipment availability.

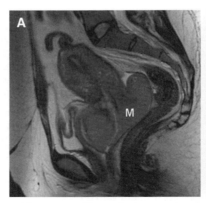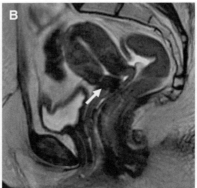

Fig. 9. A 39-year-old woman with cervical cancer treated with radiation. Initial sagittal T2-weighted MR image (*A*) shows a large cervical mass (*M*) that bulges into the vagina. After radiation treatment, sagittal T2-weighted MR imaging (*B*) shows that the tumor has resolved and the low signal intensity of the cervical stroma has been restored (*arrow*). Note radiation-induced atrophy in the uterus and fatty bone marrow replacement in the sacrum (*B*).

Acknowledgments

The authors thank Ada Muellner, BA, for her assistance in editing the manuscript.

References

[1] American Cancer Society. Cancer facts and figures: 2006. Atlanta (GA): American Cancer Society; 2006.

[2] Soliman PT, Oh JC, Schmeler KM, et al. Risk factors for young premenopausal women with endometrial cancer. Obstet Gynecol 2005;105(3): 575–80.

[3] Goldstein RB, Bree RL, Benson CB, et al. Evaluation of the woman with postmenopausal bleeding: Society of Radiologists in Ultrasound-Sponsored Consensus Conference statement. J Ultrasound Med 2001;20:1025–36.

[4] Goldstein SR, Zeltser I, Horan CK, et al. Ultrasonographically-based triage for perimenopausal patients with abnormal uterine bleeding. Am J Obstet Gynecol 1997;177:102–8.

[5] Medverd JR, Dubinsky TJ. Cost analysis model: US versus endometrial biopsy in evaluation of peri-and postmenopausal abnormal vaginal bleeding. Radiology 2002;222:619–27.

[6] Smith P, Bakos O, Heimer G, et al. Transvaginal ultrasound for identifying endometrial abnormality. Acta Obstet Gynecol Scand 1991;70: 591–4.

[7] Karlsson B, Granberg S, Wikland M, et al. Transvaginal ultrasonography of the endometrium in women with postmenopausal bleeding: a Nordic multicenter study. Am J Obstet Gynecol 1995; 172:1488–94.

[8] Smith-Bindman R, Kerlikowske K, Feldstein VA, et al. Endovaginal ultrasound to exclude endometrial cancer and other endometrial abnormalities. JAMA 1998;280:1510–7.

[9] Dubinsky TJ, Parvey HR, Maklad N. The role of transvaginal sonography and endometrial biopsy in the evaluation of peri-and postmenopausal bleeding. AJR Am J Roentgenol 1997;169:145–9.

[10] Deckardt R, Lueken RP, Gallinat A, et al. Comparison of transvaginal ultrasound, hysteroscopy and dilatation and curettage in the diagnosis of abnormal vaginal bleeding and intrauterine pathology in perimenopausal and postmenopausal women. J Am Assoc Gynecol Laparosc 2002;9: 277–82.

[11] Gerber B, Krause A, Muller H, et al. Ultrasonographic detection of asymptomatic endometrial cancer in postmenopausal patients offers no prognostic advantage over symptomatic disease discovered by uterine bleeding. Eur J Cancer 2001;37:64–71.

[12] Langer RD, Pierce JJ, O'Hanlan KA, et al. Transvaginal ultrasonography compared with endometrial biopsy for the detection of endometrial disease. N Engl J Med 1997;337:1793–8.

[13] Barakat RR. Contemporary issues in the management of endometrial cancer. CA Cancer J Clin 1998;48:299–314.

[14] Dove-Edwin I, Boks D, Goff S, et al. The outcome of endometrial carcinoma surveillance by ultrasound scan in women at risk of hereditary nonpolyposis colorectal carcinoma and familial colorectal carcinoma. Cancer 2002;15:1708–12.

[15] Benedet JL, Bender H, Jones H III, et al. FIGO staging classifications and clinical practice guidelines in the management of gynecologic cancers: FIGO Committee on Gynecologic Oncology. Int J Gynaecol Obstet 2000;70:209–62.

[16] Green FL, Page DL, Fleming ID, et al, editors. AJCC cancer staging manual. 6th edition. New York: Springer-Verlag; 2002.

[17] Sheikh M, Sawhney S, Khurana A, et al. Alteration of sonographic texture of the endometrium in post-menopausal bleeding: a guide to further management. Acta Obstet Gynecol Scand 2000;79:1006–10.

[18] Nalaboff KM, Pellerito JS, Ben-Levi E. Imaging the endometrium: disease and normal variants. Radiographics 2001;21:1409–24.

[19] Bree RL, Bowerman RA, Bohm-Velez M, et al. US evaluation of the uterus in patients with postmenopausal bleeding: a positive effect on diagnostic decision making. Radiology 2000;216:260–4.

[20] Dubinsky TJ, Stroehlein K, Abu-Ghazzeh Y, et al. Prediction of benign and malignant endometrial disease: hysterosonographic-pathologic correlation. Radiology 1999;210:393–7.

[21] Alcazar JL, Errasti T, Zornoza A. Saline infusion sonohysterography in endometrial cancer: assessment of malignant cells dissemination risk. Acta Obstet Gynecol Scand 2000;79:321–2.

[22] Sawicki V, Spiewankiewicz B, Stelmachow J, et al. Color Doppler assessment of blood flow in endometrial cancer. Eur J Gynaecol Oncol 2005; 26:279–84.

[23] Alcazar JL, Ajossa S, Floris S, et al. Reproducibility of endometrial vascular patterns in endometrial disease as assessed by transvaginal power Doppler sonography in women with postmenopausal bleeding. J Ultrasound Med 2006;25: 159–63.

[24] Timmerman D, Verguts J, Konstantinovic ML. The pedicle artery sign based on sonography with color Doppler imaging can replace second stage tests in women with abnormal vaginal bleeding. Ultrasound Obstet Gynecol 2003;22: 166–77.

[25] Bourne TH, Campbell S, Steer CV, et al. Detection of endometrial cancer by transvaginal ultrasonography with color flow imaging and blood flow analysis: a preliminary report. Gynecol Oncol 1991;40:253–9.

[26] Teefey SA, Stahl JA, Middleton WD, et al. Local staging of endometrial carcinoma: comparison of transvaginal and intraoperative sonography and gross visual inspection. AJR Am J Roentgenol 1996;166:547–52.

[27] Arko D, Takac I. High frequency transvaginal ultrasonography in preoperative assessment of myometrial invasion in endometrial cancer. J Ultrasound Med 2000;29:639–43.

[28] Fishman A, Altara M, Bernheim J, et al. The value of transvaginal sonography in the preoperative assessment of myometrial invasion in high and low grade endometrial cancer and in comparison to frozen section in grade I disease. Eur J Gynaecol Oncol 2000;21:128–30.

[29] Kinkel K, Yasushi K, Yu KK, et al. Radiologic staging in patients with endometrial cancer: a meta-analysis. Radiology 1999;212:711–8.

[30] Balfe DM, Van Dyke J, Lee JK, et al. Computed tomography in malignant endometrial neoplasms. J Comput Assist Tomogr 1983;7:677–81.

[31] Walsh JW, Goplerud DR. Computed tomography of primary, persistent, and recurrent endometrial malignancy. AJR Am J Roentgenol 1982;139:1149–54.

[32] Hardesty LA, Sumkin JH, Hakim C, et al. The ability of helical CT to preoperatively stage endometrial carcinoma. AJR Am J Roentgenol 2001;176:603–6.

[33] Creasman WT, Morrow CP, Bundy BN, et al. Surgical pathologic spread patterns of endometrial cancer: a Gynecologic Oncology Group study. Cancer 1987;60:2035–41.

[34] Hirano Y, Kubo K, Hirai Y, et al. Preliminary experience with gadolinium-enhanced dynamic MR imaging for uterine neoplasms. Radiographics 1992;12:243–56.

[35] Hricak H, Rubinstein LV, Gherman GM, et al. MR imaging evaluation of endometrial carcinoma: results of an NCI cooperative study. Radiology 1991;179:829–32.

[36] Lien HH, Blomlie V, Trope C, et al. Cancer of the endometrium: value of MR imaging in determining depth of invasion into the myometrium. AJR Am J Roentgenol 1991;157:1221–3.

[37] Manfredi R, Mirk P, Maresca G, et al. Local-regional staging of endometrial carcinoma: role of MR imaging in surgical planning. Radiology 2004;231:372–8.

[38] Frei KA, Kinkel K, Bonel HM, et al. Prediction of deep myometrial invasion in patients with endometrial cancer: clinical utility of contrast-enhanced MR imaging: a meta-analysis and Bayesian analysis. Radiology 2000;216:444–9.

[39] Kodama S, Kase H, Tanaka K, et al. Multivariate analysis of prognostic factors in patients with endometrial cancer. Int J Gynaecol Obstet 1996;53:23–30.

[40] Varpula MJ, Klemi PJ. Staging of uterine endometrial carcinoma with ultra-low field (0.02 T) MRI: a comparative study with CT. J Comput Assist Tomogr 1993;17:641–7.

[41] DelMaschio A, Vanzulli A, Sironi S, et al. Estimating the depth of myometrial involvement by endometrial carcinoma: efficacy of transvaginal sonography vs MR imaging. AJR Am J Roentgenol 1993;160:533–8.

[42] Yamashita Y, Mizutani H, Torashima M, et al. Assessment of myometrial invasion by endometrial carcinoma: transvaginal sonography vs contrast-enhanced MR imaging. AJR Am J Roentgenol 1993;161:595–9.

[43] Kinkel K, Kaji Y, Yu KK, et al. Radiologic staging in patients with endometrial cancer: a meta-analysis. Radiology 1999;212:711–8.

[44] Belhocine T, De Barsy C, Hustinx R, et al. Usefulness of (18)F-FDG PET in the post-therapy surveillance of endometrial carcinoma. Eur J Nucl Med Mol Imaging 2002;29:1132–9.

[45] Saga T, Higashi T, Ishimori T, et al. Clinical value of FDG-PET in the follow up of post-operative patients with endometrial cancer. Ann Nucl Med 2003;17:197–203.

[46] Pecorelli S, Odicino F. Cervical cancer staging. Cancer J 2003;9:390–4.

[47] Vidaurreta J, Bermudez A, di Paola G, et al. Laparoscopic staging in locally advanced cervical carcinoma: a new possible philosophy? Gynecol Oncol 1999;75:366–71.

[48] Lagasse LD, Creasman WT, Shingleton HM, et al. Results and complications of operative staging in cervical cancer: experience of the Gynecology Oncology Group. Gynecol Oncol 1980;9:90–8.

[49] LaPolla JP, Schlaerth JB, Gaddis O, et al. The influence of surgical staging on the evaluation and treatment of patients with cervical carcinoma. Gynecol Oncol 1986;24:194–9.

[50] Van Nagell JR Jr, Roddick JW Jr, Lowin DM. The staging of cervical cancer: inevitable discrepancies between clinical staging and pathologic findings. Am J Obstet Gynecol 1971;110:973–8.

[51] Hricak H, Lacey CG, Sandles LG, et al. Invasive cervical carcinoma: comparison of MR imaging and surgical findings. Radiology 1998;166:623–31.

[52] Russell AH, Anderson M, Walter J, et al. The integration of computed tomography and magnetic resonance imaging in treatment planning for gynecologic cancer. Clin Obstet Gynecol 1992;35:55–72.

[53] Subak LL, Hricak H, Powell CB, et al. Cervical carcinoma: computed tomography and magnetic resonance imaging for preoperative staging. Obstet Gynecol 1995;86:43–50.

[54] Kim SH, Choi BI, Lee HP, et al. Uterine cervical carcinoma: comparison of CT and MR findings. Radiology 1990;175:45–51.

[55] Kamura T, Tsukamoto N, Tsuruchi N, et al. Multivariate analysis of the histopathologic prognostic factors of cervical cancer in patients undergoing radical hysterectomy. Cancer 1992;69:181–6.

[56] Innocenti P, Pulli F, Savino L, et al. Staging of cervical cancer: reliability of transrectal US. Radiology 1992;185:201–5.

[57] Aoki S, Hata T, Senoh D, et al. Parametrial invasion of uterine cervical cancer assessed by transrectal ultrasound: preliminary report. Gynecol Oncol 1990;36:82–9.

[58] Kim SH, Choi BI, Kim JK, et al. Preoperative staging of uterine cervical carcinoma: comparison of CT and MRI in 99 patients. J Comput Assist Tomogr 1993;17:633–40.

[59] Pannu HK, Corl FM, Fishman EK. CT evaluation of cervical cancer: spectrum of disease. Radiographics 2001;21:1155–68.

[60] Janus CL, Mendelson DS, Moore S, et al. Staging of cervical carcinoma: accuracy of magnetic resonance imaging and computed tomography. Clin Imaging 1989;13:114–6.

[61] Walsh JW, Goplerud DR. Prospective comparison between clinical and CT staging in primary cervical carcinoma. AJR Am J Roentgenol 1981;137: 997–1003.

[62] Yang WT, Lam WW, Yu MY, et al. Comparison of dynamic helical CT and dynamic MR imaging in the evaluation of pelvic lymph nodes in cervical carcinoma. AJR Am J Roentgenol 2000;175: 759–66.

[63] Scheidler JJ, Hricak H, Yu KK, et al. Radiological evaluation of lymph node metastases in patients with cervical cancer: a meta-analysis. JAMA 1997; 278:1096–101.

[64] Hawnaur JM, Johnson RJ, Buckley CH, et al. Staging, volume estimation, and assessment of nodal status in carcinoma of the cervix: comparison of magnetic imaging with surgical findings. Clin Radiol 1994;49:443–52.

[65] Sironi S, De Cobelli F, Scarfone G, et al. Carcinoma of the cervix: value of plain and gadolinium-enhanced MR imaging in assessing degree of invasiveness. Radiology 1993;188:797–801.

[66] Sheu M, Chang C, Wang J, et al. MR staging of clinical stage I and IIa cervical carcinoma: a reappraisal of efficacy and pitfalls. Eur J Radiol 2001; 38:225–31.

[67] Hawighorst H, Knapstein PG, Weikel W, et al. Cervical carcinoma: comparison of standard and pharmacokinetic MR imaging. Radiology 1996; 201:531–9.

[68] Kim SH, Han MC. Invasion of the urinary bladder by uterine cervical carcinoma: evaluation with MR imaging. AJR Am J Roentgenol 1997; 168:393–7.

[69] Umesaki N, Tanaka T, Miyama M, et al. The role of 18F-fluoro-2-deoxy-D-glucose positron emission tomography (18F-FDG-PET) in the diagnosis of recurrence and lymph node metastasis of cervical cancer. Oncol Rep 2000;7:1261–4.

[70] Sugawara Y, Eisbruch A, Kosuda S, et al. Evaluation of FDG PET in patients with cervical cancer. J Nuc Med 1999;40:1125–31.

[71] Sironi S, Buda A, Picchio M, et al. Lymph node metastasis in patients with clinical early-stage cervical cancer: detection with integrated FDG PET/CT. Radiology 2006;238:272–9.

[72] Reinhardt MJ, Ehritt-Braun C, Vogelgesang D, et al. Metastatic lymph nodes in patients with cervical cancer: detection with MR imaging and FDG PET. Radiology 2001;218: 776–82.

[73] Rose PG, Adler LP, Rodriguez M, et al. Positron emission tomography for evaluating para-aortic nodal metastasis in locally advanced cervical cancer before surgical staging: a surgicopathologic study. J Clin Oncol 1999;17:41–5.

[74] Havrilesky LJ, Kulasingam SL, Matchar DB, et al. FDG-PET for management of cervical and ovarian cancer. Gynecol Oncol 2005;97: 183–91.

[75] Ozsarlak O, Tjalma W, Schepens E, et al. The correlation of preoperative CT, MR imaging, and clinical staging (FIGO) with histopathology findings in primary cervical carcinoma. Eur Radiol 2003;13:2338–45.

[76] Amendola MA, Hricak H, Mitchell DG, et al. Utilization of diagnostic studies in the pretreatment evaluation of invasive cervical cancer in the United States: results of intergroup protocol ACRIN 6651/GOG 183. J Clin Oncol 2005;23: 7454–9.

[77] Bipat S, Glas AS, van der Velden J, et al. Computed tomography and magnetic resonance imaging in staging of uterine cervical carcinoma: a systematic review. Gynecol Oncol 2003;91: 59–66.

[78] Hricak H, Gatsonis C, Chi DS, et al. Role of imaging in pretreatment evaluation of early invasive cervical cancer: results of the intergroup study American College of Radiology Imaging Network 6651-Gynecologic Oncology Group 183. J Clin Oncol 2005;23:9329–37.

[79] Burke TW, Hoskins WJ, Heller PB, et al. Clinical patterns of tumor recurrence after radical hysterectomy in stage IB cervical carcinoma. Obstet Gynecol 1987;69:382–5.

[80] Kaur H, Silverman PM, Iyer RB, et al. Diagnosis, staging, and surveillance of cervical carcinoma. AJR Am J Roentgenol 2003;180:1621–31.

[81] Hawighorst H, Knapstein PG, Schaeffer U, et al. Pelvic lesions in patients with treated cervical carcinoma: efficacy of pharmacokinetic analysis of dynamic MR images in distinguishing recurrent tumors from benign conditions. AJR Am J Roentgenol 1996;166:401–8.

[82] Kinkel K, Ariche M, Tardivon AA, et al. Differentiation between recurrent tumor and benign conditions after treatment of gynecologic pelvic carcinoma: value of dynamic contrast-enhanced subtraction MR imaging. Radiology 1997;204: 55–63.

[83] Yamashita Y, Harada M, Torashima M, et al. Dynamic MR imaging of recurrent postoperative cervical cancer. J Magn Reson Imaging 1996;6: 167–71.

[84] Ryu SY, Kim MH, Choi SC, et al. Detection of early recurrence with 18F-FDG PET in patients

with cervical cancer. J Nucl Med 2003;44: 347–52.

[85] Havrilesky LJ, Wong TZ, Secord AA, et al. The role of PET scanning in the detection of recurrent cervical cancer. Gynecol Oncol 2003;90: 186–90.

[86] Unger JB, Ivy JJ, Connor P, et al. Detection of recurrent cervical cancer by whole-body FDG PET scan in asymptomatic and symptomatic women. Gynecol Oncol 2004;94:212–6.

[87] Chang TC, Law KS, Hong JH, et al. Positron emission tomography for unexplained elevation of serum squamous cell carcinoma antigen levels during follow-up for patients with cervical malignancies: a phase II study. Cancer 2004;101: 164–71.

RADIOLOGIC
CLINICS
OF NORTH AMERICA

Radiol Clin N Am 45 (2007) 183–205

Imaging of Bladder Cancer

Jingbo Zhang, MD[a],*, Scott Gerst, MD[b], Robert A. Lefkowitz, MD[a], Ariadne Bach, MD[b]

- Detection and staging
  Major prognostic factors
  CT imaging
  MR imaging
  Intravenous urography
  Ultrasonography
- *Nuclear scintigraphy*
  Other diagnostic considerations
- Treatment planning
- Post-treatment imaging
- Summary
- References

Bladder cancer is the fourth most common cancer in men and the tenth most common cancer in women in the United States, with 61,420 new diagnoses and 13,060 deaths expected to occur in 2006 [1]. According to the National Cancer Institute's Surveillance, Epidemiology, and End Results (SEER) Program, between 1998 and 2002, the age-adjusted incidence and death rates for bladder cancer were 21.3 and 4.4 per 100,000 population, respectively. Between 1995 and 2001, the overall 5-year survival rate for bladder cancer was 81.8% [2]. Bladder cancers occur three to four times more often in men than in women [2,3]. The age at diagnosis is generally older than 40 years; the median age is in the mid-60s.

The urinary bladder is an extraperitoneal structure surrounded by pelvic fat. The peritoneum forms a serosal covering that is present only over the bladder dome. The bladder wall consists of four layers: uroepithelium lining the bladder lumen, the vascular lamina propria, the muscularis propria consisting of bundles of smooth detrusor muscle, and the outermost adventitia formed by connective tissue [4].

More than 95% of bladder tumors arise from the uroepithelium (epithelial tumors), including urothelial tumors (over 90%), squamous cell carcinomas (6% to 8%), and adenocarcinomas (2%) [5,6]. Urothelial tumors (or transitional cell carcinoma, TCC) exhibit a spectrum of neoplasia ranging from a benign papilloma through carcinoma in situ to invasive carcinoma [5]. Adenocarcinomas may be of urachal origin or of nonurachal origin [7], with the urachal type typically occurring in the dome of the bladder in the embryonal remnant of the urachus [8]. Squamous cell carcinoma is associated strongly with a history of recurrent urinary tract infection or bladder calculus [9]. Much rarer epithelial tumors include small cell/neuroendocrine carcinoma (1%, with or without associated paraneoplastic syndrome), carcinoid tumors, and melanoma [10]. Epithelial tumors may have a mixed histology, such as urothelial and squamous or urothelial and adenocarcinoma. These are treated as urothelial carcinomas [11].

Mesenchymal bladder tumors can be benign (leiomyoma, paraganglioma, fibroma, plasmacytoma, hemangioma, solitary fibrous tumor, neurofibroma,

[a] Memorial Sloan-Kettering Cancer Center, 1275 York Avenue, C278D, New York, NY 10021, USA
[b] Cornell University, Weill Medical College, New York, NY, USA
* Corresponding author. Memorial Sloan-Kettering Cancer Center, 1275 York Avenue, C278D, New York, NY 10021.
E-mail address: zhangj12@mskcc.org (J. Zhang).

doi:10.1016/j.rcl.2006.10.005

and lipoma) or malignant (rhabdomyosarcoma, leiomyosarcoma, lymphoma, and osteosarcoma) [10].

The pathogenesis of urothelial tumors is direct prolonged contact of the bladder urothelium with urine containing excreted carcinogens [10]. This is reflected in the propensity for urothelial carcinoma to be multicentric with synchronous and metachronous involvement of the entire urinary tract (bladder and upper tract) [10]. Approximately 30% of bladder cancer patients present with multifocal disease in the bladder and sometimes widespread associated areas of squamous metaplasia and carcinoma in situ [12]. Out of the patients who initially present with upper tract lesions, 11% to 13% percent will develop additional upper tract neoplasms, while up to 50% will develop metachronous tumors in the urinary bladder. Only approximately 5% of patients who initially present with bladder TCC, however, will develop metachronous tumors in the upper urinary tract, (this is especially likely to occur when multiple bladder lesions are present) [13–15]. Patients may start with papillary low-grade tumors, which subsequently may develop into sessile, diffuse high-grade tumors that are much more likely to be invasive at recurrence [16]. The presence of carcinoma in situ is associated with an increased incidence of recurrence and an increased likelihood of developing invasive disease [12].

The most well-established risk factor for bladder cancer is cigarette smoking [4], but chemical carcinogens (such as aniline, benzidine, aromatic amines, and azo dyes) also are thought to predispose to the development of TCC; these substances are metabolized and excreted into the urine as carcinogens that act upon the urothelium. Therefore occupation is the second most important risk factor after smoking, estimated to account for as much as 20% of all bladder cancer in the past [17]. Increased risk of bladder cancer still exists for workers and former workers in the dye, rubber, and chemical industries, and probably among painters, leather workers, and shoemakers, as well as metal workers [18–25]. Diesel exhaust also has been shown to moderately increase the risk of bladder cancer [26]. Analgesic abuse and urine stasis from structural abnormalities, such as horseshoe kidneys, also are associated with an increased incidence of these tumors [13]. A history of recurrent urinary tract infection or bladder calculus is related strongly to the development of bladder cancer, squamous cell carcinoma in particular [9]. This is also evidenced by elevated risk of bladder cancer in patients with spinal cord injury in whom chronic cystitis is inevitable [4]. Squamous cell carcinoma also is associated with *Schistosoma haematobium* infection and accounts for 40% of epithelial tumors in endemic areas [4,27]. Adenocarcinoma of nonurachal origin generally is thought to arise from metaplasia of chronically irritated transitional epithelium. Other important risk factors associated with the patient's medical history include prior radiation therapy to the pelvis [28] and prior treatment for malignancy with certain chemotherapy agents, in particular cyclophosphamide [4,29]. In addition, hormonal factors may play a role in oncogenic process of bladder cancer [4].

Although only a small fraction of patients has an affected family member, heredity may play a role in some cases of bladder cancer, as the risk of developing the disease increases almost twofold when a first-degree relative carries the diagnosis of urothelial tumor [30–33]. Familial clustering of urothelial carcinoma also has been reported [30,32]. Cytogenetic and molecular genetic analyses of tumors carried by these families may contribute substantially to the understanding of urothelial tumor pathogenesis on a molecular level [34].

Detection and staging

It is thought that patients at high risk for bladder cancer probably benefit from screening, although there are no conclusive data proving that screening reduces mortality from bladder cancer [4]. Screening has been conducted mainly by hematuria testing and urine cytology, although the optimal screening test and testing interval are uncertain [4].

The most common symptom leading to the detection of bladder cancer is hematuria, typically macroscopic and painless, in over 80% of patients [4,35]. If enough urine samples are tested, nearly all patients with cystoscopically detectable bladder cancer have at least microhematuria [36]. Among patients presenting with macroscopic hematuria, up to 13% to 28% have bladder cancer [4]. Although the incidence of bladder cancer is low in patients who have microscopic hematuria, in some investigations, it increases up to 7.5% in patients over 50 years of age [4,37]. The second most common presentation of bladder cancer is urinary frequency, urgency, and dysuria resulting from irritation and reduced bladder capacity [4]. Less commonly, patients may present with urinary tract infection, or for a more advanced lesion, urinary obstruction, pelvic pain and pressure, or a palpable pelvic mass [4]. Very rarely, patients present with symptoms of advanced disease such as weight loss and abdominal or bone pain from distant metastases [4].

When bladder cancer is suspected, numerous diagnostic tests or procedures can be performed to evaluate the patient, including urinalysis and voided urine cytology, cystoscopy, and imaging studies such as CT, MR imaging, and less frequently, intravenous urography (IVU) [38]. Typically a patient with suspicious presentations is evaluated by office cystoscopy to determine whether a lesion is present. For purely papillary lesions or cases in which only the mucosa appears abnormal, suggesting carcinoma in situ, CT is not recommended, as it rarely alters the management in these circumstances. Clinical staging for disease of stage T2 and above, however, is less accurate. It is estimated that clinical staging is inaccurate in 25% to 50% of patients who have invasive cancers [39]. Therefore if cystoscopic appearance of the bladder tumor is sessile, high-grade, or includes other signs suggestive of invasion into muscle, CT of the abdomen and pelvis is recommended for staging before the patient undergoes transurethral resection of the bladder tumor (TURBT) to confirm the diagnosis and determine the extent of tumor within the bladder. When muscle invasive disease in the bladder is found by TURBT, evaluation of upper tract collecting system, examination under anesthesia, and further staging with chest radiograph and cross-sectional imaging of the abdomen and pelvis are recommended for complete staging. A bone scan should be obtained when alkaline phosphatase is elevated or a patient presents with symptoms.

Major prognostic factors

Bladder cancer is a heterogeneous and frequently multifocal disease with a variable clinical course. The major prognostic factors in carcinoma of the bladder are the depth of invasion into the bladder wall and the degree of differentiation or pathologic grade of the tumor. Approximately 70% to 80% of patients with newly diagnosed bladder cancer will present with superficial bladder tumors (ie, stage Ta, Tis, or T1) that are mostly well differentiated and often can be cured. The pathologic grade of tumor has a greater impact on the management of these noninvasive tumors, because most muscle-invasive tumors (T2 and above) are high grade.

The most commonly used staging system is that of the American Joint Committee on Cancer (AJCC), the TNM system [40] (Box 1). The patient's overall disease stage is determined by AJCC stage groupings (Box 2). Cancer-specific survival for patients who have bladder cancer is correlated highly with the tumor stage (Table 1). The 5-year survival rate is 55% to 80% for patients with bladder cancer confined to the lamina propria treated with cystectomy, but it drops to 40% with muscular invasion, 20% with perivesical invasion, and 6% with metastatic disease [41].

Precise staging is critical for preoperative planning and prognosis. The clinical staging of bladder cancer is determined by the depth of invasion of the bladder wall, performed with a cystoscopic examination that includes a biopsy, and examination under anesthesia to assess the size and mobility of

---

Box 1: TNM staging table for bladder cancer

T—Primary tumor
TX—Primary tumor cannot be assessed.
T0—No evidence of primary tumor
Ta—Noninvasive papillary carcinoma
Tis—Carcinoma in situ
T1—Tumor invades subepithelial connective tissue.
T2—Tumor invades muscle.
- pT2a—Tumor invades superficial muscle.
- pT2b—Tumor invades deep muscle.
T3—Tumor invades perivesical tissue.
- pT3a—Tumor invades perivesical tissue microscopically.
- pT3b—Tumor invades perivesical tissue macroscopically.
T4—Tumor invades any of the following: prostate, uterus, vagina, pelvic wall, or abdominal wall.
- T4a—Tumor invades the prostate, uterus, or vagina.
- T4b—Tumor invades the pelvic wall, abdominal wall (The suffix "m" is added to the appropriate T category to indicate multiple lesions. The suffix "is" may be added to any T to indicate the presence of associated carcinoma in situ.)

N—Regional lymph nodes
NX—Regional lymph nodes cannot be assessed.
N0—No regional lymph node metastasis
N1—Metastasis in a single lymph node less than or equal to 2 cm in greatest dimension
N2—Metastasis in a single lymph node, greater than 2 cm but less than or equal to 5 cm in greatest dimension; or multiple lymph nodes, less than or equal to 5 cm in greatest dimension
N3—Metastasis in a lymph node, greater than 5 cm in greatest dimension

M—Distant metastasis
MX—Distant metastasis cannot be assessed.
M0—No distant metastasis
M1—Distant metastasis

---

palpable masses, the degree of thickening of the bladder wall, and the presence of extravesical extension or invasion of adjacent organs. Clinical staging often underestimates the extent of tumor, particularly in cancers that are less differentiated and more deeply invasive.

CT imaging

CT is the imaging modality of choice for the work-up of patients presenting with hematuria. It also is indicated in patients with high-grade bladder cancer raising suspicion for muscle invasion. Routine contrast-enhanced CT examinations are useful for detecting metastases, but they may be inadequate for detecting and staging local urothelial lesions. In the setting of hematuria, CT urography (CTU) can be used as a one-stop-shop examination to evaluate the entire urinary system and diagnose possible causes of hematuria, including lithiasis, other benign etiologies, renal parenchymal lesions, and urothelial neoplasms, thus eliminating the need for additional imaging. In the presence of urothelial tumor, the detailed evaluation of the entire urinary system provided by CTU [42] is essential, as patients with urothelial tumor may have multifocal disease. In terms of cancer staging, CTU can detect direct perirenal, periureteral, and extravesical tumor spread, as well as lymphadenopathy and distant metastases. Compared with traditional excretory urography, CTU requires a shorter examination time and has greater accuracy for detecting urothelial lesions [43]. CTU also allows more detailed evaluation of the renal parenchyma and perirenal tissues and permits better evaluation of obstructed collecting systems than does excretory urography [13]. Therefore, for evaluating urinary tract neoplasms and the work-up for hematuria, CTU is the imaging modality of choice for patients who can tolerate

Table 1: Survival rates for bladder cancer by stage

Bladder cancer stage	Relative 5-year survival (1998–2003)
0	95%
I	85%
II	55%
III	38%
IV	16%

Data from the National Cancer Database. Comission on cancer, American College of Surgeons, Chicago, IL.

iodinated intravenous contrast. The advantages of CTU are made possible by multidetector helical CT with volumetric acquisition, which provides fast acquisition of high-resolution images and allows multiplanar reconstruction.

Although some institutions use combined axial CTU with conventional overhead radiograph or CT scanned projection radiograph (tomogram/topogram) imaging [44], dedicated CTU with image postprocessing has proven to be robust and versatile, supplanting combined imaging at many institutions. Protocols differ among institutions. At the authors' institution, CTU is performed without oral contrast, using combined intravenous nonionic iodinated contrast (150 mL at 2.5 mL/s in a patient with normal renal function) and saline bolusing (400 cc). Thin-section precontrast, postcontrast, and delayed excretory phase images are obtained. Precontrast images covering the area from the top of the kidneys to the bottom of the bladder are essential for evaluating the presence of urinary calculi. They also provide a baseline attenuation measurement for evaluating the degree and pattern of enhancement for any incidentally identified lesions of the urinary tract [45]. Postcontrast images typically are performed during the renal parenchymal phase (approximately 90 seconds after initiation of the intravenous contrast injection), and they cover the entire abdomen and pelvis. These images are helpful in the identification of enhancing urothelial lesions, incidental renal cortical masses, and other abdominal/pelvic abnormalities such as hepatic metastases and lymphadenopathy Earlier phase imaging, such as arterial phase imaging targeting the kidneys or bladder, has been suggested by some investigators to be useful for evaluating TCC [46]. The excretory phase images (typically achieved with a scan delay of 10 minutes or more) provide substantial additional information, both in confirming enhancing lesions as true lesions and not pseudolesions related to focal opacified urine arising from a ureteral jet within the bladder lumen [47], and in demonstrating discrete filling defects caused by tumor not evident on earlier scans. If the urinary tract is not well distended and opacified with contrast throughout its entire course, then additional delayed images may be acquired targeting the nonopacified portion up to two times. Putting the patient in the prone position, applying abdominal compression, or both, may help distend the urinary collecting system. In the setting of frank hydronephrosis, the patient may be allowed to return to the CT department 30 or 60 minutes later for delayed imaging. The excretory phase images are reconstructed further into thin overlapping sections, which then are transferred to a workstation for three-dimensional post-

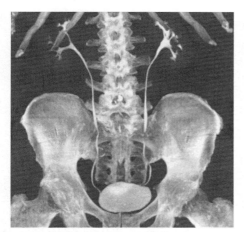

Fig. 1. A coronal maximum intensity projection image obtained from excretory phase CT urography (CTU) shows bilateral urinary collecting systems and bladder are opacified with contrast.

processing (Fig. 1). Table 2 shows a typical CTU protocol at the authors' institution for a 16-slice multidetector scanner (LightSpeed 16; General Electric, Milwaukee, Wisconsin).

Numerous different image postprocessing algorithms (either volume rendering of entire data set, thick slab averaging, or maximum intensity projections), are available for CTU to provide three-dimensional visualization of the urinary tract, or reconstruct IVP-like projectional images. The major role of postprocessed images is to provide a general overview of the anatomy and accentuate the areas of abnormality (Fig. 2). Any abnormality visualized on the postprocessed images, however, needs to be confirmed on the axial source images. In addition, three-dimensional reconstructions alone have been shown to have a suboptimal sensitivity in detecting upper tract lesions, even in retrospect [48]. Therefore they are considered supplementary only and do not replace acquired axial source images for accurate interpretation. In one study by Caoili and colleagues, 24 of 27 upper urinary tract neoplasms were detected with CTU. Of note, 21 of 27 lesions in this study were missed using the three-dimensional reconstructed images alone (especially small tumors or tumors that presented with wall thickening without distortion of the lumen; similar types of tumors frequently are missed on excretory urography). Twenty of the 24 detected lesions were visible on the axial source images using a soft tissue window that allowed visualization of ureteral or pelvic wall thickening. The remaining four lesions only could be seen using a wide window (bone window) that allowed visualization of small intraluminal lesions that were obscured on soft tissue windows by the high density of the excreted contrast material [43]. Therefore it was suggested that the axial source images should be viewed with both bone and soft tissue windows to achieve the highest diagnostic accuracy [43].

Virtual cystoscopy, obtained by manipulating CTU data acquired through the contrast-filled bladder during the excretory phase, allows navigation within a three-dimensional model, and has shown promise for detecting bladder mucosal lesions [49]. Further investigation to assess for added value of virtual cystoscopy, when compared with current

Table 2: **CT urography**			
	Precontrast	**Parenchymal**	**Excretion**
Pitch	0.9375	0.9375	1.375
Scan rotation speed	18.75 mm/rotation	18.75 mm/rotation	13.75 mm/rotation
Slice thickness/ spacing (mm)	2.5 × 2.5 mm	2.5 × 2.5 mm	2.5 × 2.5 mm
Tube rotation speed	0.8 s rotation	0.8 s rotation	0.8 s rotation
Anatomical coverage	Top of kidneys to pubic symphysis	Top of liver to pubic symphysis	Top of kidneys to pubic symphysis
Reconstructions	N/A	N/A	1.25 × 0.8 mm
Injection (rate/time/ volume)	N/A	1. 200 cc intravenous saline bolus 2. 150 cc at 2.5 cc/s 3. 200 cc intravenous saline bolus	N/A
Injection to scan delay (sec)	N/A	92 s after beginning of intravenous contrast injection	10 minutes
Oral contrast	None	None	None

Abdominal compression
Apply unless patient has known hydronephrosis/obstruction, recent surgery, or abdominal pain. Apply just before beginning injection and release at 5 minutes.

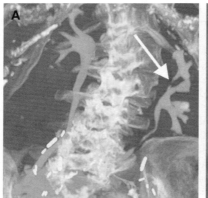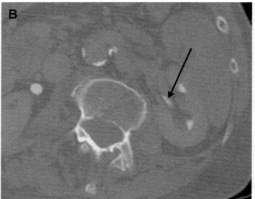

Fig. 2. 85-year-old woman who has history of bladder cancer, status postcystectomy. *(A)* Coronal MIP image from the excretory phase shows narrowing of a left upper pole infundibulum *(arrow)*. *(B)* Axial source image obtained during the excretory phase shows corresponding nodular thickening to the urothelium at this location *(arrow)*, which subsequently was proven to represent transitional cell carcinoma on surgical pathology.

axial, multiplanar, and three-dimensional model evaluation, is warranted.

Despite the superior spatial resolution and multiplanar reconstruction capabilities of CTU, evaluation for upper tract disease remains challenging. Renal pelvic TCC accounts for approximately 5% of all urothelial tumors and 7% to 10% of primary renal tumors, whereas ureteral TCC is even less common than renal pelvic TCC by a ratio of 1:3 or 1:4 [50]. Ureteral urothelial carcinomas also tend to be multifocal, and they can occur synchronously or metachronously [44]. A description and some examples of TCC of the renal pelvis are given elsewhere in this issue. Generally speaking, most common demonstrations of upper tract TCC on CT include a focal nodular, typically sessile, enhancing lesion persisting as a filling defect on excretory phase images, or segmental urothelial thickening with enhancement and luminal narrowing [51] (Fig. 3). Upper tract

TCC can be associated with varying degrees of obstruction, ranging from calyceal dilatation (Fig. 4) to hydroureteronephrosis, depending on the level of the tumor. Unfortunately, benign or inflammatory strictures may show similar findings and may be difficult to differentiate from malignancy, especially in patients who have undergone prior urinary tract surgery or instrumentation. At the authors' institution, surveillance imaging with CTU for equivocal findings frequently is performed in this clinical scenario. Irregular, nodular urothelial thickening that increases over time, particularly in the setting of positive urine cytology, raises the suspicion for urothelial carcinoma as opposed to benign changes (Fig. 5).

Adequate distension and opacification of the ureter is essential in demonstrating smaller upper tract lesions, and this has been the topic of multiple studies with several investigated techniques. Studies

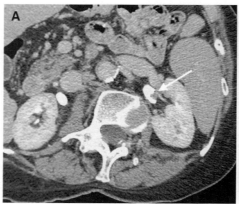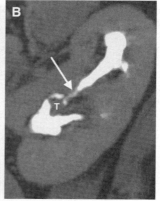

Fig. 3. 85-year-old woman who has transitional cell carcinoma (TCC) of the left renal collecting system. *(A)* Axial excretory phase CTU image demonstrates a discrete nodular filling defect *(arrow)* within the left renal pelvis. *(B)* A sagittal oblique MIP reconstruction image of the left kidney demonstrates the tumor (T) within the renal pelvis as seen on *A*, as well as focal urothelial thickening with irregular narrowing of the upper pole calyx *(arrow)*.

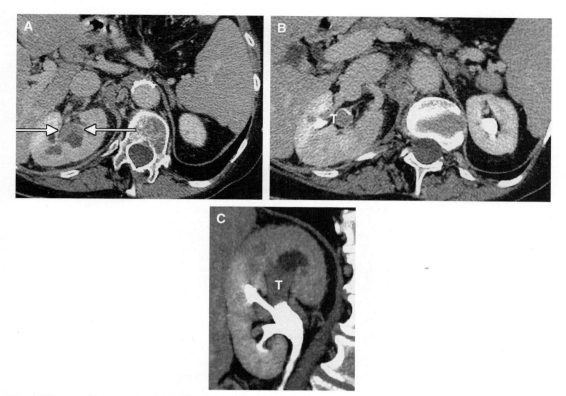

Fig. 4. 58-year-old man who has TCC of the right renal pelvis. *(A)* Axial contrast-enhanced CTU image during parenchymal phase demonstrates enhancing tumor *(arrows)* in the right renal pelvis. *(B)* On axial excretory phase CTU images, this lesion persists as a filling defect (T). *(C)* MIP reconstruction image of the right kidney in the coronal oblique plane provides an IVP-like image and demonstrates the overall extent of the tumor (T). The upper pole calyx is dilated and does not demonstrate contrast excretion, caused by tumor obstruction.

have shown variable effects of intravenous saline and external compression, used to aid opacification and distension of the upper tracts [52–54]. In addition, split-phase intravenous contrast bolusing, to allow synchronous nephrographic and excretory phase evaluation and reduce overall radiation, has been discussed [55]. Oral hydration with water just before commencing CTU scanning also has

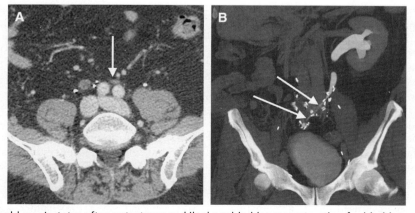

Fig. 5. 82-year-old man's status after cystectomy and ileal neobladder reconstruction for bladder cancer, presenting with negative urine cytology. *(A)* Axial parenchymal phase CTU image shows left ureteral narrowing with mild wall thickening at the level where the ureter crosses the abdominal midline *(arrow)* right ureteral stump. *(B)* A coronal thin MIP reconstructed from the excretory phase CTU images confirms the segmental narrowing of distal left ureter as shown on *A (arrows)*. This finding was stable on multiple subsequent surveillance CTUs and considered most likely to be a postoperative change.

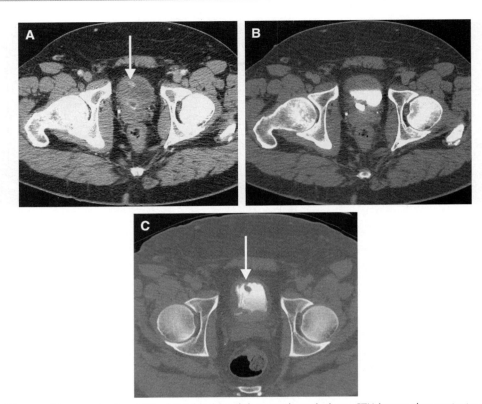

Fig. 6. 77-year-old man who has TCC of the bladder. (*A*) Parenchymal phase CTU image demonstrates a 5-mm enhancing papillary lesion (arrow) arising from the anterior bladder wall. (*B*) Excretory phase images do not readily demonstrate the lesion, as the non-dependent portion of the urine in the bladder is not opacified with contrast. (*C*). Repeat excretory phase image in the prone position demonstrates the pedunculated tumor as a discrete filling defect (arrow).

been evaluated in an effort to improve ureteral distension. Differences in scan timing, particularly for delayed excretory sequences, have shown variable results [42,53].

On CT examinations, bladder cancer may manifest various patterns of tumor growth along the bladder wall, including papillary, sessile, infiltrating, mixed, or flat intraepithelial growth [10,56]. Focal, nodular soft tissue tumor or focal asymmetric bladder wall thickening may be evident. Occasionally, more superficial papillary tumors may project within the lumen of the bladder, with a narrow pedunculation arising from the bladder wall (Fig. 6). Retraction of the bladder wall may be present. Urothelial carcinomas have been shown to demonstrate increased vascularity on more remote angiographic studies, and, more recently, on contrast-enhanced CT (Figs. 6 and 7). For example, Kim and colleagues showed that TCC tends to enhance early, with the maximal degree of enhancement occurring at approximately 60 to 80 seconds after the commencement of peripheral intravenous contrast administration at standard volumes with an injection rate of 4 mL per second [57].

For local staging of bladder cancer, perivesical fat infiltration suggests transmural extension, or T3 disease (Fig. 8). Recent TURBT, however, frequently causes linear or focal enhancement along the bladder mucosa or bladder wall, and at times bladder wall thickening, perivesical fat stranding, or fibrosis [39], thus limiting the specificity of CT. The reported accuracy in local staging of bladder cancer varies widely. Overall accuracy for local bladder cancer staging in the literature is near 60%, with a tendency to overstage [39]. Accurate diagnosis of microscopic perivesical invasion (T3a disease) is particularly difficult. Various techniques have been investigated to improve local staging. In a cohort of 65 patients with staging grouped at less than or equal to T1, T2-T3a, T3b, or T4 disease, an accuracy of 91% was achieved by distending the bladder with contrast, and an accuracy of approximately 95% was achieved when the bladder was insufflated with air [58]. More recently, sensitivity and specificity for perivesical invasion by CT, when performed 7 or more days after TURBT, were calculated at 92% and 98%, respectively [57]. But these decreased to 89% and 95%, respectively, in a larger

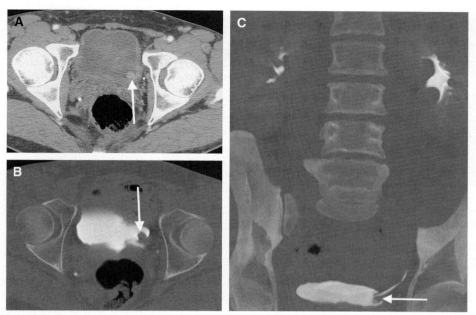

Fig. 7. 72-year-old man who has bladder cancer. *(A)* Early parenchymal phase CTU image demonstrates a bladder mass *(arrow)* with avid enhancement. *(B)* Excretory phase CTU image demonstrates the lesion as a papillary, nodular filling defect *(arrow)* in the opacified bladder adjacent to the left ureterovesicular junction (UVJ). *(C)* Coronal thin MIP image from excretory phase CTU images demonstrates the mass as a filling defect *(arrow)* adjacent to the left UVJ.

number of patients without a delay between TURBT and CT. [57] According Kim and colleagues, overall accuracy of 83% was achieved by CT for diagnosis of perivesical invasion [59].

For lymph node evaluation, the accuracy of CT ranges from 73% to 92%, with a tendency to understage nodal involvement, particularly when based on criteria for short axis nodal enlargement of near 1 cm [39]. Currently, diagnosis of nodal metastases with CTU is based on anatomic size criteria; CTU has limited ability to detect normal-sized lymph nodes that harbor low-volume metastatic disease, or to differentiate lymph nodes enlarged by a benign process from those enlarged by metastatic involvement [60,61]. Even subcentimeter perivesical nodes, particularly those that are rounded and avidly enhancing, may be noteworthy in patients with underlying bladder tumor, although they may be reactive. Discovery and investigation of functional biologic targeted imaging markers likely will be a focus of future translational research to improve sensitivity and specificity in the staging of genitourinary tumors [62].

Distant metastasis tends to occur late in the clinical course of bladder cancer and especially at the time of recurrence, with bones, lungs, brain, and liver being the most common sites [12]. Both conventional abdominal/pelvic CT and CTU, which

may be combined with chest CT if needed, can be performed to detect distant metastases (Figs. 9 and 10). CT also may suggest adjacent visceral invasion, although MR is superior because of better soft tissue contrast.

One important consideration in performing CTU is radiation exposure, which is increased because of multiphase, thin-section imaging. One recent study calculated the radiation risk for standard three-phase CTU without adjustment of tube

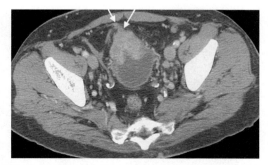

Fig. 8. 67-year-old man who has metastatic bladder cancer. Contrast-enhanced CT image demonstrates a large enhancing mass in the anterior bladder wall *(long arrow)*. The mass has grown through the bladder wall with anterior perivesical soft tissue *(short arrow)* indicative of perivesical invasion.

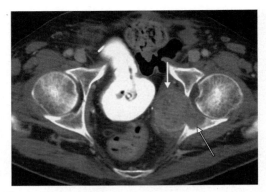

Fig. 9. 65-year-old man who has remote cystectomy for bladder cancer. Axial contrast-enhanced CT image demonstrates a lytic metastatic lesion in the left acetabulum with large soft tissue component and invasion into the adjacent internal obturator muscle *(arrows)*.

current factors and exposure technique for patient size to be approximately 1.5 times that of conventional excretory urography using standard three-phase CTU imaging without routine adjustment of tube current factors and exposure technique for patient size [63]. Other studies have confirmed an approximate 50% to 80% radiation exposure increase with helical multiphasic CTU compared with conventional excretory urography [13]. This is an important consideration, particularly in young adult populations, given that overall cumulative lifetime exposure could be increased substantially in the setting of repeat surveillance examinations in a patient who has known underlying pathology. Adjustment of tube current (tube potential, tube current–time product), scan pitch or length, and basing technique factors on patient size have been advocated as techniques to reduce overall exposure [63].

MR imaging

MR imaging has many advantages over other modalities for detecting and staging bladder neoplasms because of its intrinsic high soft tissue contrast, direct multiplanar imaging capabilities, and the availability of a non-nephrotoxic, renally excreted contrast agent. Because of these advantages, MR imaging has the potential to become the modality of choice in staging all pelvic malignancies. Currently state-of-the-art MR imaging of bladder masses includes the following sequences:

- T1 weighted spin echo images of the entire pelvis, which are helpful in identifying extravesical infiltration, pelvic adenopathy and osseous lesions [10]
- T2 weighted fast spin echo images of the bladder with small field of view and high matrix for high-resolution images in at least two different planes, which can offer a submillimeter resolution and are useful in evaluating the tumor depth and detecting invasion of surrounding organs [10,64]
- Dynamic contrast-enhanced T1 weighted images for evaluating the enhancement pattern of a bladder lesion (Fig. 11)

For dynamic contrast-enhanced images, three-dimensional fast-spoiled gradient echo sequences with fat suppression may be performed before and after contrast administration during the arterial and later phases for evaluation of the presence and pattern of enhancement in a bladder mass, and perivesical soft tissue enhancement. Multiplanar reconstruction may be performed if necessary to better delineate the spatial relationship of the bladder mass to adjacent anatomic structures. Both overdistention and underdistention of the bladder may affect diagnostic accuracy. Therefore, it has been

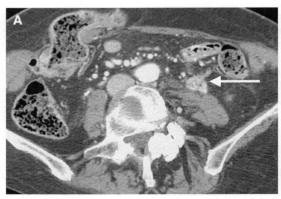
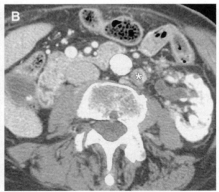

Fig. 10. 85-year-old woman who has metastatic bladder cancer. *(A)* Contrast-enhanced CT image of the abdomen shows an enhancing soft tissue nodule *(arrow)* anterior to the left psoas muscle consistent with metastatic disease. *(B)* Contrast-enhanced CT image of the abdomen shows metastatic retroperitoneal adenopathy (*).

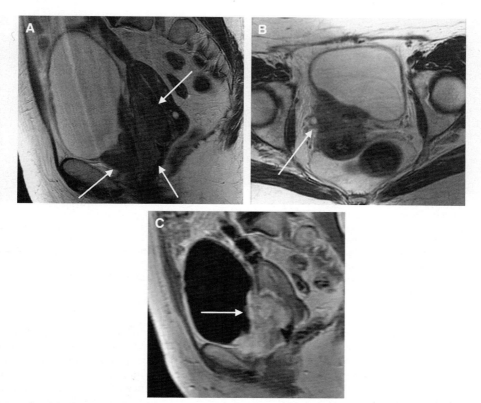

Fig. 11. 64-year-old woman who has bladder cancer. *(A)* Sagittal T2 weighted MR image (TR 5167 milliseconds, TE 107 milliseconds, field of view 20 cm, matrix 384 × 256) demonstrates a large bladder mass with invasion of the urethra, anterior uterine myometrium and vagina *(arrows)*. *(B)* Axial T2 weighted MR image (TR 4400 milliseconds, TE 108 milliseconds, field of view 20 cm, matrix 256 × 192) demonstrates the large bladder mass with gross extravesical invasion, uterine invasion, and obstruction to the right ureter *(arrow)*. *(C)* Sagittal contrast-enhanced T1 weighted MR image (TR 190 milliseconds, TE 4.2 milliseconds, field of view 28 cm, matrix 256 × 128) demonstrates avid enhancement within the large tumor *(arrow)*.

suggested by some that the patient void approximately 2 hours before the MR examination to achieve optimal bladder filling [65].

Although CT, especially CTU, is superior in the evaluation of upper tract disease because of its higher spatial resolution, MR performs equally well for detecting bladder tumors (sensitivity and positive predictive value >90%), and better in the staging of bladder tumors (accuracy of around 62% to 85% versus approximately 50% to 55%) [56,59,66–69]. Good interobserver agreement has been demonstrated in the staging of bladder cancer with MR imaging [56]. It appears that dynamic contrast-enhanced MR imaging yields higher accuracy than other imaging techniques in staging and tumor detection [59,69,70]. Both CT and MR are more accurate for staging more advanced disease [59].

For these reasons, MR imaging is considered by some to be the modality of choice for primary staging of urinary bladder cancer [61]. Bladder tumors may manifest various patterns of tumor growth including papillary, sessile, infiltrating, mixed, or flat intraepithelial growth [10,56] (Figs. 12 and 13). Most urothelial tumors are located at the bladder base (80% at initial diagnosis); they are multifocal in up to 30% to 40% of cases, and over half are less than 2.5 cm in size [10]. On T1 weighted images, the bladder tumor typically has a low-to-intermediate signal intensity that is similar to that of the bladder wall, higher than the dark urine and lower than the bright perivesical fat [56,70,71] (see Figs. 12 and 13). On T2 weighted images, the tumor tends to have intermediate signal intensity that is mildly brighter than the dark bladder wall muscle and lower than the high-signal urine [56,65,71] (see Figs. 12 and 13).

An intact, low-signal intensity muscle layer at the base of the tumor is indicative of nonmuscle invasive bladder tumor of stage Ta or T1 [56] (see Fig. 12). Current MR imaging cannot differentiate stage Ta from stage T1 tumors [56].

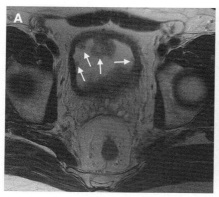 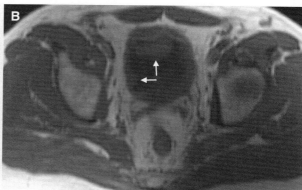

Fig. 12. 58-year-old man who has bladder cancer. *(A)* Axial T2 weighted image (TR 5000 milliseconds, TE 112 milliseconds, field of view 20 cm, matrix 448 × 256) demonstrates multifocal papillary lesions *(arrows)* projecting into the bladder lumen. The bladder lesions demonstrate slightly higher T2 signal compared with the bladder wall. Note that an intact, low-signal intensity muscle layer is present at the bases of the tumors. The patient was confirmed to have stage T1 bladder cancer on pathology. *(B)* On axial T1 weighted image (TR 550 milliseconds, TE 11 milliseconds, field of view 34 cm, matrix 256 × 128), the bladder tumors *(arrows)* demonstrate intermediate signal intensity similar to that of the bladder wall.

Muscle invasive tumor is suggested when the normal low signal of bladder wall muscle is interrupted by intermediate tumor signal [56,72] (see Fig. 13). In the evaluation of the depth of mural invasion, when proper technique is used, the accuracy of MR is reported to be as high as 96%, superior to that of CT; [64,73,74] however, the results reported in the literature are quite variable. One study reported that in about half of the patients, a three-layer architecture could be seen in the normal bladder wall on T2 weighted images, with the inner and outer dark layers corresponding to muscle layers, and the middle T2 bright layer corresponding to loose connective tissue [64]. This finding was helpful in the local staging of bladder tumor but was not present in all patients included in the latter study or in other studies.

Soft tissue extension into the perivesical fat can be seen on both T1 and T2 weighted images and is suggestive of stage 3 disease (see Fig. 13). The diagnosis of stage T3a (microscopic perivesical invasion) is difficult. A bladder wall lesion with an irregular, shaggy outer border and streaky areas of the same signal intensity as the tumor in perivesical fat are suggestive of stage T3b disease [56] (see Fig. 13). Overstaging, however, is a common error in local bladder cancer evaluation because of the frequent presence of postbiopsy inflammation, fibrosis, and granulation tissue mimicking perivesical invasion, especially soon after transurethral resection [59]. On dynamic contrast-enhanced images, tumor demonstrates earlier, and more avid enhancement than normal bladder wall and postbiopsy changes [10,56,70,75] (see Fig. 13). Therefore, gadolinium enhancement may have the

potential to determine the depth of tumor penetration into the bladder wall, differentiate perivesical tumor invasion from postbiopsy change, and better define invasion into adjacent organs [71]. The difference in enhancement pattern between bladder tumor and postbiopsy changes, however, can be quite subtle and may be detected only by fast dynamic first-pass MR imaging [61]. For example, Barentsz and colleagues found that bladder cancer started to enhance 6.5 seconds +/− 3.5 (standard deviation) after the beginning of arterial enhancement in the pelvis, which was only a few seconds earlier than most other structures (for example, postbiopsy tissue, 13.6 seconds +/− 4.2) [61]. Based on these findings, accuracy in differentiating postbiopsy tissue from malignancy improved from 79% to 90%, and specificity improved from 33% to 92%. Overall, tumor staging accuracy improved significantly from 67% to 84% (*P*<.01) [61].

As in the evaluation of other pelvic malignancies, MR is the modality of choice in assessing involvement of adjacent organs and structures, including the prostate in men, the uterus and vagina in women, and the pelvic sidewall or abdominal wall. Multiplanar T2 weighted and contrast-enhanced sequences provide the most informative images (see Fig. 11). In terms of bladder cancer involving the prostate, there are two different scenarios: direct extension through the bladder wall (contiguous involvement of the prostate), or noncontiguous simultaneous transitional cell carcinomas involving the prostate urethra and bladder [76,77]. The prognosis of the latter (46% to 55% 5-year survival rate) is significantly better than that of the former (7% to 21% 5-year survival

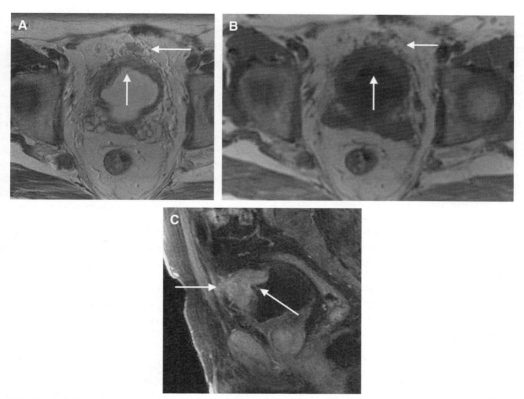

Fig. 13. 67-year-old man who has metastatic bladder cancer. *(A)* Axial T2 weighted image (TR 4567 milliseconds, TE 98 milliseconds, field of view 18 cm, matrix 256 × 224) demonstrates a large infiltrating tumor *(vertical arrow)* in the anterior bladder wall. The normal low signal of anterior bladder wall muscle is replaced by the intermediate tumor signal throughout its entire thickness, indicative of deep muscle invasion. The outer border is irregular and shaggy, with an ill-defined soft tissue nodule *(horizontal arrow)* in the prevesical fat, indicating perivesical invasion. *(B)* On axial T1 weighted image (TR 600 milliseconds, TE 14 milliseconds, field of view 32 cm, matrix 256 × 192), the bladder tumor *(vertical arrow)* demonstrates intermediate signal intensity similar to that of the bladder wall. Perivesical invasion also is seen on this T1 weighted image *(horizontal arrow)*. *(C)* Sagittal contrast-enhanced T1 weighted image with fat suppression (TR 3.9 milliseconds, TE 1.9 milliseconds, field of view 24cm, matrix 256 × 192) demonstrates early and avid enhancement in the anterior bladder mass *(oblique arrow)*. Also note the enhancing soft tissue in prevesical fat indicating perivesical tumor invasion *(horizontal arrow)*.

rate) [76,77]. In addition, among patients who have noncontiguous prostate involvement, outcomes differ between those with urethral mucosal involvement, ductal/acinar involvement, or stromal invasion [76]. Therefore, contiguous and noncontiguous involvement of the prostate carries distinct clinico–pathological features, and some investigators suggest that they should not be included in the same stage [76]. In the noncontiguous involvement of prostate by transitional cell carcinoma, prostate involvement also should be staged according to invasion degree [76]. Cross-sectional imaging, particularly MR imaging, is helpful in distinguishing these pathways and determining the degree of prostate invasion.

The incidence of lymph node metastasis is approximately 30% in cases of deep muscle invasion and 60% when extravesical invasion is present [12,78]. Lymphatic spread is initially to perivesical and presacral nodes, followed by the internal iliac, obturator, and external iliac nodes. Subsequent spread is by means of the common iliac and retroperitoneal nodes, and attention to these regions should be paid on imaging evaluation in any patient presenting with invasive disease [12].

The accuracy of MR imaging in staging nodal metastases based on anatomic size criteria ranges from 73% to 90% and is comparable to that of CT [61,65,74]. A commonly used criterion to diagnose pathologic adenopathy is a minimal axial diameter of 10 mm in oval-shaped nodes or 8 mm in round nodes [61]. Microscopic metastatic deposits in normal-sized nodes can be missed, however, when only size criteria are used for diagnosis [61], thus leading to false-negative diagnoses. Better results have been reported with intravenous administration of ferumoxtran-10, a type of ultrasmall iron particle that is taken up by macrophages and causes signal loss in normal, but not in metastatic lymph nodes on T2* weighted images [60]. Significant improvement in detection of metastatic nodal disease by MR (sensitivity, 96%; specificity, 95%; and negative predictive value, 98%) was achieved using this new contrast agent [60]. When nodal metastasis is suspected based on imaging, the patient may need to undergo imaging-guided biopsy of the suspicious lymph node for a definitive diagnosis [61]. This is because patients with nodal metastases have a poor prognosis and generally do not benefit from cystectomy. Those patients with invasive tumors with no nodal involvement have a 5-year survival rate of 28%, and those with nodal involvement have a 5-year survival of 11% [12,79]. Therefore positive biopsy results can prevent unnecessary invasive surgeries [80].

In patients who have bladder cancer, distant metastases are rare at the time of presentation; therefore specific imaging tests generally are not required unless there are pertinent clinical symptoms and signs [12]. Occasionally bone metastases occur in patients who have aggressive high-grade tumors at the time of presentation [12]. Investigations for distant metastases should be directed by clinical symptomatology [12].

Although MR imaging has certain advantages over CT, including suitability for patients with poor renal function and a lack of ionizing radiation, it also has numerous disadvantages in the evaluation of the urinary system. These include poor detection of calcifications and air, limiting its ability to evaluate patients with hematuria, and inferior spatial resolution compared with CT, limiting the ability to detect small, subtle lesions [13]. Because of these disadvantages, MR has played only a limited role in evaluating upper tract urothelial tumors. With the advent of newer, faster sequences allowing for higher imaging speed and better spatial resolution, however, the quality of MR urography (MRU) may be improved significantly. MRU can be performed in a static or a dynamic form; the former uses heavily T2 weighted sequences to delineate the fluid-filled collecting systems, while the latter uses T1 weighted sequences to image the excretion of gadolinium into the collecting systems. A diuretic often is needed for optimal opacification of the collecting system on T1 weighted excretory MRU. Transitional cell carcinoma of the upper tract is lower in signal than water on T2 weighted images and is nearly isointense to renal parenchyma on both T1 and T2 weighted images. In a pattern similar to the one they show on

CT, these lesions demonstrate moderate early enhancement after the administration of intravenous contrast material.

Intravenous urography

Many patients who have bladder cancer present with hematuria and traditionally would undergo excretory urography, which used to be the most common imaging test for the evaluation of hematuria. A bladder tumor may be recognized as a pedunculated, radiolucent filling defect projecting into the lumen or a focal irregularity of the bladder wall. In a study by Hillman and colleagues, only 60% of known bladder tumors could be detected on intravenous urography (IVU) [81]. Therefore CT, especially CTU, is being used increasingly for the workup for hematuria and suspected urothelial tumors. Cystoscopy and biopsy remain the standard of reference in confirming the diagnosis of bladder cancer. Once the diagnosis of bladder cancer is made, CT or MR is performed for staging and treatment planning, and routine IVU generally is not indicated [4,82].

Ultrasonography

Sonographic detection of bladder tumors depends on the size and location of the neoplasm [83]. Bladder tumors less than 0.5 cm in size and tumors located in the bladder neck or dome areas are difficult to detect [83]. On the other hand, diagnostic accuracy may approach 95% for tumors more than 0.5 cm in size situated on the posterior or lateral walls of the bladder [83]. Bladder cancer on ultrasound appears as an intraluminal nonmobile mass or focal area of bladder wall thickening (Fig. 14). Doppler flow should be used to establish flow within the mass, differentiating the mass from sludge and clot (Figs. 15 and 16). It is important to evaluate the bladder when it is fully distended [84]. The extent of invasion of the bladder wall and extravesicular extension cannot be assessed accurately by transabdominal ultrasound. Edema, intravesicular clot, and tumor calcification can cause overstaging of tumors [84]. A few earlier studies reported efficacy of transurethral ultrasonography in evaluation of bladder tumors [85,86].

Nuclear scintigraphy

Evaluation of bladder cancer by fluorine 18 fluorodeoxyglucose (FDG) positron emission tomography (PET) is limited by the renal excretion of the radioisotope into the collecting system and bladder. Currently, the role of PET or PET-CT is in the detection of metastases [87,88]. Preliminary work has been performed with tracers not excreted in the urine, such as 11C methionine [89] and 11C choline

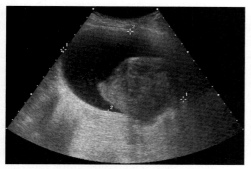

Fig. 14. 75-year-old man who has bladder cancer. Longitudinal ultrasound image of the bladder demonstrates a large intraluminal bladder mass. Biopsy of the mass revealed invasive high-grade urothelial carcinoma with sarcomatoid features, myxoid background, and extensive necrosis.

[90], which may be useful for detecting the primary bladder tumor.

Other diagnostic considerations

Bladder diverticula present with unique clinical problems. They have an increased risk of developing cancer because of urinary stasis (approximately 7% of bladder tumors occur within diverticula) [10,39]. As in conventional bladder cancers, urothelial cancer is the most common type, although all major epithelial types may involve bladder diverticula [10]. Tumors occurring in diverticula tend to invade perivesical fat early because of the lack of the muscularis mucosal layer in the diverticular wall, thus leading to a poorer prognosis [4,10,91] (Fig. 17). Moreover, the thinner wall makes accurate staging difficult. It has been suggested that in cases of diverticular tumor, stage T2 should be omitted, and that staging should progress from T1

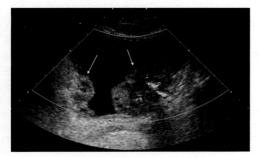

Fig. 15. 47-year-old man who has bladder cancer. Transverse ultrasound image of the bladder demonstrates bilateral intraluminal bladder masses *(arrows)*. Feeding blood vessels in the masses are documented by color Doppler. Radical cystectomy was performed, and urothelial carcinoma was found with perivesical invasion.

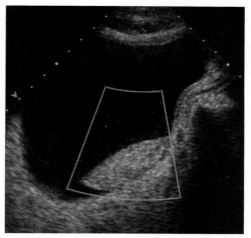

Fig. 16. 65-year-old man who has multiple myeloma presenting with hematuria. Oblique ultrasound image of the bladder demonstrated a well-defined echogenic mass in the dependent portion of the bladder. Doppler ultrasound did not detect any vascularity within this mass. This mass resolved in a few days with bladder irrigation, consistent with a blood clot.

(tumor is confined to the diverticulum) directly to T3 (extradiverticular disease is present) [92]. Management is similar to that of vesical tumor of the same stage, except that diverticulectomy may be performed in appropriate cases [4,91,92]. The thin diverticular wall also increases the risk of perforation during treatment, especially when complete resection of tumor is attempted by a transurethral approach [4].

In addition to the most common urothelial tumors, other benign or malignant tumors, and non-neoplastic lesions may be encountered in the bladder. Therefore, a differential diagnosis always should be considered when filling defects or irregularity in the bladder wall are detected. Possible causes include cystitis (Fig. 18), air, blood clot, calculi, bezoar, inflammatory masses, or an extrinsic or intrinsic bladder tumor. Air and calculi can be identified readily on CT. Intraluminal blood clots of the bladder tend to be dependent, with high precontrast attenuation, and without significant enhancement after administration of intravenous contrast. Post-treatment inflammatory masses such as Bacillus Calmette-Guerin (BCG) granulomas can result in diagnostic dilemmas and may require further evaluation with cystoscopy, biopsy, or radiographic follow-up (Fig. 19).

Intrinsic bladder tumors include mucosal and mesenchymal tumors. Extrinsic tumors from the prostate and uterus can involve the bladder wall and result in diagnostic difficulties. The relatively

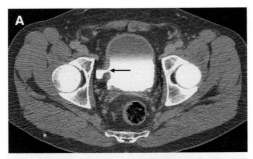

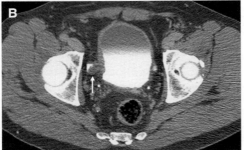

Fig. 17. 68-year-old man who has TCC arising from bladder diverticulum with perivesical invasion. *(A)* Excretory phase CTU image demonstrates a right bladder diverticulum *(arrow)*. *(B)* More superior portion of the bladder diverticulum demonstrates a filling defect indicative of a soft tissue mass *(arrow)*. This was confirmed to be TCC with perivesical invasion on surgical pathology. Mild asymmetric thickening of the right bladder wall also was noted, proven to represent postbiopsy reactive changes on pathology.

more common bladder malignancies other than urothelial carcinoma include squamous cell carcinoma, adenocarcinoma, small cell carcinoma, and lymphoma.

In areas of the world where schistosomiasis is endemic, squamous cell carcinoma is a major health problem, accounting for up to 50% of bladder cancers [93]. In the United States, squamous cell carcinoma accounts for less than 5% of bladder neoplasms. It is predominately nonbilharzial and generally is associated with a poor prognosis because of advanced disease stage at presentation [5]. Risk factors in nonbilharzial regions include indwelling catheters, bladder calculi, diverticula, or chronic infection. Other possible risk factors include cyclophosphamide, smoking, and intravesical BCG [5,94]. On imaging, squamous carcinoma may appear as a single enhancing mass or as diffuse or focal wall thickening [95]. It tends to be sessile, and may be associated with small calcifications, particularly in the setting of chronic inflammation [96,97]. Most manifest as large solitary masses, and more than 80% demonstrate muscle wall invasion. Metastases are identified in at least 10% at the time of diagnosis [98].

Adenocarcinoma of the bladder can be primary (two thirds are nonurachal and one third urachal) or secondary (metastases) in origin. Adenocarcinoma is associated with bladder exstrophy and a persistent urachus. The urachal tumors characteristically are located at the dome of the bladder (Fig. 20). These tumors are typically large and have a prominent extravesicular component with calcification [99]. They may have mucinous components that do not enhance. Metastatic adenocarcinoma is more common than primary adenocarcinoma, most commonly from the colon, prostate, rectum, stomach, breast, or lung. Metastatic adenocarcinoma usually occurs at a late phase [100].

Small cell bladder cancer is an uncommon bladder tumor with poor long-term survival [101]. Tumors are typically large and polypoid or nodular and may have an ulcerated surface [102]. They have been reported to exhibit patchy tumor enhancement, very rapid growth, and extensive local invasion [103].

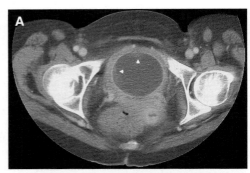

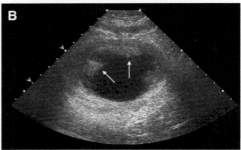

Fig. 18. 20-year-old woman who has Hodgkin's and non-Hodgkin's lymphoma status after bone marrow transplant, presenting with gross hematuria. Hemorrhagic cystitis was diagnosed on cystoscopy. *(A)* Contrast-enhanced CT image of the pelvis demonstrated circumferentially thickened bladder wall with vague intraluminal areas of increased attenuation *(arrows)*. *(B)* Ultrasound image obtained 4 days after the CT demonstrated thickened bladder wall and intraluminal echogenic areas *(arrows)* consistent with blood clots, corresponding to the areas of increased attenuation on CT.

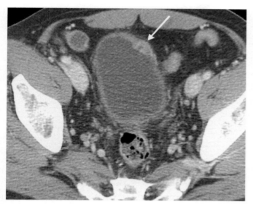

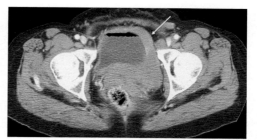

Fig. 21. 47-year-old woman who has lymphoma. Contrast-enhanced CT image of the abdomen demonstrated diffuse asymmetric left bladder wall thickening *(arrow)*. Note the presence of air in nondependent portion of the bladder from recent instrumentation.

Fig. 19. 64-year-old man's status after resection of stage T1 high-grade bladder TCC, presenting with chills, arthralgias, and myalgias after commencing second course of intravesical BCG treatment. *(A)* Contrast-enhanced CT image of the pelvis demonstrated focal nodular thickening with enhancement of the left anterior bladder wall *(arrow)*, which was new compared with prior examinations. After treatment with antituberculosis medications, this completely resolved. Subsequent biopsy showed only inflammatory cells.

Generally, nontransitional cell carcinomas of the bladder tend to be aggressive tumors that present as locally advanced disease at the time of initial diagnosis [56]. For these locally advanced cases, MR imaging facilitates accurate staging for treatment planning [56].

Lymphoma of the bladder may mimic urothelial carcinoma, but it is rare and secondary, as there is no lymphoid tissue in the bladder [97]. In the authors' experience, lymphoma may show somewhat diffuse, albeit sometimes asymmetric thickening and enhancement of the bladder wall, with a homogeneous appearance (Fig. 21).

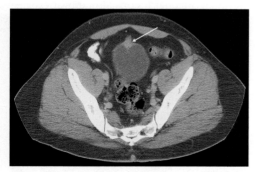

Fig. 20. 49-year-old man who has urachal adenocarcinoma. Axial contrast-enhanced CT demonstrated a 2 cm focal area of soft tissue thickening *(arrow)* at the bladder dome with extension into the adjacent perivesical fat. Patient underwent a partial cystectomy, excision of urachus, and umbilicus. Pathology revealed an urachal adenocarcinoma.

Because of the significant overlap in the clinical history and imaging findings of the various bladder tumors and other conditions that mimic bladder tumor, a definitive diagnosis generally requires biopsy [10] (**Figs. 22 and 23**).

Treatment planning

Nonmuscle invasive tumors (also referred to as superficial tumors) include noninvasive carcinomas (Ta), carcinoma in situ (Tis), and tumors invading the lamina propria (T1). The standard treatment for noninvasive bladder cancer is transurethral resection with fulguration, which can be repeated when necessary. Depending on the depth of invasion and histologic grade, intravesical medication such as BCG may be used to reduce the chances of recurrence or prevent progression to a higher grade or stage. Patients who have extensive multifocal recurrent disease or other unfavorable prognostic features may require more aggressive forms of definitive treatment such as radical cystectomy [104]. Imaging rarely changes clinical management in this group of patients.

For muscle-invasive bladder cancer, additional workup procedures including a CT or MR imaging examination of the abdomen and pelvis are needed for accurate staging. For stage T2 and T3 disease, and selected T4a disease without nodal metastasis, radical cystectomy is considered standard treatment. It involves removal of the bladder, perivesical tissues, prostate, and seminal vesicles in men and the uterus, fallopian tubes, ovaries, anterior vaginal wall, and urethra in women and may or may not be accompanied by pelvic lymph node dissection [105]. There is evidence that neoadjuvant therapy before cystectomy may improve survival of patients with muscle-invasive bladder cancer [106]. The prognosis is poor for patients with stage IV bladder carcinoma (defined by the presence of pelvic or

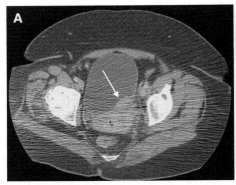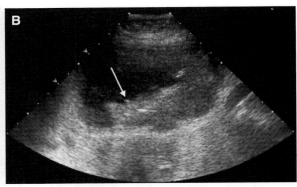

Fig. 22. 57-year-old woman with high-grade sarcomatoid carcinoma of the bladder. Contrast-enhanced CT image of the pelvis *(A)* and ultrasound image of the bladder *(B)* demonstrate a poorly defined large mass *(arrows)* involving the left lateral wall of the bladder with left hydronephrosis (not shown), and invading the vagina and lower uterine segment.

abdominal wall invasion, or nodal or distant metastasis). The potential for cure in stage IV disease is restricted to patients with involvement of pelvic organs by direct extension or small volume metastases to regional lymph nodes [107]. Radical cystectomy with or without preoperative irradiation or chemotherapy may be considered in these patients if no nodal disease is identified on imaging. If enlarged lymph nodes are documented by imaging, a biopsy may be needed for a definitive confirmation before chemotherapy or radiation therapy is initiated. Findings suspicious for distant metastases on imaging also typically need to be confirmed by biopsy. If confirmed, these patients generally are treated with systemic chemotherapy.

Post-treatment imaging

Imaging of bladder cancer after recent treatment is particularly challenging. Intravesical medication and transurethral resection or biopsy of the tumor often cause inflammation and edema, leading to avid mucosal and submucosal enhancement after administration of intravenous contrast [56] (Fig. 24). Using CT or MR imaging, it is difficult to discriminate between recent post-treatment changes and tumor recurrence by signal characteristics alone, but the presence of a mass with signal characteristics typical of tumor may indicate the presence of tumor recurrence [12]. Radiation and surgery also may cause prolonged nonspecific thickening of the bladder wall, and the rest of the urinary collecting system (see Fig. 5). These changes are difficult to distinguish from tumor based on imaging. Interval changes over time on imaging, such as increased thickening or development of mass-like lesions may be helpful for diagnosing recurrence or progression of disease.

CTU offers a comprehensive evaluation of the urinary system and has value in assessment for complications related to various treatments, from radiation therapy to intravesical therapy such as BCG administration and TURBT, to cystectomy and neobladder reconstruction. Cystitis, with resultant bladder wall thickening, may be seen after radiation therapy (see Fig. 20). After intravesical administration of BCG for treatment of superficial bladder cancer, some patients may develop a systemic reaction referred to as BCG granulomatosis, which may include fever and systemic symptoms, with masses involving urinary organs such as the kidneys, bladder, and prostate gland (Figs. 19, 25, and 26). The renal masses tend to be hypoattenuating on CT examination, with less avid enhancement, which may or may not appear heterogeneous [108,109] (see Fig. 25). Experience at the authors' institution in a limited number of patients has suggested that, similar to renal BCG granulomas, bladder lesions also appear expansile, and typically appear intramural in location. Bladder

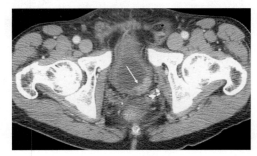

Fig. 23. 74-year-old man who has invasive neuroendocrine small cell carcinoma of the bladder. Contrast-enhanced CT of the pelvis demonstrates an enhancing 2 × 1 cm soft tissue mass *(arrow)* in the left posterolateral bladder wall.

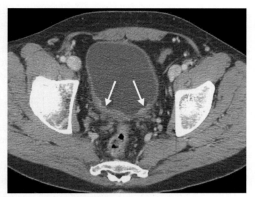

Fig. 24. 64-year-old man's status after recent transurethral resection of noninvasive bladder tumor. Contrast-enhanced CT image of the pelvis demonstrated posterior bladder wall thickening with superficial enhancement along the bladder mucosa *(arrows)*, and the presence of perivesical inflammatory change.

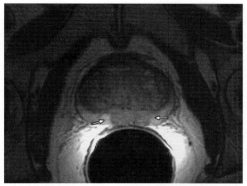

Fig. 26. 67-year-old man's status after intravesical BCG treatment of bladder cancer, presenting with elevated prostate-specific antigen and palpable prostate nodule on digital rectal examination. Axial T2 weighted endorectal MR image of the prostate (TR 5017 milliseconds, TE 100 milliseconds, field of view 14 cm, matrix 256 × 192) demonstrates a large nodule *(arrows)* at the base of the posterior peripheral zone with capsular bulging, corresponding to the nodule palpated on digital examination. Subsequent ultrasound-guided prostate biopsy confirmed granulomatous prostatitis.

wall lesions may show avid enhancement (see Fig. 19). BCG granulomas involving the prostate may mimic prostate cancer on both physical examination and blood biochemical tests (Fig. 26). These lesions may be difficult to differentiate from primary or metastatic urinary tumors. The awareness of this entity in the appropriate clinical setting is critical in making the diagnosis, and the patient should be treated medically with antimycobacterial therapy. Follow-up imaging to confirm response to therapy is important.

Perforation of the bladder wall is one of the most common complications associated with transurethral resection of cancer (incidence 5%) [110]. It is associated with increased postoperative hemorrhage and infection [110]. Recognition of this

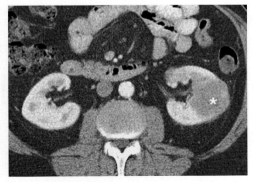

Fig. 25. 52-year-old man who has worsening fever, chills, and night sweats after intravesical BCG therapy for bladder cancer. (A) Contrast-enhanced CT image of the abdomen demonstrated a large hypoattenuating mass (*) in the midportion of the left kidney. After several weeks of antituberculosis therapy, the lesion significantly decreased in size (not shown), and the patient's constitutional symptoms resolved.

complication is important for timely initiation of proper treatment. Complications related with various surgical techniques, such as cystectomy with orthotopic neobladder reconstruction, diversions with continent reservoirs, or other diversions, are well evaluated by CTU. Common complications include postoperative urinary leak, stricture with obstruction, extrinsic compression of the diverted ureter, and development of abscesses [111].

It is challenging to find the appropriate method for long-term surveillance of bladder cancer. Because these patients have increased risk of cancer in the entire urothelial surface, they often require lifelong surveillance, which is essential to clinical management, as most recurrences are superficial and can be managed by endoscopic means. Cystoscopy with biopsy remains the gold standard for detecting bladder cancer recurrence, but it is invasive and expensive [10]. In addition, it cannot detect upper tract tumor. Urinary cytology is noninvasive and relatively inexpensive. It has been used routinely for tumor detection and long-term surveillance [10]. It has high specificity (>90%) but low sensitivity for low-grade tumors (<50%) [112]. Investigations are being performed to find new urinary markers to improve sensitivity while maintaining specificity in the detection of urinary tumors. Imaging is a routine part of surveillance in patients who have bladder cancer. The imaging modality of choice is CTU for the reasons discussed previously. With the advancement in MR technique and faster imaging acquisition, MR imaging of both bladder and the upper tract may be done in one comprehensive examination for patients in whom contrast-enhanced CT is contraindicated. Detailed discussion of MR imaging of the upper tract is beyond the scope of this article. Generally speaking, MR of the upper tract is hindered by its relatively-low spatial resolution compared with CT, much longer examination time, and the need for additional injections (diuretics, saline bolus, or both) to distend the collecting system.

MR imaging, however, is promising for predicting treatment response in patients with advanced bladder cancer early in the course of chemotherapy [113,114]. It has been shown that using changes in the time to the start of tumor or lymph node enhancement at fast dynamic contrast-enhanced MR imaging, the accuracy, sensitivity, and specificity in distinguishing responders from nonresponders were 95%, 93%, and 100%, respectively, significantly higher than the values achieved using conventional tumor size parameters with conventional MR imaging (73%, 79%, and 63%, respectively) [113].

The prognosis for any patient with progressive or recurrent invasive bladder cancer is generally poor, despite reports of relatively high rates of response, and occasional complete responses, to combination chemotherapy [115,116].

Summary

CT urography can be used as a one-stop-shop examination to evaluate the entire urinary system in the presence of hematuria, thus eliminating the need for additional imaging. It also serves as a great tool for staging and post-treatment follow-up in patients who have bladder cancer. MR imaging is an excellent tool for local staging of bladder cancer because of its intrinsic high soft tissue contrast, submillimeter spatial resolution, and direct multiplanar imaging capabilities. Differentiation of post-treatment changes in the bladder from tumor, however, still can be difficult.

References

[1] American Cancer Society. Cancer facts and figures. Atlanta (GA): American Cancer Society; 2006.

[2] Ries LAG, Eisner MP, Kosary CL, et al. SEER cancer statistics review, 1975–2002: based on a November 2004 SEER data submission. Posted to the SEER website 2005. Bethesda (MD): National Cancer Institute. Available at: http:// seer.cancer.gov/csr/1975_2002. Accessed November 10, 2006.

[3] Jemal A, Murray T, Ward E, et al. Cancer statistics, 2005. CA Cancer J Clin 2005;55(1):10–30.

[4] Kirkali Z, Chan T, Manoharan M, et al. Bladder cancer: epidemiology, staging and grading, and diagnosis. Urology 2005;66:4–34.

[5] Murphy WM, Grignon DJ, Perlman EJ. Tumors of the kidney, bladder, and related urinary structures. Washington, DC: American Registry of Pathology; 2004. p. 394.

[6] Mostofi FK, Davis CJ, Sesterhenn IA. Pathology of tumors of the urinary tract. In: Skinner DG, Lieskovsky G, editors. Diagnosis and management of genitourinary cancer. Philadelphia: WB Saunders; 1988. p. 83–117.

[7] Wilson TG, Pritchett TR, Lieskovsky G, et al. Primary adenocarcinoma of bladder. Urology 1991;38(3):223–6.

[8] Kakizoe T, Matsumoto K, Andoh M, et al. Adenocarcinoma of urachus. Report of 7 cases and review of literature. Urology 1983;21(4):360–6.

[9] Kantor AF, Hartge P, Hoover RN, et al. Urinary tract infection and risk of bladder cancer. Am J Epidemiol 1984;119(4):510–5.

[10] Wong-You-Cheong JJ, Woodward PJ, Manning MA, et al. From the Archives of the AFIP: neoplasms of the urinary bladder: radiologic-pathologic correlation. Radiographics 2006;26(2):553–80.

[11] Reuter VE. Pathology of bladder cancer: assessment of prognostic variables and response to therapy. Semin Oncol 1990;17(5):524–32.

[12] MacVicar AD. Bladder cancer staging. BJU Int 2000;86(Suppl 1):111–22.

[13] Browne RF, Meehan CP, Colville J, et al. Transitional cell carcinoma of the upper urinary tract: spectrum of imaging findings. Radiographics 2005;25(6):1609–27.

[14] Huguet-Perez J, Palou J, Millan-Rodriguez F, et al. Upper tract transitional cell carcinoma following cystectomy for bladder cancer. Eur Urol 2001;40(3):318–23.

[15] Millan-Rodriguez F, Chechile-Toniolo G, Salvador-Bayarri J, et al. Upper urinary tract tumors after primary superficial bladder tumors: prognostic factors and risk groups. J Urol 2000; 164(4):1183–7.

[16] Heney NM, Nocks BN, Daly JJ, et al. Ta and T1 bladder cancer: location, recurrence and progression. Br J Urol 1982;54(2):152–7.

[17] Vineis P, Simonato L. Proportion of lung and bladder cancers in males resulting from occupation: a systematic approach. Arch Environ Health 1991;46(1):6–15.

[18] Markowitz SB, Levin K. Continued epidemic of bladder cancer in workers exposed to ortho-toluidine in a chemical factory. J Occup Environ Med 2004;46(2):154–60.

[19] Popp W, Schmieding W, Speck M, et al. Incidence of bladder cancer in a cohort of workers exposed to 4-chloro-o-toluidine while synthesising chlordimeform. Br J Ind Med 1992; 49(8):529–31.

[20] Schulte PA, Ringen K, Hemstreet GP, et al. Risk assessment of a cohort exposed to aromatic

amines. Initial results. J Occup Med 1985; 27(2):115–21.

[21] Schulte PA, Ringen K, Hemstreet GP, et al. Risk factors for bladder cancer in a cohort exposed to aromatic amines. Cancer 1986;58(9):2156–62.

[22] Steenland K, Palu S. Cohort mortality study of 57,000 painters and other union members: a 15-year update. Occup Environ Med 1999; 56(5):315–21.

[23] Marrett LD, Hartge P, Meigs JW. Bladder cancer and occupational exposure to leather. Br J Ind Med 1986;43(2):96–100.

[24] Gaertner RR, Theriault GP. Risk of bladder cancer in foundry workers: a meta-analysis. Occup Environ Med 2002;59(10):655–63.

[25] Theriault G, Tremblay C, Cordier S, et al. Bladder cancer in the aluminum industry. Lancet 1984;1(8383):947–50.

[26] Boffetta P, Silverman DT. A meta-analysis of bladder cancer and diesel exhaust exposure. Epidemiology 2001;12(1):125–30.

[27] Bedwani R, Renganathan E, El Kwhsky F, et al. Schistosomiasis and the risk of bladder cancer in Alexandria, Egypt. Br J Cancer 1998;77(7): 1186–9.

[28] Kaldor JM, Day NE, Kittelmann B, et al. Bladder tumours following chemotherapy and radiotherapy for ovarian cancer: a case–control study. Int J Cancer 1995;63(1):1–6.

[29] Travis LB, Curtis RE, Glimelius B, et al. Bladder and kidney cancer following cyclophosphamide therapy for non-Hodgkin's lymphoma. J Natl Cancer Inst 1995;87(7):524–30.

[30] Kiemeney LA, Schoenberg M. Familial transitional cell carcinoma. J Urol 1996;156(3): 867–72.

[31] Kramer AA, Graham S, Burnett WS, et al. Familial aggregation of bladder cancer stratified by smoking status. Epidemiology 1991;2(2):145–8.

[32] Aben KK, Witjes JA, Schoenberg MP, et al. Familial aggregation of urothelial cell carcinoma. Int J Cancer 2002;98(2):274–8.

[33] Czene K, Lichtenstein P, Hemminki K. Environmental and heritable causes of cancer among 9.6 million individuals in the Swedish Family Cancer Database. Int J Cancer 2002;99(2): 260–6.

[34] Motzer RJ, Bander NH, Nanus DM. Renal cell carcinoma. N Engl J Med 1996;335(12): 865–75.

[35] Pashos CL, Botteman MF, Laskin BL, et al. Bladder cancer: epidemiology, diagnosis, and management. Cancer Pract 2002;10(6):311–22.

[36] Messing EM, Vaillancourt A. Hematuria screening for bladder cancer. J Occup Med 1990; 32(9):838–45.

[37] Sultana SR, Goodman CM, Byrne DJ, et al. Microscopic haematuria: urological investigation using a standard protocol. Br J Urol 1996; 78(5):691–6 [discussion 697–698].

[38] Grossfeld GD, Litwin MS, Wolf JS Jr, et al. Evaluation of asymptomatic microscopic hematuria in adults: the American Urological Association best practice policy—part II: patient evaluation, cytology, voided markers, imaging, cystoscopy, nephrology evaluation, and follow-up. Urology 2001;57(4):604–10.

[39] Hall TB, MacVicar AD. Imaging of bladder cancer. Imaging 2001;13(1):1–10.

[40] American Joint Committee on Cancer. AJCC cancer staging manual. 6th edition. New York: Springer; 2002.

[41] Reuter VE, Bladder. Risk and prognostic factors—a pathologist's perspective. Urol Clin North Am 1999;26(3):481–92.

[42] Kawamoto S, Horton KM, Fishman EK. Opacification of the collecting system and ureters on excretory-phase CT using oral water as contrast medium. AJR Am J Roentgenol 2006;186(1): 136–40.

[43] Caoili EM, Cohan RH, Inampudi P, et al. MDCT urography of upper tract urothelial neoplasms. AJR Am J Roentgenol 2005;184(6):1873–81.

[44] Kawashima A, Vrtiska TJ, LeRoy AJ, et al. CT urography. Radiographics 2004;24(Suppl 1): S35–54.

[45] Schreyer HH, Uggowitzer MM, Ruppert-Kohlmayr A. Helical CT of the urinary organs. Eur Radiol 2002;12(3):575–91.

[46] Lang EK, Thomas R, Davis R, et al. Multiphasic helical computerized tomography for the assessment of microscopic hematuria: a prospective study. J Urol 2004;171(1):237–43.

[47] Olcott EW, Nino-Murcia M, Rhee JS. Urinary bladder pseudolesions on contrast-enhanced helical CT: frequency and clinical implications. AJR Am J Roentgenol 1998;171(5):1349–54.

[48] Caoili EM, Cohan RH, Inampudi P, et al. MDCT urography of upper tract urothelial neoplasms. AJR Am J Roentgenol 2005;184(6):1873–81.

[49] Kim JK, Park SY, Kim HS, et al. Comparison of virtual cystoscopy, multiplanar reformation, and source CT images with contrast material-filled bladder for detecting lesions. AJR Am J Roentgenol 2005;185(3):689–96.

[50] Hall MC, Womack S, Sagalowsky AI, et al. Prognostic factors, recurrence, and survival in transitional cell carcinoma of the upper urinary tract: a 30-year experience in 252 patients. Urology 1998;52(4):594–601.

[51] Milestone B, Friedman AC, Seidmon EJ, et al. Staging of ureteral transitional cellcarcinoma by CT and MRI. Urology 1990;36(4):346–9.

[52] McTavish JD, Jinzaki M, Zou KH, et al. Multidetector row CT urography: comparison of strategies for depicting the normal urinary collecting system. Radiology 2002;225(3):783–90.

[53] Caoili EM, Inampudi P, Cohan RH, et al. Optimization of multidetector row CT urography: effect of compression, saline administration, and prolongation of acquisition delay. Radiology 2005;235(1):116–23.

[54] Sudakoff GS, Dunn DP, Hellman RS, et al. Opacification of the genitourinary collecting system

during MDCT urography with enhanced CT digital radiography: nonsaline versus saline bolus. AJR Am J Roentgenol 2006;186(1):122–9.

[55] Chow LC OE, Sommer FG. Multidetector row CT urography (CTU) with synchronous nephrographic and excretory phase enhancement [abstract]. AJR Am J Roentgenol 2003;180:71.

[56] Tekes A, Kamel I, Imam K, et al. Dynamic MRI of bladder cancer: evaluation of staging accuracy. AJR Am J Roentgenol 2005;184(1):121–7.

[57] Kim JK, Park SY, Ahn HJ, et al. Bladder cancer: analysis of multidetector row helical CT enhancement pattern and accuracy in tumor detection and perivesical staging. Radiology 2004;231(3):725–31.

[58] Caterino M, Giunta S, Finocchi V, et al. Primary cancer of the urinary bladder: CT evaluation of the T parameter with different techniques. Abdom Imaging 2001;26(4):433–8.

[59] Kim B, Semelka RC, Ascher SM, et al. Bladder tumor staging: comparison of contrast-enhanced CT, T1 and T2 weighted MR imaging, dynamic gadolinium-enhanced imaging, and late gadolinium-enhanced imaging. Radiology 1994;193(1):239–45.

[60] Deserno WM, Harisinghani MG, Taupitz M, et al. Urinary bladder cancer: preoperative nodal staging with ferumoxtran-10-enhanced MR imaging. Radiology 2004;233(2):449–56.

[61] Barentsz JO, Jager GJ, van Vierzen PB, et al. Staging urinary bladder cancer after transurethral biopsy: value of fast dynamic contrast-enhanced MR imaging. Radiology 1996;201(1):185–93.

[62] Hricak H. New horizons in genitourinary oncologic imaging. Abdom Imaging 2006;31(2):182–7.

[63] Nawfel RD, Judy PF, Schleipman AR, et al. Patient radiation dose at CT urography and conventional urography. Radiology 2004;232(1):126–32.

[64] Maeda H, Kinukawa T, Hattori R, et al. Detection of muscle layer invasion with submillimeter pixel MR images: staging of bladder carcinoma. Magn Reson Imaging 1995;13(1):9–19.

[65] Barentsz JO, Ruijs SH, Strijk SP. The role of MR imaging in carcinoma of the urinary bladder. AJR Am J Roentgenol 1993;160(5):937–47.

[66] Barentsz JO, Witjes JA, Ruijs JH. What is new in bladder cancer imaging. Urol Clin North Am 1997;24(3):583–602.

[67] Tachibana M, Baba S, Deguchi N, et al. Efficacy of gadolinium-diethylenetriaminepentaacetic acid-enhanced magnetic resonance imaging for differentiation between superficial and muscle-invasive tumor of the bladder: a comparative study with computerized tomography and transurethral ultrasonography. J Urol 1991;145(6):1169–73.

[68] Fisher MR, Hricak H, Tanagho EA. Urinary bladder MR imaging. Part II. Neoplasm. Radiology 1985;157(2):471–7.

[69] Tanimoto A, Yuasa Y, Imai Y, et al. Bladder tumor staging: comparison of conventional and gadolinium-enhanced dynamic MR imaging and CT. Radiology 1992;185(3):741–7.

[70] Neuerburg JM, Bohndorf K, Sohn M, et al. Staging of urinary bladder neoplasms with MR imaging: is Gd-DTPA helpful? J Comput Assist Tomogr 1991;15(5):780–6.

[71] Siegelman ES, Schnall MD. Contrast-enhanced MR imaging of the bladder and prostate. Magn Reson Imaging Clin N Am 1996;4(1):153–69.

[72] Rholl KS, Lee JK, Heiken JP, et al. Primary bladder carcinoma: evaluation with MR imaging. Radiology 1987;163(1):117–21.

[73] Buy JN, Moss AA, Guinet C, et al. MR staging of bladder carcinoma: correlation with pathologic findings. Radiology 1988;169(3):695–700.

[74] Tavares NJ, Demas BE, Hricak H. MR imaging of bladder neoplasms: correlation with pathologic staging. Urol Radiol 1990;12(1):27–33.

[75] Sohn M, Neuerburg J, Teufl F, et al. Gadolinium-enhanced magnetic resonance imaging in the staging of urinary bladder neoplasms. Urol Int 1990;45(3):142–7.

[76] Pagano F, Bassi P, Ferrante GL, et al. Is stage pT4a (D1) reliable in assessing transitional cell carcinoma involvement of the prostate in patients with a concurrent bladder cancer? A necessary distinction for contiguous or noncontiguous involvement. J Urol 1996;155(1):244–7.

[77] Esrig D, Freeman JA, Elmajian DA, et al. Transitional cell carcinoma involving the prostate with a proposed staging classification for stromal invasion. J Urol 1996;156(3):1071–6.

[78] van der Werf-Messing B, Schroeder RH, Bush H. Part II. Clinical practice: bladder. In: Halnan KE, editor. Treatment of cancer. London: Chapman & Hall; 1982. p. 457–74.

[79] Raghavan D, Shipley WU, Garnick MB, et al. Biology and management of bladder cancer. N Engl J Med 1990;322(16):1129–38.

[80] Barentsz JO, Jager GJ, Witjes JA. MR imaging of the urinary bladder. Magn Reson Imaging Clin N Am 2000;8(4):853–67.

[81] Hillman BJ, Silvert M, Cook G, et al. Recognition of bladder tumors by excretory urography. Radiology 1981;138(2):319–23.

[82] Sharir S. Update on clinical and radiological staging and surveillance of bladder cancer. Can J Urol 2006;13(Suppl 1):71–6.

[83] Itzchak Y, Singer D, Fischelovitch Y. Ultrasonographic assessment of bladder tumors. I. Tumor detection. J Urol 1981;126(1):31–3.

[84] Dershaw DD, Scher HI. Sonography in evaluation of carcinoma of bladder. Urology 1987;29:454–7.

[85] Akdas A, Turkeri L, Ersev D, et al. Transurethral ultrasonography, fiberoptic cystoscopy and bladder washout cytology in the evaluation of bladder tumours. International Urology and Nephrology 1992;24(5):503–8.

[86] Holm HH, Juul N, Torp-Pedersen S, et al. Bladder tumor staging by transurethral ultrasonic scanning. Eur Urol 1988;15(1–2):31–3.

[87] Jana S, Blaufox MD. Nuclear medicine studies of the prostate, testes, and bladder. Semin Nucl Med 2006;36(1):51–72.

[88] Schoder H, Larson SM. Positron emission tomography for prostate, bladder, and renal cancer. Semin Nucl Med 2004;34(4):274–92.

[89] Ahlstrom H, Malmstrom PU, Letocha H, et al. Positron emission tomography in the diagnosis and staging of urinary bladder cancer. Acta Radiol 1996;37(2):180–5.

[90] de Jong IJ, Pruim J, Elsinga PH, et al. Visualisation of bladder cancer using (11)C-choline PET: first clinical experience. Eur J Nucl Med Mol Imaging 2002;29(10):1283–8.

[91] Melekos MD, Asbach HW, Barbalias GA. Vesical diverticula: etiology, diagnosis, tumorigenesis, and treatment. Analysis of 74 cases. Urology 1987;30(5):453–7.

[92] Golijanin D, Yossepowitch O, Beck SD, et al. Carcinoma in a bladder diverticulum: presentation and treatment outcome. J Urol 2003; 170(5):1761–4.

[93] Shokeir AA. Squamous cell carcinoma of the bladder: pathology, diagnosis and treatment. BJU Int 2004;93(2):216–20.

[94] Stein JP, Skinner EC, Boyd SD, et al. Squamous cell carcinoma of the bladder associated with cyclophosphamide therapy for Wegener's granulomatosis: a report of 2 cases. J Urol 1993; 149(3):588–9.

[95] Wong JT, Wasserman NF, Padurean AM. Bladder squamous cell carcinoma. Radiographics 2004; 24(3):855–60.

[96] Narumi Y, Sato T, Hori S, et al. Squamous cell carcinoma of the uroepithelium: CT evaluation. Radiology 1989;173(3):853–6.

[97] Wong-You-Cheong JJ, Woodward PJ, Manning MA, et al. From the archives of the AFIP: neoplasms of the urinary bladder. Radiologic–pathologic correlation. Radiographics 2006;26(2):553–80.

[98] Tekes A, Kamel IR, Chan TY, et al. MR imaging features of non-transitional cell carcinoma of the urinary bladder with pathologic correlation. AJR Am J Roentgenol 2003;180(3): 779–84.

[99] Thali-Schwab CM, Woodward PJ, Wagner BJ. Computed tomographic appearance of urachal adenocarcinomas: review of 25 cases. Eur Radiol 2005;15(1):79–84.

[100] Bates AW, Baithun SI. Secondary neoplasms of the bladder are histological mimics of nontransitional cell primary tumours: clinico–pathological and histological features of 282 cases. Histopathology 2000;36(1):32–40.

[101] Cheng L, Pan CX, Yang XJ, et al. Small cell carcinoma of the urinary bladder: a clinico–pathologic analysis of 64 patients. Cancer 2004; 101(5):957–62.

[102] Sved P, Gomez P, Manoharan M, et al. Small cell carcinoma of the bladder. BJU Int 2004; 94(1):12–7.

[103] Kim JC, Kim KH, Jung S. Small cell carcinoma of the urinary bladder: CT and MR imaging findings. Korean J Radiol 2003;4(2):130–5.

[104] Amling CL, Thrasher JB, Frazier HA, et al. Radical cystectomy for stages Ta, Tis and T1 transitional cell carcinoma of the bladder. J Urol 1994;151(1):31–5 [discussion 35–6].

[105] Richie JP. Surgery for invasive bladder cancer. Hematol Oncol Clin North Am 1992;6(1): 129–45.

[106] Grossman HB, Natale RB, Tangen CM, et al. Neoadjuvant chemotherapy plus cystectomy compared with cystectomy alone for locally advanced bladder cancer. N Engl J Med 2003; 349(9):859–66.

[107] Vieweg J, Gschwend JE, Herr HW, et al. The impact of primary stage on survival in patients with lymph node positive bladder cancer. J Urol 1999;161(1):72–6.

[108] Soda T, Hori D, Onishi H, et al. Granulomatous nephritis as a complication of intrarenal Bacille Calmette-Guerin therapy. Urology 1999;53(6): 1228.

[109] Tavolini IM, Gardiman M, Benedetto G, et al. Unmanageable fever and granulomatous renal mass after intracavitary upper urinary tract Bacillus Calmette-Guerin therapy. J Urol 2002; 167(1):244–5.

[110] Dick A, Barnes R, Hadley H, et al. Complications of transurethral resection of bladder tumors: prevention, recognition and treatment. J Urol 1980;124(6):810–1.

[111] Sudakoff GS, Guralnick M, Langenstroer P, et al. CT urography of urinary diversions with enhanced CT digital radiography: preliminary experience. AJR Am J Roentgenol 2005;184(1): 131–8.

[112] Planz B, Synek C, Robben J, et al. Diagnostic accuracy of DNA image cytometry and urinary cytology with cells from voided urine in the detection of bladder cancer. Urology 2000; 56(5):782–6.

[113] Barentsz JO, Berger-Hartog O, Witjes JA, et al. Evaluation of chemotherapy in advanced urinary bladder cancer with fast dynamic contrast-enhanced MR imaging. Radiology 1998; 207(3):791–7.

[114] Barentsz JO, Engelbrecht M, Jager GJ, et al. Fast dynamic gadolinium-enhanced MR imaging of urinary bladder and prostate cancer. J Magn Reson Imaging 1999;10(3):295–304.

[115] Harker WG, Meyers FJ, Freiha FS, et al. Cisplatin, methotrexate, and vinblastine (CMV): an effective chemotherapy regimen for metastatic transitional cell carcinoma of the urinary tract. A Northern California Oncology Group study. J Clin Oncol 1985;3(11):1463–70.

[116] Sternberg CN, Yagoda A, Scher HI, et al. Methotrexate, vinblastine, doxorubicin, and cisplatin for advanced transitional cell carcinoma of the urothelium. Efficacy and patterns of response and relapse. Cancer 1989;64(12):2448–58.

RADIOLOGIC
CLINICS
OF NORTH AMERICA

Radiol Clin N Am 45 (2007) 207–222

ELSEVIER
SAUNDERS

Imaging of Prostate Cancer

Oguz Akin, MD[a,b,*], Hedvig Hricak, MD, PhD[a,b]

- Screening
- Diagnosis
- Tumor detection and staging
  Transrectal ultrasonography
  CT
  *MR imaging and MR spectroscopic
    imaging*
- Nuclear medicine studies
  *Capromab pendetide
    immunoscintigraphy*

  Radionuclide bone scintigraphy
  Positron emission tomography
- Treatment planning
- Post-treatment follow-up
  Follow-up after radical prostatectomy
  Follow-up after radiation therapy
- Summary
- Acknowledgments
- References

Prostate cancer is the most common cancer and one of the leading causes of cancer death in American men. The American Cancer Society estimates that in 2006, 234,460 new cases of prostate cancer will be diagnosed and 27,350 men will die from this disease in the United States [1]. The management of prostate cancer is challenging because the disease has variable clinical and pathologic behavior. The choice of treatment should be patient specific and risk adjusted, aimed at improving cancer control while reducing the risks of treatment-related complications. There is a growing demand for further individualization of treatment plans, which requires the accurate characterization of the location and extent of cancer. This characterization necessitates the optimal use of imaging methods that play an integral role in prostate cancer management.

Risk factors for developing prostate cancer are advanced age, ethnicity, and family history of the disease. More than 65% of all prostate cancers occur in men older than 65 years. African American men have the highest incidence of prostate cancer in the world. Familial predisposition is seen in 5% to 10% of prostate cancers. A diet high in saturated fat may also play a role.

Measurement of prostate-specific antigen (PSA) in blood and digital rectal examination (DRE) are offered for early detection of the disease for men at average risk beginning at age 50 years and for men at high risk beginning at age 45 years.

Treatment options for prostate cancer vary depending on age, disease stage, potential side effects of the treatment, and other medical conditions of the patient. Surgery, external beam radiation therapy, and brachytherapy can be used for treatment of early-stage prostate cancer. Hormonal therapy, chemotherapy, radiation therapy, or a combination of these can be used to treat metastatic disease or as supplemental therapies in early-stage disease. Watchful waiting without immediate treatment can be offered in some older patients who have limited life expectancy or less-aggressive tumors.

[a] Weill Medical College of Cornell University, New York, NY, USA
[b] Department of Radiology, Memorial Sloan-Kettering Cancer Center, 1275 York Avenue, New York, NY 10021, USA
* Corresponding author. Department of Radiology, Memorial Sloan-Kettering Cancer Center, 1275 York Avenue, New York, NY 10021.
E-mail address: akino@mskcc.org (O. Akin).

doi:10.1016/j.rcl.2006.10.008
radiologic.theclinics.com

Today, more than 90% of prostate cancers are diagnosed during early stages. Over the past 20 years, the 5-year survival rate for all stages increased from 67% to 100% [1]. This improvement in 5-year survival rate is mainly due to early diagnosis.

This article reviews the role of imaging in the diagnosis and management of prostate cancer. Transrectal ultrasonography (TRUS), which can be used to guide biopsy, is the most frequently used imaging technique in cancer detection. For determining the extent of disease, CT and MR imaging are the most commonly used modalities; bone scintigraphy and positron emission tomography (PET) have roles only in advanced disease. Currently, the role of imaging in prostate cancer is evolving to improve disease detection and staging, to determine the aggressiveness of disease, and to predict outcomes in different patient populations.

Screening

Prostate cancer screening is performed with DRE and measurement of serum PSA level. Since the advent of PSA screening, the incidence of prostate cancer has increased, but most prostate cancers are now diagnosed at an early stage.

There are certain limitations to PSA screening. PSA is not specific for prostate cancer and can be elevated in other conditions including benign prostatic hyperplasia, inflammation, trauma, and urinary retention. Although cancerous prostate tissue produces far more PSA in the serum than hyperplastic tissue, benign prostatic hyperplasia is the most common cause of elevated serum PSA concentration [2].

Patients who have abnormal DRE findings or elevated PSA levels are further evaluated with prostate biopsy. Establishing a threshold at which prostate biopsy should be performed in asymptomatic patients is very difficult. Using a cutoff value that is too low may cause unnecessary biopsies or detection of clinically insignificant cancers, whereas using a cutoff value that is too high may prevent detection of early-stage but aggressive tumors. A PSA level of 4.0 ng/mL is generally accepted as the lower limit for biopsy consideration [3].

Although PSA screening is a valuable tool in the early detection of prostate cancer, it is only one of the factors used to assess the likelihood that a patient has prostate cancer. Evaluation of other risk factors and DRE results may necessitate prostate biopsy in some patients who have normal PSA levels.

Diagnosis

Needle biopsy, which is often guided by TRUS, continues to be the "gold standard" for the diagnosis of prostate cancer. TRUS provides reasonably good-quality images of the prostate and adjacent structures and facilitates needle placement and tissue sampling.

The fact that prostate cancer is often a multifocal and heterogeneous disease makes diagnosis by biopsy difficult. Only a small amount of tissue is obtained with needle biopsy. Thus, sampling errors are common. Initial TRUS-guided biopsy detects prostate cancer in only 22% to 34% of the cases [4–6]. Thus, many patients require repeat biopsy. In patients who have initial negative results from TRUS-guided prostate biopsy, prostate cancer is detected in 10% to 19% on the second, in 5% to 14% on the third, and in 4% to 11% on the fourth repeat biopsy [4–6]. The traditional sextant biopsy schema, in which six parallel core samples are obtained, is now considered inadequate. Newer prostate biopsy strategies include higher numbers of biopsy samples from different regions of the prostate to improve cancer detection and risk assessment [7,8].

Tumor detection and staging

The TNM staging system is widely used to stage prostate cancer (Table 1) [9]. Although imaging techniques are sometimes useful in the detection of prostate cancer, their main use is in the staging of the disease. A combination of the currently available imaging modalities is usually necessary to help determine appropriate treatment strategies.

Transrectal ultrasonography

In addition to its role in biopsy guidance, TRUS is a commonly used imaging method for the detection and local staging of prostate cancer because of its widespread availability and ease of use.

TRUS provides good-quality images of the prostate gland because a high-frequency (5- to 7.5-MHz) probe can be placed in the rectum close to the prostate. Prostate cancer is most often seen as a hypoechoic area within the peripheral zone. Up to 40% of prostate cancers, however, are isoechoic, limiting their detection with TRUS [10,11]. The finding of a hypoechoic area within the peripheral zone is not specific for prostate carcinoma and can also be seen in benign processes such as prostatitis and focal atrophy [11]. Therefore, TRUS has a limited role in the detection of prostate cancer [12].

Capsular bulging and irregularity and the obliteration of the fat plane posterior to the prostate and of the rectoprostatic angle are findings suggestive of extracapsular extension on TRUS. In addition, seminal vesicle invasion by the tumor can be observed on TRUS. The accuracy of TRUS in the

Table 1: **TNM staging system for staging prostate cancer**

T – Primary tumor

TX	Primary tumor cannot be assessed
T0	No evidence of primary tumor
T1	Clinically inapparent tumor neither palpable nor visible by imaging
T1a	Tumor incidental histologic finding in 5% or less of tissue resected
T1b	Tumor incidental histologic finding in more than 5% of tissue resected
T1c	Tumor identified by needle biopsy (eg, because of elevated PSA)
T2	Tumor confined within prostate
T2a	Tumor involves one half of one lobe or less
T2b	Tumor involves more than one half of one lobe but not both lobes
T2c	Tumor involves both lobes
T3	Tumor extends through the prostate capsule
T3a	Extracapsular extension (unilateral or bilateral)
T3b	Tumor invades seminal vesicle(s)
T4	Tumor is fixed or invades adjacent structures other than seminal vesicles: bladder neck, external sphincter, rectum, levator muscles, and/or pelvic wall

N – Regional lymph nodes

NX	Regional lymph nodes were not assessed
N0	No regional lymph node metastasis
N1	Metastasis in regional lymph node(s)

M – Distant metastasis

MX	Distant metastasis cannot be assessed (not evaluated by any modality)
M0	No distant metastasis
M1	Distant metastasis
M1a	Nonregional lymph node(s)
M1b	Bone(s)
M1c	Other site(s) with or without bone disease

Adapted from Green FL, Page DL, Fleming ID, et al, editors. AJCC cancer staging manual. 6th edition. New York: Springer-Verlag; 2002.

prediction of extracapsular extension of prostate cancer varies widely, with sensitivities ranging from 50% to 92% and specificities ranging from 58% to 86% [13–15]. For the diagnosis of seminal vesicle invasion, reported sensitivities range from 22% to 60%, and the specificity is about 88% [14,16].

The major limitation of TRUS is its limited soft tissue resolution. Color Doppler and power Doppler, which can show vascular changes in tissues, can be added to improve the detection of prostate cancer on TRUS [17,18]. Even with these techniques, however, accuracy of TRUS in the local staging of prostate cancer remains limited. Contrast-enhanced TRUS is a new technique that is under investigation for the assessment of prostate cancer [19]. A study showed that contrast-enhanced TRUS improved the sensitivity of TRUS in tumor detection from 38% to 65%, with no significant change in its specificity, which was about 80% [20].

CT

CT for local staging of prostate cancer is of little value because even with contrast enhancement, CT lacks the soft tissue resolution necessary for the detection of prostate cancer within normal prostate.

When there is marked extracapsular extension, soft tissue extending into the periprostatic fat and adjacent structures can be diagnosed with CT (Fig. 1). Unilateral enlargement of a seminal vesicle by soft tissue–density tumor with obliteration of the fat plane between the seminal vesicle and prostatic base is suggestive of seminal vesicle invasion. With its accuracy of about 65% to 67%, however, CT is of limited clinical use for the local staging of prostate cancer [21,22]. CT may be helpful in the evaluation of patients who have advanced disease with adjacent organ invasion and distant lymphadenopathy [23], although patients presenting

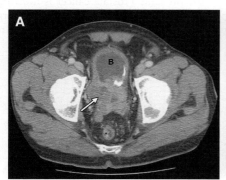
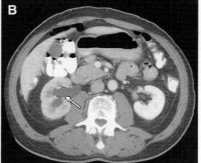

Fig. 1. Contrast-enhanced CT images of a 69-year-old man who had Gleason grade 4 + 5 prostate cancer. (*A*) Image shows a large prostatic mass (*arrow*) invading the bladder (B) and extending to the right pelvic wall. (*B*) Image shows hydronephrosis (*arrow*) in the right kidney due to obstruction of the right ureter by the mass.

with advanced disease are becoming less and less common.

Recently developed multidetector CT technology allows estimation of prostate perfusion and localization of prostate cancer. One report indicated that this technique was able to detect only localized, high-volume, poorly differentiated prostate cancers [24]. Further research is needed to define the role of multidetector CT in the evaluation of prostate cancer.

MR imaging and MR spectroscopic imaging

MR imaging and proton MR spectroscopic imaging are rapidly evolving as the most sensitive tools for the noninvasive, anatomic, and metabolic evaluation of prostate cancer [25,26]. Therefore, this article places special emphasis on these techniques.

MR imaging demonstrates the zonal anatomy of the prostate with excellent soft tissue resolution and allows assessment of local extent of disease. The addition of MR spectroscopy can improve prostate cancer detection and localization. Furthermore, MR spectroscopy provides metabolic information correlating with pathologic Gleason grade and thus may offer a noninvasive means to better predict prostate cancer aggressiveness [25,26].

A magnet strength of at least 1.5 T is required for high-quality MR imaging and MR spectroscopic imaging study of the prostate. The combined use of an endorectal coil with a pelvic phased-array coil markedly improves image quality. In general, T1-weighted axial images of the entire pelvis are obtained for the detection of nodal disease. Thinsection (3-mm) T2-weighted images with a small field of view (~14 cm) in the transverse, sagittal, and coronal planes are used for tumor detection, localization, and staging. The use of a dynamic

contrast-enhanced MR sequence is optional and may aid in tumor detection. Postbiopsy hemorrhage may cause under- or overestimation of the tumor presence and local extent. Therefore, MR imaging must be delayed for at least 4 to 8 weeks after prostate biopsy.

The MR spectroscopic imaging techniques that are commercially available include chemical shift imaging with point resolved spectroscopy (PRESS) voxel excitation and band selective inversion with gradient dephasing for water and lipid suppression. The PRESS technique generates a cubic or rectangular voxel by the acquisition of three orthogonal slice selective pulses (ie, a 90° pulse followed by two 180° pulses). Currently, three-dimensional proton MR spectroscopic mapping of the entire prostate is possible with a resolution of 0.24 mL or smaller, depending on the parameters used. The setup for spectroscopic imaging is the same as for morphologic imaging, and both datasets are usually acquired in the same examination to overlay metabolic information directly on the corresponding anatomic display (Fig. 2).

On MR imaging, prostate cancer is most easily seen on T2-weighted images as a focus of decreased signal intensity (Fig. 3). Low signal intensity can also be seen in several other conditions such as hemorrhage, prostatitis, atrophy, benign prostatic hyperplasia nodules, or sequelae resulting from radiation therapy or hormonal treatment.

MR spectroscopy provides metabolic information about prostatic tissue by displaying the relative concentrations of citrate, creatine, choline, and polyamines within contiguous voxels. Normal prostate tissue contains high levels of citrate—higher in the peripheral zone than in the central and transition zones. Glandular hyperplastic nodules,

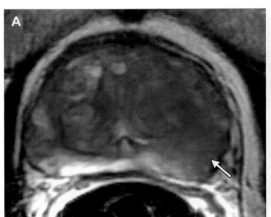
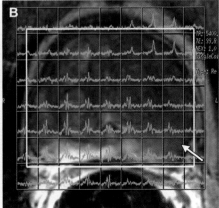

Fig. 2. Gleason grade 4 + 3 prostate cancer in a 65-year-old man. Transverse T2-weighted MR image (*A*) and corresponding MR spectroscopic data (*B*) superimposed on the anatomic image show the tumor (*arrow*) on the left side.

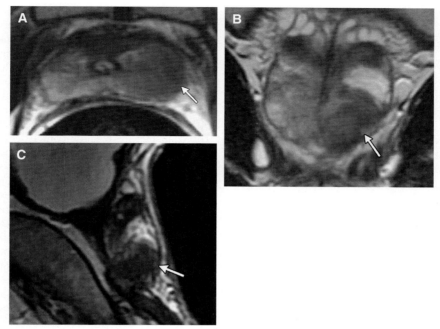

Fig. 3. Gleason grade 4 + 3 prostate cancer in a 66-year-old man. Transverse (*A*), coronal (*B*), and sagittal (*C*) T2-weighted MR images show a low–signal intensity focus consistent with tumor (*arrow*) in the peripheral zone of the prostate extending from left midgland to apex.

however, can demonstrate citrate levels as high as those observed in the peripheral zone. In the presence of prostate cancer, the citrate level is diminished or not detectable because of a conversion from citrate-producing to citrate-oxidating metabolism. The choline is elevated due to a high phospholipid cell membrane turnover in the proliferating malignant tissue. Therefore, voxels containing prostate cancer depict an increased choline-to-citrate ratio (Fig. 4). Because the creatine peak is very close to the choline peak in the spectral trace, the two may be inseparable; therefore, for practical purposes, the ratio of choline plus creatine to citrate ([Cho + Cr]/Cit) is used for the spectral analysis in the clinical setting. With the latest spectroscopic sequences, polyamine peaks can also be resolved. The polyamine peak decreases in the presence of prostate cancer.

The classification system described by Kurhanewicz and colleagues [27] is often used for spectral interpretation. A voxel is classified as normal, as suspicious for cancer, or as very suspicious for cancer. Furthermore, a voxel may contain nondiagnostic levels of metabolites or artifacts that obscure the metabolite frequency range. Voxels are considered suspicious for cancer when (Cho + Cr)/Cit is at least 2 SD above the average ratio for the normal peripheral zone, and voxels are considered very suspicious for cancer when (Cho + Cr)/Cit is more than

3 SD above the average ratio [28]. Voxels considered nondiagnostic contain no metabolites with signal-to-noise ratios greater than 5. In voxels in which only one metabolite is detectable, the other metabolites are assigned a value equivalent to the noise SD.

It has been shown that the (Cho + Cr)/Cit ratio in a lesion correlates with the Gleason grade [29]. Thus, a potential advantage of MR spectroscopy is that it may allow noninvasive assessment of prostate cancer aggressiveness.

One study found that in prostate cancer detection and tumor localization, MR imaging had 61% and 77% sensitivity, respectively, and 46% and 81% specificity, respectively, with moderate inter-reader agreement; MR spectroscopy had significantly higher specificity (75%, *P*<.05) but lower sensitivity (63%, *P*<.05). The investigators reported high specificity (91%) when combined MR imaging and MR spectroscopy indicated a positive result, and high sensitivity (95%) when either test alone did so [30]. A recent study comparing DRE, TRUS-guided biopsy, and MR imaging in the detection and localization of prostate cancer showed that MR imaging significantly increased the accuracy of prostate cancer localization compared with DRE or TRUS-guided biopsy (*P*<.0001 for each). The area under the receiver operating characteristic (ROC) curve for tumor localization was higher for MR imaging

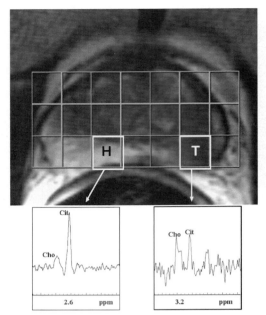

Fig. 4. Gleason grade 5 + 4 prostate cancer in a 59-year-old man. MR spectroscopy shows normal spectra in the healthy (H) right peripheral zone and suspicious spectra with elevated choline and reduced citrate in the left peripheral zone tumor (T).

than for DRE at the prostatic apex (0.72 versus 0.66), the midgland (0.80 versus 0.69), and the base (0.83 versus 0.69); it was also higher for MR imaging than for TRUS-biopsy at the midgland (0.75 versus 0.68) and the base (0.81 versus 0.61) but not the apex (0.67 versus 0.70) [31].

Most MR imaging studies focus on tumor detection in the peripheral zone of the prostate, where most cancers originate. The transition zone, however, harbors cancer in up to 25% of radical prostatectomy specimens [32]. A recent study showed that MR imaging can be used to assess transition zone prostate cancers. In detecting the location of transition zone cancer, the areas under the ROC curves of two readers were 0.75 and 0.73. Both readers' accuracy in detecting transition zone cancer foci increased significantly ($P = .001$) as tumor volume increased [33].

Dynamic contrast-enhanced MR imaging has been proposed as a means of achieving higher accuracy in prostate cancer localization and staging than can be obtained with conventional T2-weighted MR imaging [34]. It has been postulated that on dynamic contrast-enhanced imaging, increased microvascular density in prostate cancer results in different contrast enhancement than that seen in normal prostate. Numerous contrast enhancement parameters can be used to differentiate cancerous from benign tissue, including onset time, time to

peak enhancement, peak enhancement, relative peak enhancement, and washout time. A recent study suggested that the peak enhancement of cancer relative to that of surrounding benign tissue is the most accurate parameter for cancer localization [35]. Another suggested approach to cancer detection is the identification of areas of enhancement on early postcontrast images (within the first 30–60 seconds after contrast material injection) [36]. The challenge in dynamic contrast-enhanced MR imaging is to provide an optimal balance between temporal and spatial resolution. More studies are necessary to optimize the technology and define the clinical value of this technique.

As mentioned before, biopsy remains the gold standard for the diagnosis of prostate cancer. In patients who have elevated PSA levels or clinical findings suggestive of prostate cancer and negative TRUS-guided biopsy results, MR imaging and MR spectroscopy can be used to localize areas that may harbor prostate cancer and can help direct targeted biopsies and limit multiple repeat biopsies [37,38]. MR imaging-guided transrectal prostate biopsy is technically possible; however, the uses of and indications for MR imaging in prostate biopsy and other types of prostate interventions such as brachytherapy seed placement are under investigation [39–41].

MR imaging criteria for extracapsular extension include a contour deformity with a step-off or angulated margin, an irregular capsular bulge or retraction, a breach of the capsule with evidence of direct tumor extension, obliteration of the rectoprostatic angle, and asymmetry of the neurovascular bundles. MR imaging criteria for seminal vesicle invasion include contiguous low–signal intensity tumor extension from the base of the gland into the seminal vesicles, disruption or loss of the normal architecture of the seminal vesicle and decreased conspicuity of the seminal vesicle wall, tumor extension along the ejaculatory duct (nonvisualization of the ejaculatory duct), asymmetric decrease in the signal intensity of the seminal vesicles with mass effect, and obliteration of the angle between the prostate and the seminal vesicle on sagittal images. MR imaging is also helpful for diagnosing the invasion of adjacent organs (eg, the urinary bladder and rectum). Combined transverse, coronal, and sagittal planes of section facilitate evaluation of extracapsular extension, seminal vesicle invasion, and adjacent organ invasion [25,26] (**Figs. 5–8**).

The accuracy of MR imaging in the local staging of prostate cancer varies widely (from 50% to 92%) [34]. MR imaging has been reported to have 13% to 95% sensitivity and 49% to 97% specificity for the detection of extracapsular extension and 23% to 80% sensitivity and 81% to 99% specificity

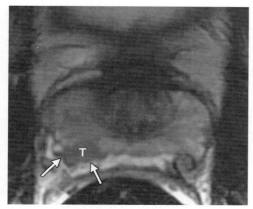

Fig. 5. Gleason grade 4 + 4 prostate cancer in a 54-year-old man. This tumor was clinically staged as T1c; however, a transverse T2-weighted MR image showed a small tumor (T) with gross extracapsular extension (*arrows*) and the tumor was staged as T3a, which was confirmed at pathologic examination after prostatectomy.

for the detection of seminal vesicle invasion [42–50]. A recent study showed that for two readers, the areas under the ROC curves were 0.93 and 0.81 for the detection of seminal vesicle invasion at MR imaging; the features that had the highest sensitivity and specificity were low signal intensity within the seminal vesicle and lack of preservation of seminal vesicle architecture. Tumor at the prostate base that extended beyond the capsule and low signal intensity within a seminal vesicle that had lost its normal architecture were highly predictive of seminal vesicle invasion [51].

MR spectroscopy may have a role in reducing the wide variation in the accuracy of MR imaging for local staging of prostate cancer, which may be attributed to the lack of standardized diagnostic criteria and interobserver variability in image interpretation. In a study on the detection of extracapsular extension by two independent readers, the addition of MR spectroscopy to MR imaging reduced interobserver variability and significantly improved accuracy for the less experienced reader, whose area under the ROC curve increased from 0.62 to 0.75 ($P<.05$); for the more experienced reader, the addition of MR spectroscopy also improved accuracy, but not significantly (the area under the ROC curve increased from 0.78 to 0.86) [52].

A study has shown that for the prediction of extracapsular extension, MR imaging findings contribute significant incremental value to clinical variables (areas under the ROC curves for detection of extracapsular extension with and without endorectal MR imaging findings were 0.838 and 0.772, respectively, $P = .022$) [53]. A related study that analyzed the same data demonstrated that the incremental value of MR imaging in predicting extracapsular extension was only significant when interpretation was performed by genitourinary

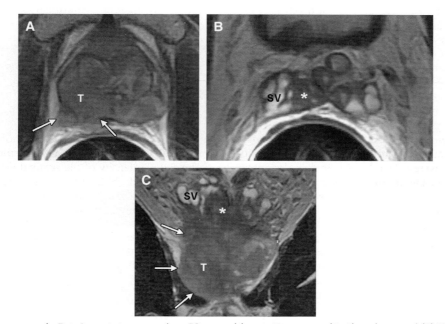

Fig. 6. Gleason grade 5 + 4 prostate cancer in a 58-year-old man. Transverse (*A, B*) and coronal (*C*) T2-weighted MR images show a large tumor (T) predominantly involving the right side of the prostate and seminal vesicles (SV). Note that disruption of the capsule and gross extracapsular extension of tumor (*arrows*) (*A, C*) and bilateral seminal vesicle (SV) invasion (*asterisk*) (*B, C*) are seen.

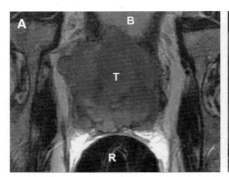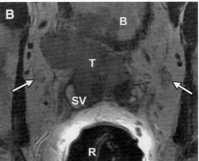

Fig. 7. Gleason grade 4 + 5 prostate cancer in a 69-year-old man. Transverse T2-weighted MR images (*A*, *B*) show a large tumor (T) that invades the urinary bladder (B) anteriorly and abuts the rectum (R) posteriorly. Bilateral obturator lymphadenopathy (*arrows*) and bilateral seminal vesicle (SV) invasion are also seen (*B*).

radiologists with experience in endorectal MR imaging [54]. In another study, MR imaging and combined MR imaging and MR spectroscopic imaging contributed significant incremental value ($P \leq .02$) to the staging nomograms in predicting organ-confined prostate cancer; the contribution of MR findings was significant in all risk groups but was greatest in the intermediate- and high-risk groups ($P<.01$ for both) [55].

For the assessment of lymph node metastases, MR imaging, like CT, has low sensitivity (0%–69%) [47,56–61]. The low sensitivity of MR imaging and CT is mainly due to the inability of cross-sectional imaging to detect metastases in normal-sized nodes. High-resolution MR imaging with lymphotropic superparamagnetic nanoparticles, however, is a promising technique in the detection of occult lymph node metastases because it allows detection of metastases in normal-sized lymph nodes. In one study, MR imaging with lymphotropic superparamagnetic nanoparticles had a significantly higher sensitivity than conventional MR imaging in the detection of metastasis on a node by node basis (90.5% versus 35.4%, $P<.001$); the new technique also had a sensitivity of 100% and a specificity of 95.7 in detecting nodal metastasis on a per patient basis [62].

Although these results are promising, the low incidence of lymph node metastasis in patients who have prostate cancer does not warrant the routine use of lymphotropic superparamagnetic nanoparticles. A recent study showed that incorporation of the Partin nomogram results and standard MR imaging findings regarding extracapsular extension and seminal vesicle invasion improves the prediction of lymph node metastasis on MR imaging in patients who have prostate cancer [63]. Only 22 (5%) of 411 patients in the study had lymph node metastases at surgical pathology, and MR imaging was an independent, statistically significant

predictor of lymph node metastasis ($P = .002$), with positive and negative predictive values of 50% and 96.36%, respectively. On multivariate analysis, prediction of lymph node status using a model that included all MR imaging variables (extracapsular extension, seminal vesicle invasion, and lymph node metastases) along with the Partin nomogram results had a significantly greater area under the ROC curve than the univariate model that included only MR imaging lymph node metastasis findings (areas under the ROC curves were 0.892 and 0.633, respectively, $P<.01$). The investigators suggested that because MR imaging offers high negative predictive value for lymph node metastasis in addition to anatomic information useful for

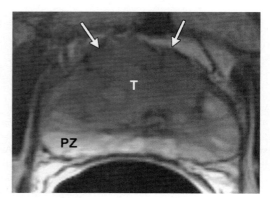

Fig. 8. Gleason grade 4 + 5 prostate cancer in the transition zone in a 68-year-old man. This anterior tumor involving the entire transition zone was clinically staged as T1c; however, a transverse T2-weighted MR image showed a large transition zone tumor (T) with gross anterior extraprostatic extension (*arrows*) and the tumor was staged as T3a, which was confirmed at pathologic examination after prostatectomy. Although the tumor was large, its anterior location far from the rectum made clinical evaluation difficult. PZ, peripheral zone.

treatment planning, MR imaging and the Partin no-mogram could be used together to determine whether imaging with lymphotropic superpara-magnetic nanoparticles is warranted.

Nuclear medicine studies

Capromab pendetide immunoscintigraphy

Capromab pendetide immunoscintigraphy is a mu-rine monoclonal antibody that reacts with prostate membrane–specific antigen, which is highly ex-pressed in prostate cancer. Immunoscintigraphy is accomplished by labeling the antibody with indium 111. After infusion of the antibody, whole-body pla-nar and single-photon emission CT images are ob-tained. Capromab pendetide immunoscintigraphy can be used for the detecting lymph node metasta-ses, the site of relapse in a patient who has a detect-able PSA after prostatectomy, and occult metastasis before primary therapy [64]. One study found that capromab pendetide immunoscintigraphy scan-ning had 67% to 94% sensitivity and 42% to 80% specificity for the detection of lymph node metasta-ses [65,66]. Another study on the use of capromab pendetide immunoscintigraphy scanning to evalu-ate patients who had recurrent prostate cancer showed that the technique had a sensitivity of 89%, a specificity of 67%, and an overall accuracy of 89% [67]. Coregistration of capromab pendetide immunoscintigraphy images with MR imaging or CT could improve the specificity of the examination [68]; however, there are many reasons for false-pos-itive uptake of this antibody, and the image quality is often suboptimal. In the era of PET, the imaging of prostate cancer with capromab pendetide immu-noscintigraphy should no longer be encouraged.

Radionuclide bone scintigraphy

Radionuclide bone scan is a sensitive imaging method used to detect bone metastases in patients who have prostate cancer (**Fig. 9**) [69]. Bone scans are commonly obtained even for patients in low- and intermediate-risk categories [70]; however, studies have shown that patients who have PSA levels of 20 ng/mL or less and a Gleason score lower than 8 have a 1% to 13% rate of positive bone scans [71,72]. Other studies have confirmed that in pa-tients who have low PSA levels (<10 ng/mL) and no skeletal symptoms, the yield of bone scanning is too low to warrant its routine use unless the pa-tient has stage T3 or T4 disease or a high Gleason score [73–75]. Therefore, a PSA level of greater than 15 to 20 ng/mL is usually used as the cutoff point for obtaining a bone scan, but patients who have skeletal symptoms and those who have a high Gleason score or advanced stage should also be assessed with bone scans.

Positron emission tomography

The role of PET is still under investigation in the staging workup of patients who have prostate can-cer (see **Fig. 9**) [76–80]. Fluorodeoxyglucose (FDG), the most commonly used PET tracer, was re-ported to be ineffective for the initial staging of prostate cancer because most primary prostate can-cer lesions were not detected by FDG-PET [81]. FDG-PET, however, could have a role in the detec-tion of local recurrence or distant metastases with increasing PSA after initial treatment failure [55,76,80,82].

Other radiotracers are being studied for their use in prostate cancer, including C 11 or F 18 choline and acetate, methionine C 11, fluorine 18, fluorodi-hydrotestosterone, and gallium 68–labeled pep-tides [77,79,80,83–86]. These agents, however, are not widely available and their use remains experimental.

Treatment planning

The therapeutic options for patients who have pros-tate cancer vary widely and include watchful wait-ing, androgen ablation (chemical or surgical castration), hormone therapy, radical surgery, and various forms of radiation therapy (brachytherapy, external beam irradiation). The choice of optimal treatment strategy in patients who have prostate cancer is patient specific and risk adjusted. The ther-apeutic goal is to maximize cancer control while minimizing the risks of complications. The optimal treatment option for prostate cancer is chosen based on clinical TNM stage, Gleason grade, and the level of PSA. Other factors such as patient age, associated medical illnesses, and the patient's per-sonal preferences also have an effect on the treat-ment planning process. The findings from imaging studies assist in this patient-specific treat-ment planning approach. Imaging may also have a role in the guidance and assessment of emerging local prostate cancer therapies.

Post-treatment follow-up

After treatment, patients who have prostate cancer are followed with periodic measurement of PSA levels and DRE. Imaging is necessary after treatment for clinically localized prostate cancer only if there are suspicious findings on DRE, PSA is elevated, or the patient has symptoms such as bone pain.

Follow-up after radical prostatectomy

Radical prostatectomy includes resection of the prostate, the seminal vesicles, and the pelvic lymph nodes. After radical prostatectomy, PSA decreases to undetectable levels (<0.1 ng/mL) within a few

A

B

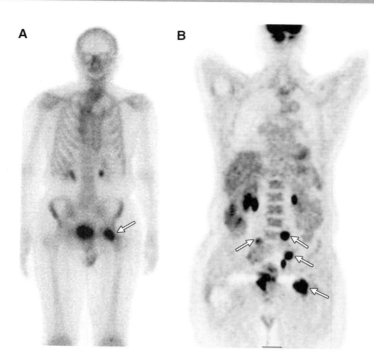

Fig. 9. Gleason grade 5 + 4 prostate cancer in a 76-year-old man. Bone scan (*A*) and PET (*B*) show a metastatic focus in the left femur (*large arrows*). Metastatic lymph nodes (*small arrows*) are also seen on PET (*B*).

weeks of surgery and should remain undetectable thereafter [87,88]. Detectable levels of PSA in patients who have undergone radical prostatectomy indicate that there is residual prostate tissue because PSA is specific to the prostate. A rise in a previously undetectable or stable PSA level after surgery is suggestive of residual, recurrent, or metastatic disease. In these cases, the role of imaging is to help distinguish locally recurrent disease (which can be managed with local therapy) from distant metastatic disease (which requires systemic therapy). The type of recurrence is difficult to determine clinically because an increasing PSA level is rarely associated with symptoms or findings at physical examination.

Radionuclide bone scintigraphy

Radionuclide bone scan is often the first examination obtained. If the bone scan is negative or inconclusive, then further imaging studies are performed. The probability of a positive bone scan in patients who have biochemical failure following radical prostatectomy is very low until PSA levels increase above 30 to 40 ng/mL [89]. Therefore, bone scans are recommended only when the patient has symptoms of bone pain, a rapid rise in PSA, or markedly elevated PSA [90].

Transrectal ultrasonography

TRUS is the most commonly used imaging modality in the detection of local recurrence following prostatectomy. TRUS is also used for biopsy

guidance of the vesicourethral anastomosis and prostatic fossa to document local recurrence. A negative result on TRUS-guided biopsy, however, does not definitely rule out recurrent disease due to possible sampling errors. Only about 25% of men who have prostatectomy and PSA levels lower than 1 ng/mL have positive biopsy results [91]. The yield for detection of locally recurrent tumor with TRUS-guided biopsy, however, rises significantly with increasing PSA levels [91,92].

CT

CT is not effective for detecting early recurrent tumor in the surgical bed. A study showed that CT detected only 36% of recurrences, and all of these were larger than 2 cm [93]. CT can be useful in the evaluation of nodal recurrence (Fig. 10); however, CT relies only on size criteria for the detection of positive lymph nodes. CT can also be useful in detecting bone and visceral metastases, although bone scan and MR imaging are superior in the diagnosis and follow-up of bone metastases [94].

MR imaging

Due to its excellent soft tissue resolution, MR imaging is superior to TRUS and CT in the detection of clinically evident locally recurrent disease after radical prostatectomy (Fig. 11). Two studies reported that MR imaging had 95% to 100% sensitivity and 100% specificity for detecting local recurrence

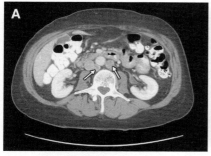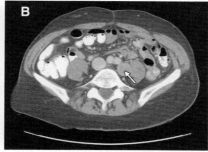

Fig. 10. Recurrent prostate cancer in a 76-year-old man. (*A, B*) Transverse contrast-enhanced CT images show distal para-aortic and left common iliac lymphadenopathy (*arrows*).

[95,96]. In one of these studies, local recurrences seen on MR imaging were perianastomotic in 29% of patients and retrovesical in 40%, within retained seminal vesicles in 22%, and at anterior or lateral surgical margins in 9%; the mean diameter of tumors was 1.4 cm (range, 0.8–4.5 cm), and PSA levels ranged from undetectable to 10 ng/mL (mean, 2.18 ng/mL) [95].

MR imaging can also be used in the detection of nodal disease; however, the accuracy of MR imaging for staging pelvic lymph nodes by size criteria is similar to that of CT.

MR imaging is more sensitive and specific in the diagnosis of bone metastases compared with bone scan; however, it is more feasible to use bone scan to cover the entire skeleton. In addition, bone scan is more cost-effective than MR imaging. Therefore, MR imaging should be used when other imaging modality findings are indeterminate.

Positron emission tomography

The role of PET in detecting recurrence, assessing prognosis, monitoring therapy, and studying the biology of prostate cancer is still under investigation.

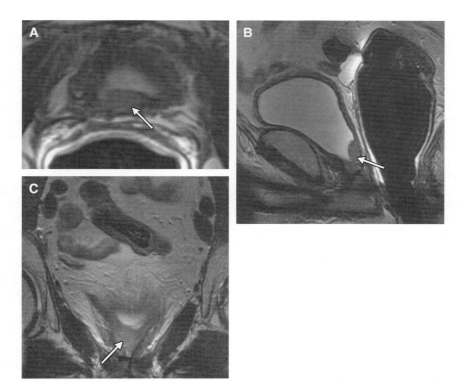

Fig. 11. Recurrent prostate cancer after radical prostatectomy in a 76-year-old man. Transverse (*A*), sagittal (*B*), and coronal (*C*) T2-weighted MR images demonstrate nodular intermediate–signal intensity tumor (*arrows*) consistent with local recurrence in the bladder neck.

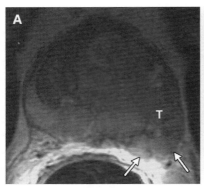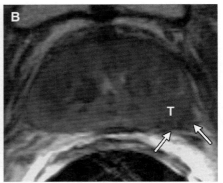

Fig. 12. Gleason grade 4 + 5 prostate cancer in a 66-year-old man. Transverse T2-weighted MR image (*A*) shows a large tumor (T) with gross extracapsular extension (*arrows*). After radiation treatment, transverse T2-weighted image (*B*) shows that the tumor (T) and extracapsular extension markedly decreased (*arrows*). Note that the rest of the prostate demonstrates diffuse low signal intensity consistent with radiation changes (*B*).

FDG-PET could have a role in the detection of local recurrence or distant metastases with increasing PSA after initial treatment failure [76,80,82]. A study showed that FDG-PET detected local or systemic disease in 31% of 91 patients who had PSA relapse following prostatectomy. In this study, the probability for disease detection increased with PSA level [82].

Follow-up after radiation therapy

Following radiation therapy, the PSA level decreases in most patients during the first year. Recurrence following radiation therapy is defined as three consecutive rises in PSA after a postradiation PSA nadir [97]. Detection of local recurrence after failed radiation therapy is a clinical challenge because an increase in the PSA level is not a reliable variable for differentiating local from distant recurrence. After radiation therapy, the prostate becomes atrophic and fibrotic, making detection of local recurrent disease within the irradiated prostate difficult by DRE. If bone scan is positive, then further imaging is not necessary. If the bone scan is negative, then TRUS-directed biopsy of the prostate can be performed. Lymph nodes can be evaluated by CT or by MR imaging.

It is commonly believed that assessment of location and extent of prostate cancer on MR imaging is hindered by tissue changes related to radiation therapy (Fig. 12). A recent study showed, however, that MR imaging and MR spectroscopy could be more sensitive than sextant biopsy and DRE for sextant localization of cancer recurrence after external beam radiation therapy [98]. In this study, MR imaging and MR spectroscopy had sensitivities of 68% and 77%, respectively, whereas the sensitivities of biopsy and DRE were 48% and 16%, respectively. MR spectroscopy appears to be less specific (78%) than the other three tests, which each had a specificity higher than 90%. Another recent study also showed that in patients who underwent salvage prostatectomy after failed radiation therapy, MR imaging could help identify tumor sites and depict local extent of disease. In this study, areas under the ROC curves for two readers were 0.61 and 0.75 for tumor detection, 0.76 and 0.87 for prediction of extracapsular extension, and 0.70 and 0.76 for prediction of seminal vesicle invasion [99].

Summary

Imaging modalities are rapidly evolving to provide improved evaluation of prostate cancer. Our understanding of imaging criteria and experience in image interpretation are also growing. In addition to the traditional roles of imaging in prostate cancer (ie, localization and staging), extensive research is being done on metabolic imaging to predict cancer aggressiveness. Future directions in prostate cancer imaging include more precise patient stratification for different management options and new methods for guidance and assessment of emerging local prostate cancer therapies.

Acknowledgments

The authors thank Ada Muellner, BA, for her assistance in editing the manuscript.

References

[1] American Cancer Society. Cancer facts & figures 2006. Atlanta (GA): American Cancer Society; 2006. Publication 500806.

[2] Gretzer MB, Partin AW. PSA markers in prostate cancer detection. Urol Clin North Am 2003;30: 677–86.

[3] Catalona WJ, Richie JP, Ahmann FR, et al. Comparison of digital rectal examination and serum prostate specific antigen in the early detection of prostate cancer: results of a multicenter clinical trial of 6,630 men. J Urol 1994; 151:1283–90.

[4] Djavan B, Ravery V, Zlotta A, et al. Prospective evaluation of prostate cancer detected on biopsies 1, 2, 3 and 4: when should we stop? J Urol 2001;166:1679–83.

[5] Keetch DW, Catalona WJ, Smith DS. Serial prostatic biopsies in men with persistently elevated serum prostate specific antigen values. J Urol 1994;151:1571–4.

[6] Roehl KA, Antenor JA, Catalona WJ. Serial biopsy results in prostate cancer screening study. J Urol 2002;167:2435–9.

[7] Djavan B, Remzi M, Marberger M. When to biopsy and when to stop biopsying. Urol Clin North Am 2003;30:253–62.

[8] Macchia RJ. Biopsy of the prostate—an ongoing evolution. J Urol 2004;171:1487–8.

[9] Green FL, Page DL, Fleming ID, et al, editors. AJCC cancer staging manual. 6th edition. New York: Springer-Verlag; 2002.

[10] Shinohara K, Wheeler TM, Scardino PT. The appearance of prostate cancer on transrectal ultrasonography: correlation of imaging and pathological examinations. J Urol 1989;142:76–82.

[11] Shinohara K, Scardino PT, Carter SS, et al. Pathologic basis of the sonographic appearance of the normal and malignant prostate. Urol Clin North Am 1989;16:675–91.

[12] Gustafsson O, Carlsson P, Norming U, et al. Cost-effectiveness analysis in early detection of prostate cancer: an evaluation of six screening strategies in a randomly selected population of 2,400 men. Prostate 1995;26:299–309.

[13] Lorentzen T, Nerstrom H, Iversen P, et al. Local staging of prostate cancer with transrectal ultrasound: a literature review. Prostate Suppl 1992; 4:11–6.

[14] Rifkin MD, Zerhouni EA, Gatsonis CA, et al. Comparison of magnetic resonance imaging and ultrasonography in staging early prostate cancer. Results of a multi-institutional cooperative trial. N Engl J Med 1990;323:621–6.

[15] Smith JA Jr, Scardino PT, Resnick MI, et al. Transrectal ultrasound versus digital rectal examination for the staging of carcinoma of the prostate: results of a prospective, multi-institutional trial. J Urol 1997;157:902–6.

[16] Hardeman SW, Causey JQ, Hickey DP, et al. Transrectal ultrasound for staging prior to radical prostatectomy. Urology 1989;34:175–80.

[17] Cornud F, Hamida K, Flam T, et al. Endorectal color Doppler sonography and endorectal MR imaging features of nonpalpable prostate cancer: correlation with radical prostatectomy findings. AJR Am J Roentgenol 2000;175:1161–8.

[18] Sedelaar JP, van Leenders GJ, Goossen TE, et al. Value of contrast ultrasonography in the detection of significant prostate cancer: correlation with radical prostatectomy specimens. Prostate 2002;53:246–53.

[19] Halpern EJ, Ramey JR, Strup SE, et al. Detection of prostate carcinoma with contrast-enhanced sonography using intermittent harmonic imaging. Cancer 2005;104:2373–83.

[20] Halpern E, Rosenberg M, Gomella LG. Prostate cancer: contrast-enhanced US for detection. Radiology 2001;219:219–25.

[21] Hricak H, Dooms GC, Jeffrey RB, et al. Prostatic carcinoma: staging by clinical assessment, CT, and MR imaging. Radiology 1987;162:331–6.

[22] Platt JF, Bree RL, Schwab RE. The accuracy of CT in the staging of carcinoma of the prostate. AJR Am J Roentgenol 1987;149:315–8.

[23] Yu KK, Hricak H. Imaging prostate cancer. Radiol Clin North Am 2000;38:59–85.

[24] Ives EP, Burke MA, Edmonds PR, et al. Quantitative computed tomography perfusion of prostate cancer: correlation with whole-mount pathology. Clin Prostate Cancer 2005;4:109–12.

[25] Claus FG, Hricak H, Hattery RR. Pretreatment evaluation of prostate cancer: role of MR imaging and 1H MR spectroscopy. Radiographics 2004; 24:S167–80.

[26] Hricak H. MR imaging and MR spectroscopic imaging in the pre-treatment evaluation of prostate cancer. Br J Radiol 2005;78:S103–11.

[27] Kurhanewicz J, Vigneron DB, Hricak H, et al. Three-dimensional 1H spectroscopic imaging of the in situ human prostate with high spatial (0.24 to 0.7 cm3) spatial resolution. Radiology 1996;198:795–805.

[28] Males R, Vigneron DB, Star-Lack J, et al. Clinical application of BASING and spectral/spatial water and lipid suppression pulses for prostate cancer staging and localization by in vivo 3D 1H magnetic resonance spectroscopic imaging. Magn Reson Med 2000;43:17–22.

[29] Zakian KL, Sircar K, Hricak H, et al. Correlation of proton MR spectroscopic imaging with Gleason score based on step-section pathologic analysis after radical prostatectomy. Radiology 2005; 234:804–14.

[30] Scheidler J, Hricak H, Vigneron DB, et al. Prostate cancer: localization with three-dimensional proton MR spectroscopic imaging—clinicopathologic study. Radiology 1999;213:473–80.

[31] Mullerad M, Hricak H, Kuroiwa K, et al. Comparison of endorectal magnetic resonance imaging, guided prostate biopsy and digital rectal examination in the preoperative anatomical localization of prostate cancer. J Urol 2005;174:2158–63.

[32] McNeal JE, Redwine EA, Freiha FS, et al. Zonal distribution of prostatic adenocarcinoma: correlation with histologic pattern and direction of spread. Am J Surg Pathol 1988;12:897–906.

[33] Akin O, Sala E, Moskowitz CS, et al. Transition zone prostate cancers: features, detection, localization, and staging at endorectal MR imaging. Radiology 2006;28. [Epub ahead of print].

[34] Engelbrecht MR, Jager GJ, Laheij RJ, et al. Local staging of prostate cancer using magnetic resonance imaging: a meta-analysis. Eur Radiol 2002; 12:2294–302.

[35] Engelbrecht MR, Huisman HJ, Laheij RJ, et al. Discrimination of prostate cancer from normal peripheral zone and central gland tissue by using dynamic contrast-enhanced MR imaging. Radiology 2003;229:248–54.

[36] Ogura K, Maekawa S, Okubo K, et al. Dynamic endorectal magnetic resonance imaging for local staging and detection of neurovascular bundle involvement of prostate cancer: correlation with histopathologic results. Urology 2001;57: 721–6.

[37] Beyersdorff D, Taupitz M, Winkelmann B, et al. Patients with a history of elevated prostate-specific antigen levels and negative transrectal US-guided quadrant or sextant biopsy results: value of MR imaging. Radiology 2002;224:701–6.

[38] Terris MK. Prostate biopsy strategies: past, present, and future. Urol Clin North Am 2002;29: 205–12.

[39] Atalar E, Menard C. MR-guided interventions for prostate cancer. Magn Reson Imaging Clin N Am 2005;13:491–504.

[40] Beyersdorff D, Winkel A, Hamm B, et al. MR imaging-guided prostate biopsy with a closed MR unit at 1.5 T: initial results. Radiology 2005;234: 576–81.

[41] Susil RC, Menard C, Krieger A, et al. Transrectal prostate biopsy and fiducial marker placement in a standard 1.5T magnetic resonance imaging scanner. J Urol 2006;175:113–20.

[42] Bartolozzi C, Menchi I, Lencioni R, et al. Local staging of prostate carcinoma with endorectal coil MRI: correlation with whole-mount radical prostatectomy specimens. Eur Radiol 1996;6: 339–45.

[43] Cornud F, Flam T, Chauveinc L, et al. Extraprostatic spread of clinically localized prostate cancer: factors predictive of pT3 tumor and of positive endorectal MR imaging examination results. Radiology 2002;224:203–10.

[44] Ikonen S, Karkkainen P, Kivisaari L, et al. Magnetic resonance imaging of clinically localized prostatic cancer. J Urol 1998;159:915–9.

[45] Ikonen S, Karkkainen P, Kivisaari L, et al. Endorectal magnetic resonance imaging of prostatic cancer: comparison between fat-suppressed T2-weighted fast spin echo and three-dimensional dual-echo, steady-state sequences. Eur Radiol 2001;11:236–41.

[46] May F, Treumann T, Dettmar P, et al. Limited value of endorectal magnetic resonance imaging and transrectal ultrasonography in the staging of clinically localized prostate cancer. BJU Int 2001; 87:66–9.

[47] Perrotti M, Kaufman RP Jr, Jennings TA, et al. Endo-rectal coil magnetic resonance imaging in clinically localized prostate cancer: is it accurate? J Urol 1996;156:106–9.

[48] Presti JC, Hricak H, Narayan PA, et al. Local staging of prostatic carcinoma: comparison of transrectal sonography and endorectal MR imaging. AJR Am J Roentgenol 1996;166:103–8.

[49] Rorvik J, Halvorsen OJ, Albrektsen G, et al. MRI with an endorectal coil for staging of clinically localised prostate cancer prior to radical prostatectomy. Eur Radiol 1999;9:29–34.

[50] Yu KK, Hricak H, Alagappan R, et al. Detection of extracapsular extension of prostate carcinoma with endorectal and phased-array coil MR imaging: multivariate feature analysis. Radiology 1997;202: 697–702.

[51] Sala E, Akin O, Moskowitz CS, et al. Endorectal MR imaging in the evaluation of seminal vesicle invasion: diagnostic accuracy and multivariate feature analysis. Radiology 2006;238:929–37.

[52] Yu KK, Scheidler J, Hricak H, et al. Prostate cancer: prediction of extracapsular extension with endorectal MR imaging and three-dimensional proton MR spectroscopic imaging. Radiology 1999;213:481–8.

[53] Wang L, Mullerad M, Chen HN, et al. Prostate cancer: incremental value of endorectal MR imaging findings for prediction of extracapsular extension. Radiology 2004;232:133–9.

[54] Mullerad M, Hricak H, Wang L, et al. Prostate cancer: detection of extracapsular extension by genitourinary and general body radiologists at MR imaging. Radiology 2004;232:140–6.

[55] Wang L, Hricak H, Kattan MW, et al. Prediction of organ-confined prostate cancer: incremental value of MR imaging and MR spectroscopic imaging to staging nomograms. Radiology 2006; 238:597–603.

[56] Beer M, Schmidt H, Riedl R. The clinical value of preoperative staging of bladder and prostatic cancers with nuclear magnetic resonance and computerized tomography [in German]. Urologe A 1989;28:65–9.

[57] Bezzi M, Kressel HY, Allen KS, et al. Prostatic carcinoma: staging with MR imaging at 1.5 T. Radiology 1988;169:339–46.

[58] Jager GJ, Barentsz JO, Oosterhof GO, et al. Pelvic adenopathy in prostatic and urinary bladder carcinoma: MR imaging with a three-dimensional TI-weighted magnetization-prepared-rapid gradient-echo sequence. AJR Am J Roentgenol 1996; 167:1503–7.

[59] Kier R, Wain S, Troiano R. Fast spin-echo MR images of the pelvis obtained with a phased-array coil: value in localizing and staging prostatic carcinoma. AJR Am J Roentgenol 1993;161:601–6.

[60] Nicolas V, Beese M, Keulers A, et al. MR tomography in prostatic carcinoma: comparison of conventional and endorectal MRT [in German]. Rofo. 1994;161:319–26.

[61] Tuzel E, Sevinc M, Obuz F, et al. Is magnetic resonance imaging necessary in the staging of prostate cancer? Urol Int 1998;61:227–31.

[62] Harisinghani MG, Barentsz J, Hahn PF, et al. Noninvasive detection of clinically occult

lymph-node metastases in prostate cancer. N Engl J Med 2003;348(25):2491–9. Erratum in N Engl J Med 2003;349(10):1010.

[63] Wang L, Hricak H, Kattan MW, et al. Combined endorectal and phased-array MRI in the prediction of pelvic lymph node metastasis in prostate cancer. AJR Am J Roentgenol 2006;186:743–8.

[64] Lange PH. PROSTASCINT scan for staging prostate cancer. Urology 2001;57:402–6.

[65] Bermejo CE, Coursey J, Basler J, et al. Histologic confirmation of lesions identified by Prostascint scan following definitive treatment. Urol Oncol 2003;21:349–52.

[66] Polascik TJ, Manyak MJ, Haseman MK, et al. Comparison of clinical staging algorithms and 111indium-capromab pendetide immunoscintigraphy in the prediction of lymph node involvement in high risk prostate carcinoma patients. Cancer 1999;85:1586–92.

[67] Elgamal AA, Troychak MJ, Murphy GP. ProstaScint scan may enhance identification of prostate cancer recurrences after prostatectomy, radiation, or hormone therapy: analysis of 136 scans of 100 patients. Prostate 1998;37:261–9.

[68] Schettino CJ, Kramer EL, Noz ME, et al. Impact of fusion of indium-111 capromab pendetide volume data sets with those from MRI or CT in patients with recurrent prostate cancer. AJR Am J Roentgenol 2004;183:519–24.

[69] Gerber G, Chodak GW. Assessment of value of routine bone scans in patients with newly diagnosed prostate cancer. Urology 1991;37:418–22.

[70] Cooperberg MR, Lubeck DP, Grossfeld GD, et al. Contemporary trends in imaging test utilization for prostate cancer staging: data from the cancer of the prostate strategic urologic research endeavor. J Urol 2002;168:491–5.

[71] O'Sullivan JM, Norman AR, Cook GJ, et al. Broadening the criteria for avoiding staging bone scans in prostate cancer: a retrospective study of patients at the Royal Marsden Hospital. BJU Int 2003;92:685–9.

[72] Oesterling JE. Using PSA to eliminate the staging radionuclide bone scan. Significant economic implications. Urol Clin North Am 1993;20: 705–11.

[73] Albertsen PC, Hanley JA, Harlan LC, et al. The positive yield of imaging studies in the evaluation of men with newly diagnosed prostate cancer: a population based analysis. J Urol 2000; 163:1138–43.

[74] Kosuda S, Yoshimura I, Aizawa T, et al. Can initial prostate specific antigen determinations eliminate the need for bone scans in patients with newly diagnosed prostate carcinoma? A multicenter retrospective study in Japan. Cancer 2002;94:964–72.

[75] Wymenga LF, Boomsma JH, Groenier K, et al. Routine bone scans in patients with prostate cancer related to serum prostate-specific antigen and alkaline phosphatase. BJU Int 2001;88: 226–30.

[76] Hofer C, Kubler H, Hartung R, et al. Diagnosis and monitoring of urological tumors using positron emission tomography. Eur Urol 2001;40: 481–7.

[77] Kumar R, Zhuang H, Alavi A. PET in the management of urologic malignancies. Radiol Clin North Am 2004;42:1141–53.

[78] Peterson JJ, Kransdorf MJ, O'Connor MI. Diagnosis of occult bone metastases: positron emission tomography. Clin Orthop 2003;415: S120–8.

[79] Sanz G, Rioja J, Zudaire JJ, et al. PET and prostate cancer. World J Urol 2004;22:351–2.

[80] Schoder H, Larson SM. Positron emission tomography for prostate, bladder, and renal cancer. Semin Nucl Med 2004;34:274–92.

[81] Liu IJ, Zafar MB, Lai YH, et al. Fluorodeoxyglucose positron emission tomography studies in diagnosis and staging of clinically organ-confined prostate cancer. Urology 2001;57:108–11.

[82] Schoder H, Herrmann K, Gonen M, et al. 2-[18F]fluoro-2-deoxyglucose positron emission tomography for the detection of disease in patients with prostate-specific antigen relapse after radical prostatectomy. Clin Cancer Res 2005;11: 4761–9.

[83] Maecke HR, Hofmann M, Haberkorn U. (68)Ga-labeled peptides in tumor imaging. J Nucl Med 2005;46:S172–8.

[84] Mathews D, Oz OK. Positron emission tomography in prostate and renal cell carcinoma. Curr Opin Urol 2002;12:381–5.

[85] Oyama N, Akino H, Kanamaru H, et al. 11C-acetate PET imaging of prostate cancer. J Nucl Med 2002;43:181–6.

[86] Toth G, Lengyel Z, Balkay L, et al. Detection of prostate cancer with 11C-methionine positron emission tomography. J Urol 2005;173:66–9.

[87] Laufer M, Pound CR, Carducci MA, et al. Management of patients with rising prostate-specific antigen after radical prostatectomy. Urology 2000;55:309–15.

[88] Partin AW, Oesterling JE. The clinical usefulness of prostate specific antigen: update 1994. J Urol 1994;152:1358–68.

[89] Cher ML, Bianco FJ Jr, Lam JS, et al. Limited role of radionuclide bone scintigraphy in patients with prostate specific antigen elevations after radical prostatectomy. J Urol 1998;160:1387–91.

[90] Kane CJ, Amling CL, Johnstone PA, et al. Limited value of bone scintigraphy and computed tomography in assessing biochemical failure after radical prostatectomy. Urology 2003;61:607–11.

[91] Connolly JA, Shinohara K, Presti JC Jr, et al. Local recurrence after radical prostatectomy: characteristics in size, location, and relationship to prostate-specific antigen and surgical margins. Urology 1996;47:225–31.

[92] Leventis AK, Shariat SF, Slawin KM. Local recurrence after radical prostatectomy: correlation of US features with prostatic fossa biopsy findings. Radiology 2001;219:432–9.

[93] Kramer S, Gorich J, Gottfried HW, et al. Sensitivity of computed tomography in detecting local recurrence of prostatic carcinoma following radical prostatectomy. Br J Radiol 1997;70:995–9.

[94] Hricak H, Schoder H, Pucar D, et al. Advances in imaging in the postoperative patient with a rising prostate-specific antigen level. Semin Oncol 2003; 30:616–34.

[95] Sella T, Schwartz LH, Swindle PW, et al. Suspected local recurrence after radical prostatectomy: endorectal coil MR imaging. Radiology 2004;23:379–85.

[96] Silverman JM, Krebs TL. MR imaging evaluation with a transrectal surface coil of local recurrence of prostatic cancer in men who have undergone radical prostatectomy. AJR Am J Roentgenol 1997;168:379–85.

[97] Horwitz EM, Vicini FA, Ziaja EL, et al. The correlation between the ASTRO Consensus Panel definition of biochemical failure and clinical outcome for patients with prostate cancer treated with external beam irradiation. American Society of Therapeutic Radiology and Oncology. Int J Radiat Oncol Biol Phys 1998;41: 267–72.

[98] Pucar D, Shukla-Dave A, Hricak H, et al. Prostate cancer: correlation of MR imaging and MR spectroscopy with pathologic findings after radiation therapy-initial experience. Radiology 2005;236: 545–53.

[99] Sala E, Eberhardt SC, Akin O, et al. Endorectal MR imaging before salvage prostatectomy: tumor localization and staging. Radiology 2006; 238:176–83.

RADIOLOGIC
CLINICS
OF NORTH AMERICA

Radiol Clin N Am 45 (2007) 223–230

Index

Note: Page numbers of article titles are in **boldface** type.

doi:10.1016/S0033-8389(06)00147-3

Moving?

Make sure your subscription moves with you!

To notify us of your new address, find your **Clinics Account Number** (located on your mailing label above your name), and contact customer service at:

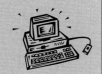

E-mail: elspcs@elsevier.com

800-654-2452 (subscribers in the U.S. & Canada)
407-345-4000 (subscribers outside of the U.S. & Canada)

Fax number: 407-363-9661

Elsevier Periodicals Customer Service
6277 Sea Harbor Drive
Orlando, FL 32887-4800

*To ensure uninterrupted delivery of your subscription, please notify us at least 4 weeks in advance of move.